PROGRESS IN BRAIN RESEARCH

VOLUME 42

HORMONES, HOMEOSTASIS AND THE BRAIN

PROGRESS IN BRAIN RESEARCH

PROGRESS IN BRAIN RESEARCH

VOLUME 42

HORMONES, HOMEOSTASIS
AND THE BRAIN

Proceedings of the Vth International Congress of the International
Society of Psychoneuroendocrinology

EDITED BY

W. H. GISPEN

Tj. B. van WIMERSMA GREIDANUS

B. BOHUS

AND

D. de WIED

Rudolf Magnus Institute for Pharmacology, Medical Faculty, University of Utrecht, Utrecht (The Netherlands)

ELSEVIER SCIENTIFIC PUBLISHING COMPANY

AMSTERDAM/OXFORD/NEW YORK

1975

ELSEVIER SCIENTIFIC PUBLISHING COMPANY
335 JAN VAN GALENSTRAAT
P.O. BOX 211, AMSTERDAM, THE NETHERLANDS

AMERICAN ELSEVIER PUBLISHING COMPANY, INC.
52 VANDERBILT AVENUE
NEW YORK, NEW YORK 10017

LIBRARY OF CONGRESS CARD NUMBER: 74-29681

ISBN 0-444-41292-1

WITH 146 ILLUSTRATIONS AND 42 TABLES

PRINTED IN THE NETHERLANDS

List of Contributors

R. ADER, Department of Psychiatry, University of Rochester School of Medicine and Dentistry, Rochester, N.Y. 14642, U.S.A.

E. ARNAULD, Laboratoire de Neurophysiologie, Université de Bordeaux II, 24 rue Paul Broca, 33000 Bordeaux, France

P. M. ARNOLD, Max-Planck-Institute for Biophysical Chemistry, and Institute of Psychology, Göttingen, G.F.R.

J. R. BASSETT, School of Biological Sciences, Macquarie University, North Ryde, N.S.W. 2113, Australia

A. BAUDUIN, Institute of Medicine and Institute of Pediatrics, University of Liège, Liège, Belgium

M. J. BAUM, Department of Endocrinology, Growth and Reproduction, Medical Faculty, Erasmus University, Rotterdam, The Netherlands

D. BECKER, Max-Planck-Institute for Biophysical Chemistry, and Institute of Psychology, Göttingen, G.F.R.

O. BENKERT, Psychiatrische Klinik der Universität München, Nussbaumstrasse 7, 8 Munich 2, G.F.R.

B. BISWAS, Department of Biochemistry, University College of Science, Calcutta University, Calcutta-19, India

B. BOHUS, Rudolf Magnus Institute for Pharmacology, University of Utrecht, Medical Faculty, Vondellaan 6, Utrecht, The Netherlands

E. R. H. BOS, Department of Biological Psychiatry, Isotope Laboratory, Department of Internal Medicine, Division of Endocrinology, Medical Faculty, University of Groningen, Groningen, The Netherlands

R. M. BOYAR, Departments of Neurology, Oncology and the Institute of Steroid Research, Montefiore Hospital and Medical Center and The Albert Einstein College of Medicine, Bronx, N.Y. 10467, U.S.A.

F. BRAMBILLA, Ospedale Psichiatrico Paolo Pini, Milan and Ospedale Psichiatrico Antonini, Milan, Limbiate and Patologia Medica II, Università di Milano, Milan, Italy

G. R. BREESE, Departments of Psychiatry and Pharmacology and The Biological Sciences Research Center, The Child Development Institute, University of North Carolina School of Medicine, Chapel Hill, N.C. 27514, U.S.A.

B. W. L. BROOKSBANK, Department of Psychology, The Queen's University, Belfast, N. Ireland

W. VAN DEN BURG, Department of Biological Psychiatry, Isotope Laboratory, Department of Internal Medicine, Division of Endocrinology, Medical Faculty, University of Groningen, Groningen, The Netherlands

M. S. BUSH, Nestlé Products Technical Assistance Co. Ltd., Vevey, Switzerland

R. VAN BUSKIRK, Department of Psychobiology, School of Biological Sciences, University of California, Irvine, Calif. 92664, U.S.A.

K. D. CAIRNCROSS, School of Biological Sciences, Macquarie University, North Ryde, N.S.W. 2113, Australia

A. CAYER, Biology Department, New York University, Washington Square, New York, N.Y. 10003, U.S.A.

M.-F. CHENG, Rutgers–The State University, Institute of Animal Behavior, Newark, N.J. 07102, U.S.A.

E. CHIARAVIGLIO, Instituto de Investigación Médica M.y M. Ferreyra, Córdoba, Argentina

G. CHOUVET, Département de Médecine Expérimentale, Université Claude Bernard, 8 Avenue Rockefeller, 69373 Lyon, France

G. D. COOVER, Institutes of Physiology and Psychology, University of Bergen, Bergen, Norway

J. J. COWLEY, Department of Psychology, The Queen's University, Belfast, N. Ireland

O. D. CREUTZFELDT, Max-Planck-Institute for Biophysical Chemistry, and Institute of Psychology, Göttingen, G.F.R.

M. DERYCK, Institutes of Physiology and Psychology, University of Bergen, Bergen, Norway

H. DOORENBOS, Department of Biological Psychiatry, Isotope Laboratory, Department of Internal Medicine, Division of Endocrinology, Medical Faculty, University of Groningen, Groningen, The Netherlands

C. A. DUDLEY, Department of Physiology, University of Texas Health Science Center at Dallas, Southwestern Medical School, Dallas, Texas 75235, U.S.A.

R. E. J. DYBALL, ARC Institute of Animal Physiology, Babraham, Cambridge CB2 4AT, Great Britain

R. G. Dyer, ARC Institute of Animal Physiology, Babraham, Cambridge CB2 4AT, Great Britain

J. E. Dyksterhuis, Department of Pediatrics, University of Nebraska Medical Center, Omaha, Nebr., U.S.A.

R. Elbertse, Pharmacology Department, Scientific Development Group, Organon, Oss, The Netherlands

E. Endröczi, Research Division, Postgraduate Medical School, Budapest, Hungary

M. Fekete, Institute of Physiology, University Medical School, Pécs, Hungary

S. Feldman, Department of Neurology, Hadassah University Hospital, Jerusalem, Israel

J. T. Fitzsimons, The Physiological Laboratory, Cambridge, Great Britain

A. W. K. Gaillard, Institute for Perception TNO, Soesterberg, The Netherlands

P. Garrud, Department of Experimental Psychology, University of Oxford, South Parks Road, Oxford OX1 3PS, Great Britain

M. Gaylor, Division of Hypertension and Clinical Pharmacology, Department of Medicine, University of Pittsburgh School of Medicine, Pittsburgh, Pa. 15261, U.S.A.

J. J. Ghosh, Department of Biochemistry, University College of Science, Calcutta University, Calcutta-19, India

W. H. Gispen, Division of Molecular Neurobiology, Rudolf Magnus Institute for Pharmacology, and Laboratory of Physiological Chemistry, Medical Faculty, Institute of Molecular Biology, University of Utrecht, Padualaan 8, Utrecht-De Uithof, The Netherlands

E. Glassman, Division of Chemical Neurobiology, Department of Biochemistry, School of Medicine, The University of North Carolina, Chapel Hill, N. C. 27514, U.S.A.

P. E. Gold, Department of Psychobiology, School of Biological Sciences, University of California, Irvine, Calif. 92664, U.S.A.

P. R. Gouin, Department of Psychiatry and Pharmacology, U.C.L.A. School of Medicine, Harbor General Hospital Campus, Torrance, Calif. 90509, U.S.A.

A. N. Granitsas, Department of General Biology, Medical School, Aristotelian University, Thessaloniki, Greece

M. D. Green, Department of Pharmacology, School of Medicine and the Brain Research Institute, University of California, Los Angeles, Calif. 90024, U.S.A.

B. I. Grosser, Departments of Psychiatry, Pharmacology and Anatomy, University of Utah College of Medicine, Salt Lake City, Utah, U.S.A.

A. Guastalla, Ospedale Pischiatrico Paolo Pini, Milan and Ospedale Psichiatrico Antonini, Milan, Limbiate and Patologia Medica II, Università di Milano, Milan, Italy

A. Guerrini, Ospedale Pischiatrico Paolo Pini, Milan and Ospedale Psichiatrico Antonini, Milan, Limbiate and Patologia Medica II, Università di Milano, Milan, Italy

G. Hartmann, Institute of Physiology, University Medical School, Pécs, Hungary

J. Haycock, Department of Psychobiology, School of Biological Sciences, University of California, Irvine, Calif. 92664, U.S.A.

I. Hegedüs, Central Research Division, Postgraduate Medical School, Budapest, Hungary

L. Hellman, Departments of Neurology, Oncology and the Institute of Steroid Research, Montefiore Hospital and Medical Center and The Albert Einstein College of Medicine, Bronx, N.Y. 10467, U.S.A.

S. A. Hitoglou, Department of General Biology, Medical School, Aristotelian University, Thessaloniki, Greece

Á. Hraschek, Central Research Division, Postgraduate Medical School, Budapest, Hungary

J. B. Hutchison, MRC Unit on the Development and Integration of Behaviour, University of Cambridge, Madingley, Cambridge, Great Britain

R. E. Hutchison, MRC Unit on the Development and Integration of Behaviour, University Sub-Department of Animal Behaviour Madingley, Cambridge, Great Britain

M. Hyyppä, Departments of Endocrinology and Pharmacology, University of Milan, Milan, Italy

W. de Jong, Rudolf Magnus Institute for Pharmacology, University of Utrecht, Medical Faculty, Vondellaan 6, Utrecht, The Netherlands

M. Jouvet, Département de Médecine Expérimentale, Université Claude Bernard, 8 Avenue Rockefeller, 69373 Lyon, France

S. Justo, Departments of Endocrinology and Pharmacology, University of Milan, Milan, Italy

S. Kapen, Departments of Neurology, Oncology and the Institute of Steroid Research, Montefiore Hospital and Medical Center and The Albert Einstein College of Medicine, Bronx, N.Y. 10467, U.S.A.

A. J. Kastin, Veterans Administration Hospital and Tulane University School of Medicine, and University of New Orleans, New Orleans, La., Ohio State University, Columbus, Ohio and Temple University, Philadelphia, Pa., U.S.A.

M. Kawakami, Department of Physiology, Yokohama City University School of Medicine, Yokohama, Japan

C. Køhler, Institutes of Physiology and Psychology, University of Bergen, Bergen, Norway

G. L. Kovács, Department of Physiology, University Medical School, Pécs, Hungary

Zs. Kovács, Central Research Division, Postgraduate Medical School, Budapest, Hungary

D. T. Krieger, Division of Endocrinology, Department of Medicine, Mount Sinai School of Medicine, City University of New York, New York City, N.Y., U.S.A.

I. T. Kurtsin, I.P. Pavlov Institute of Physiology, Academy of Sciences U.S.S.R., Leningrad, U.S.S.R.

A. Lajtha, New York State Research Institute for Neurochemistry and Drug Addiction, Ward's Island, New York, N.Y. 10035, U.S.A.

S. Langenstein, Max-Planck-Institute for Biophysical Chemistry, and Institute of Psychology, Göttingen, G.F.R.

L. Lazarus, Garvan Institute of Medical Research, St. Vincent's Hospital, Sydney 2010, Australia

P. D. Leathwood, Nestlé Products Technical Assistance Co. Ltd., Vevey, Switzerland

J. J. Legros, Institute of Medicine and Institute of Pediatrics, University of Liège, Liège, Belgium

S. Levine, Department of Psychiatry, Stanford University, Stanford, Calif. 94305, U.S.A.

M. A. Lipton, Departments of Psychiatry and Pharmacology and The Biological Sciences Research Center, The Child Development Institute, University of North Carolina School of Medicine, Chapel Hill, N.C. 27514, U.S.A.

K. Lissák, Institute of Physiology, University Medical School, Pécs, Hungary

P. Lomax, Department of Pharmacology, School of Medicine and the Brain Research Institute, University of California, Los Angeles, Calif. 90024, U.S.A.

J. T. Martin, Department of Animal Science, University of Minnesota, St. Paul, Minn. 55101, U.S.A.

L. Martini, Departments of Endocrinology and Pharmacology, University of Milan, Milan, Italy

I. Marton, Central Research Division, Postgraduate Medical School, Budapest, Hungary

S. M. McCann, Department of Physiology, University of Texas Health Science Center at Dallas, Southwestern Medical School, Dallas, Texas 75235, U.S.A.

R. H. McDonald, Jr., Division of Hypertension and Clinical Pharmacology, Department of Medicine, University of Pittsburgh School of Medicine, Pittsburgh, Pa. 15261, U.S.A.

J. L. McGaugh, Department of Psychobiology, School of Biological Sciences, University of California, Irvine, Calif. 92664, U.S.A.

L. H. Miller, Veterans Administration Hospital and Tulane University School of Medicine, and University of New Orleans, New Orleans, La., Ohio State University, Columbus, Ohio and Temple University, Philadelphia, Pa. U.S.A.

R. L. Moss, Department of Physiology, University of Texas Health Science Center at Dallas, Southwestern Medical School, Dallas, Texas 75235, U.S.A.

M. Motta, Departments of Endocrinology and Pharmacology, University of Milan, Milan, Italy

A. H. Mulder, Department of Pharmacology, Medical Faculty, Free University, Amsterdam, The Netherlands

D. Nag, Department of Biochemistry, University College of Science, Calcutta University, Calcutta-19, India

A. Neidle, New York State Research Institute for Neurochemistry and Drug Addiction, Ward's Island, New York, N.Y. 10035, U.S.A.

B. C. Nisula, Reproduction Research Branch, National Institute of Child Health and Human Development, National Institutes of Health, Bethesda, Md. 20014, U.S.A.

Cs. Nyakas, Central Research Division, Postgraduate Medical School, Budapest, Hungary

R. Perumal, Department of Biochemistry, University of Malaya, Kuala-Lumpur, Malaysia

Y. Pfeifer, Bioclimatology Unit, Department of Applied Pharmacology, School of Pharmacy, Hebrew University, Jerusalem, Israel

D. A. Piers, Department of Biological Psychiatry, Isotope Laboratory, Department of Internal Medicine, Division of Endocrinology, Medical Faculty, University of Groningen, Groningen, The Netherlands

N. P. Plotnikoff, Experimental Therapy Division, Abbott Laboratories, North Chicago, Ill., U.S.A.

M. K. Poddar, Department of Biochemistry, University College of Science, Calcutta University, Calcutta-19, India

R. E. POLAND, Department of Psychiatry and Pharmacology, U.C.L.A. School of Medicine, Harbor General Hospital Campus, Torrance, Calif. 90509, U.S.A.

S. PÖPPL, Max-Planck-Institute for Biophysical Chemistry, and Institute of Psychology, Göttingen, G.F.R.

H. M. VAN PRAAG, Department of Biological Psychiatry, Isotope Laboratory, Department of Internal Medicine, Division of Endocrinology, Medical Faculty, University of Groningen, Groningen, The Netherlands

A. J. PRANGE, JR., Departments of Psychiatry and Pharmacology and The Biological Sciences Research Center, The Child Development Institute, University of North Carolina School of Medicine, Chapel Hill, N.C. 27514, U.S.A.

F. RAVESSOUD, Department of Psychiatry and Pharmacology, U.C.L.A. School of Medicine, Harbor General Hospital Campus, Torrance, Calif. 90509, U.S.A.

D. P. REDMOND, Division of Hypertension and Clinical Pharmacology, Department of Medicine, University of Pittsburgh School of Medicine, Pittsburgh, Pa. 15261, U.S.A.

D. J. REED, Departments of Psychiatry, Pharmacology and Anatomy, University of Utah College of Medicine, Salt Lake City, Utah, U.S.A.

M. E. A. REITH, Division of Molecular Neurobiology, Rudolf Magnus Institute for Pharmacology, and Laboratory of Physiological Chemistry, Medical Faculty, Institute of Molecular Biology, University of Utrecht, Padualaan 8, Utrecht-De Uithof, The Netherlands

H. VAN RIEZEN, Pharmacology Department, Scientific Development Group, Organon, Oss, The Netherlands

F. RIGGI, Ospedale Pischiatrico Paolo Pini, Milan and Ospedale Psichiatrico Antonini, Milan, Limbiate and Patologia Medica II, Università di Milano, Milan, Italy

H. RIGTER, Pharmacology Department, Scientific Development Group, Organon, Oss, The Netherlands

C. ROVERE, Ospedale Psichiatrico Paolo Pini, Milan and Ospedale Psichiatrico Antonini, Milan, Limbiate and Patologia Medica II, Università di Milano, Milan, Italy

R. T. RUBIN, Department of Psychiatry, U.C.L.A. School of Medicine, Harbor General Hospital Campus, Torrance, Calif. 90509, U.S.A.

E. J. SACHAR, Department of Psychiatry, Albert Einstein College of Medicine, 1300 Morris Park Avenue, Bronx, N.Y. 10461, U.S.A.

T. SAGVOLDEN, Institutes of Physiology and Psychology, University of Bergen, Bergen, Norway

Y. SAKUMA, Department of Physiology, Yokohama City University School of Medicine, Yokohama, Japan

A. F. SANDERS, Institute for Perception TNO, Soesterberg, The Netherlands

C. A. SANDMAN, Veterans Administration Hospital and Tulane University School of Medicine, and University of New Orleans, New Orleans, La., Ohio State University, Columbus, Ohio and Temple University, Philadelphia, Pa., U.S.A.

V. R. SARA, Garvan Institute of Medical Research, St. Vincent's Hospital, Sydney 2010, Australia

A. V. SCHALLY, Veterans Administration Hospital and Tulane University School of Medicine, and University of New Orleans, New Orleans, La., Ohio State University, Columbus, Ohio and Temple University, Philadelphia, Pa., U.S.A.

A. E. SCHINDLER, Universitäts-Frauenklinik, 74 Tübingen, G.F.R.

P. SCHOTMAN, Division of Molecular Neurobiology, Rudolf Magnus Institute for Pharmacology, and Laboratory of Physiological Chemistry, Medical Faculty, Institute of Molecular Biology, University of Utrecht, Padualaan 8, Utrecht-De Uithof, The Netherlands

P. SCHRETLEN, Department of Endocrinology, Growth and Reproduction, Medical Faculty, Erasmus University, Rotterdam, The Netherlands

A. P. SHAPIRO, Division of Hypertension and Clinical Pharmacology, Department of Medicine, University of Pittsburgh School of Medicine, Pittsburgh, Pa. 15261, U.S.A.

P. G. SMELIK, Department of Pharmacology, Medical Faculty, Free University, Amsterdam, The Netherlands

M. L. SOULAIRAC, Department of Psychophysiology, Faculty of Sciences, University of Paris VI, Paris, France

W. STEVENS, Departments of Psychiatry, Pharmacology and Anatomy, University of Utah College of Medicine, Salt Lake City, Utah, U.S.A.

J. M. STOLK, Departments of Psychiatry and Pharmacology, Dartmouth Medical School, Hanover, N.H. 03755, U.S.A.

F. L. STRAND, Biology Department, New York University, Washington Square, New York, N. Y. 10003, U.S.A.

L. O. STRATTON, Veterans Administration Hospital and Tulane University School of Medicine, and University of New Orleans, New Orleans, La., Ohio State University, Columbus, Ohio and Temple University, Philadelphia, Pa., U.S.A.

F. G. SULMAN, Bioclimatology Unit, Department of Applied Pharmacology, School of Pharmacy, Hebrew University, Jerusalem, Israel

E. SUPERSTINE, Bioclimatology Unit, Department of Applied Pharmacology, School of Pharmacy, Hebrew University, Jerusalem, Israel

G. SZABÓ, Central Research Division, Postgraduate Medical School, Budapest, Hungary

F. TALLIÁN, Central Research Division, Postgraduate Medical School, Budapest, Hungary

P. TEITELBAUM, Psychology Department, University of Illinois, Champaign, Ill. 61820, U.S.A.

G. TELEGDY, Department of Physiology, University Medical School, Pécs, Hungary

W. TIRSCH, Max-Planck-Institute for Biophysical Chemistry, and Institute of Psychology, Göttingen, G.F.R.

C. M. TIWARY, Department of Pediatrics, University of Nebraska Medical Center, Omaha, Nebr., U.S.A.

E. TOMORUG, Hospital "Gh. Marinescu", Bucharest, Rumania

B. B. TOWER, Department of Psychiatry and Pharmacology, U.C.L.A. School of Medicine, Harbor General Hospital Campus, Torrance, Calif. 90509, U.S.A.

H. URSIN, Institutes of Physiology and Psychology, University of Bergen, Bergen, Norway

J.-L. VALATX, Département de Médecine Expérimentale, Université Claude Bernard, 8 Avenue Rockefeller, 69373 Lyon, France

M. VERFAILLE, Institute of Medicine and Institute of Pediatrics, University of Liège, Liège, Belgium

I. VERMES, Department of Physiology, University Medical School, Pécs, Hungary

J. D. VINCENT, Laboratoire de Neurophysiologie, Université de Bordeaux II, 24 rue Paul Broca, 33000 Bordeaux, France

E. D. WEITZMAN, Department of Neurology, Montefiore Hospital and Medical Center, and The Albert Einstein College of Medicine, Bronx, N.Y. 10467, U.S.A.

D. DE WIED, Rudolf Magnus Institute for Pharmacology, University of Utrecht, Medical Faculty, Vondellaan 6, Utrecht, The Netherlands

I. C. WILSON, Division of Research, The North Carolina Department of Mental Health, Raleigh, N.C. 27611, U.S.A.

J. E. WILSON, Division of Chemical Neurobiology, Department of Biochemistry, School of Medicine, The University of North Carolina, Chapel Hill, N.C. 27514, U.S.A.

Tj. B. VAN WIMERSMA GREIDANUS, Rudolf Magnus Institute for Pharmacology, University of Utrecht, Medical Faculty, Vondellaan 6, Utrecht, The Netherlands

D. L. WOLGIN, Psychology Department, University of Illinois, Champaign, Ill. 61820, U.S.A.

W. WUTTKE, Max-Planck-Institute for Biophysical Chemistry, and Institute of Psychology, Göttingen, G.F.R.

P. ZANDBERG, Rudolf Magnus Institute for Pharmacology, University of Utrecht, Medical Faculty, Vondellaan 6, Utrecht, The Netherlands

A. ZANOBONI, Ospedale Psichiatrico Paolo Pini, Milan and Ospedale Psichiatrico Antonini, Milan, Limbiate and Patologia Medica II, Università di Milano, Milan, Italy

W. ZANOBONI-MUCIACCIA, Ospedale Psichiatrico Paolo Pini, Milan and Ospedale Psichiatrico Antonini, Milan, Limbiate and Patologia Medica II, Università di Milano, Milan, Italy

A. K. VAN ZANTEN, Department of Biological Psychiatry, Isotope Laboratory, Department of Internal Medicine, Division of Endocrinology, Medical Faculty, University of Groningen, Groningen, The Netherlands

Preface

Hormones, Homeostasis and the Brain was the topic of the Vth International Meeting of the International Society of Psychoneuroendocrinology held at Utrecht from 24 to 27 July 1974. The meeting brought clinical investigators and laboratory researchers together to discuss the implication of hormones in brain function.

The therapeutic potential of new psychoactive drugs is still difficult to predict from animal experiments. However, the mode of action of hormones on their target tissues is much better known than that of drugs in general and on the basis of this knowledge, sophisticated animal models to study the influence of hormones in the brain are gradually becoming available. Behavioral, electrophysiological and biochemical parameters are used and much can be learned in this way from laboratory and clinical studies on the central action of hormones.

Thanks are due to the University of Utrecht for their cooperation, the Dr. Saal van Zwanenberg Foundation and the International Society of Psychoneuroendocrinology for financial assistance and the Organon Company for additional support.

The staff of the Rudolf Magnus Institute was responsible for the excellent organization of the meeting. In particular I wish to thank Miss Tine Baas, Miss Sylvia van Bijlevelt, Dr. M. E. A. Reith and Mr. J. C. van den Berg for their secretarial and administrative contributions.

D. DE WIED
Utrecht (The Netherlands)

Contents

Session V — Amines, Steroids and the Brain

Free Communications (abstracts)

Session VI — Early Hormonal Influences on Ontogenesis of Behavior and Brain Development

Free Communications (abstracts)

RELEASING HORMONES ON THE CENTRAL NERVOUS SYSTEM

Chairmen: L. MARTINI (Milan)
A. J. PRANGE (Chapel Hill, N.C.)

Behavioral Effects of Hypothalamic Releasing Hormones in Animals and Men

ARTHUR J. PRANGE, JR., IAN C. WILSON*,
GEORGE R. BREESE AND MORRIS A. LIPTON

Departments of Psychiatry and Pharmacology and The Biological Sciences Research Center of The Child Development Institute, University of North Carolina School of Medicine, Chapel Hill, N.C. 27514 (U.S.A.)

Hypothalamic polypeptide releasing factors and release inhibiting factors appear to exert effects on brain other than their effects on the pituitary gland. These brain effects may have direct behavioral consequences. They may have indirect consequences by altering responses to centrally active drugs. The exploitation of these properties of hypothalamic hormones for the treatment of illness has hardly begun. Presently this work is engaged on two fronts. The first is clinical empiricism, wherein positive, null, or untoward effects of one or another hormone in one or another condition suggest a trial of the hormone in another condition or of some other hormone in the same condition. The other front is the laboratory quest for mechanisms. The description of mechanism clarifies empirical facts already known. More importantly, it may suggest additional investigations. In this communication we shall report preliminary work accomplished in both the clinic and the laboratory. Whenever possible we shall try to relate the two.

Thyrotropin-releasing hormone (TRH)

TRH, L-pyroglutamyl-L-histidyl-L-proline amide, is a potent releaser of pituitary thyrotropin (thyroid stimulating hormone, TSH) (Fleischer *et al.*, 1970) and prolactin (Bowers *et al.*, 1971). It was the first of three, perhaps four, hypothalamic polypeptide releasing factors thus far identified and synthesized (Burgus *et al.*, 1969; Bowers *et al.*, 1970). Jackson and Reichlin (1974a) have reviewed the phylogenetic distribution of TRH. It is widely distributed throughout the phylum *Chordata*. However, in beasts such as axolotl it seems incapable of producing metamorphosis (Taurog *et al.*, 1974), suggesting that it lacks thyroid stimulating properties. This observation implies that TRH may have other functions. A similar implication proceeds from the discovery

---

* Division of Research, The North Carolina Department of Mental Health, Raleigh, N.C. 27611, U.S.A.

References p. 7–9

that TRH is widely distributed in brain except in cerebellum (Winokur and Utiger, 1974; Jackson and Reichlin, 1974b).

The findings listed above lent plausibility to our earlier report that TRH caused a rapid, though brief, antidepressant effect in humans (Prange and Wilson, 1972; Prange *et al.*, 1972). This first demonstration of a behavioral effect of a hypothalamic polypeptide in man was quickly confirmed by T. M. Itil (personal communication), Kastin *et al.* (1972), and Van der Vis-Melsen and Wiener (1972). Takahashi *et al.* (1973), however, found no advantage for TRH over the standard agent imipramine in the treatment of severe, relapsing patients. Deniker *et al.* (1974) found only a partial response to TRH, and this was limited to patients with the bipolar form of the disorder. It would appear possible that TRH response may help identify a subgroup of patients whose biochemical substrate for depression is not shared by all members of the phenotype. We are more impressed by the fact that TRH is remarkably effective in some depressed patients than by the fact that it is not a sovereign remedy for all.

The frequent, though not invariable, antidepressant response produced by TRH may not be its most valuable contribution to progress in treating and understanding depressive disorders. All investigators who have studied the matter have found that in depressed patients pituitary secretion of TSH after TRH stimulation is deficient when compared to the response of normal subjects (Van der Vis-Melsen and Wiener, 1972; Kastin *et al.*, 1972; Prange *et al.*, 1972; Takahashi *et al.*, 1973). In our initial study we found this to be the case; when we later obtained data from our own normal subjects the difference was statistically insignificant; more recently with the accumulation of more patients and subjects the difference is found to be valid. The statistical difficulty was caused in part by large variance in the patient group and this in turn was due to the fact that some depressed patients showed no discernible TSH response whatever after TRH injection.

The poverty of the pituitary response to TRH in depressed patients cannot be attributed to increased negative feedback from elevated thyroid hormones. In our patients we proved euthyroidism by usual chemical criteria, and in the patients of other investigators there was no reason to suspect hyperthyroidism. Thus, we have interpreted the finding as an implication that in depression the tonic stimulation of the pituitary by hypothalamic TRH is deficient, leading to a paucity of releasable TSH (Prange *et al.*, 1972). While this notion may be correct, it is not the simplest idea that will govern the most neuroendocrine information pertaining to depression. In this condition there is also a deficiency of growth hormone response evoked by insulin hypoglycemia (Sachar *et al.*, 1971; Mueller *et al.*, 1972). Somatotropin-release inhibiting factor (SRIF, somatostatin), of course, inhibits the release of growth hormone (Siler *et al.*, 1973; Brazeau *et al.*, 1974); more recently it has been shown also to inhibit TRH-induced release of TSH (Vale *et al.*, 1973a). It is reasonable to suggest, therefore, that in depression there is excessive activity of SRIF. This notion fits nicely with what is known about the behavioral effects of this substance (see below). We are currently investigating the aptitude of the SRIF-injected animal as a pharmacological model of depression.

In our early work with TRH in depression we noted that withdrawal and emotional flatness, when present, were often improved along with other symptoms. This suggested a trial of the hormone in schizophrenia, and we were further inclined toward this venture by the observation of Tiwary *et al.* (1972) that a dose of TRH given for diagnostic purposes to a mentally deficient boy had greatly improved his disorganized behavior. We have reported our favorable, preliminary, single-blind experience with TRH in 4 schizophrenic women (Wilson *et al.*, 1973a), and our double-blind experience with 8 more patients has been similar. Our patients have been highly selected: each has had several hospital admissions for schizophrenia, has shown good response to phenothiazines, but has relapsed after interrupting medication against advice; none has been in an excited state; all have been withdrawn from drugs for several weeks before being given intravenous TRH or nicotinic acid as a control for side effects. Only one patient has failed to show an excellent response to TRH, 0.5 mg, and she showed an excellent response when given 1.0 mg at a later date in a double-blind fashion. In general, improvement has become apparent within 6 hr after injection. It has lasted on average about a week before relapse has become complete, though a few patients have been discharged in full remission and have then been managed with supportive psychotherapy alone. Improvement has been as notable in the sphere of thought disorder as in the sphere of affect. Patients have remarked about the clarity of thought they have experienced. They have usually shown an eagerness to establish meaningful relationships. These results require attempted replications. TRH, and perhaps other selected hypothalamic polypeptides, should be tested in all categories of the schizophrenias and in childhood autism.

Tiwary *et al.* (1973) have reported an immediate focusing of attention after TRH in two hyperkinetic children, and our group, with L.A. O'Tuama's leadership, found a lessening of random activity in two children in a preliminary study. In a continuing trial we are trying to relate previous drug responses with TRH response.

TRH in our clinic has also shown promise in preliminary work in producing a relaxed state with moderate relief of depression in men with alcohol withdrawal syndrome. We have treated patients with only mild forms of this syndrome and only patients lacking a history of delirium tremens. We are ignorant of the pathophysiology of this condition and, therefore, also of what may precipitate it.

T. N. Chase and M. A. Lipton (personal communication) have given very large doses of TRH by slow intravenous infusion to patients with Parkinson's disease and have found it to be completely without effect. They agree with our view that slow administration may not produce blood levels of hormone that may be needed for adequate penetration of the blood–brain barrier. Although the point is moot, it should be entertained not only in regard to slow i.v. administration, but also in regard to oral use of TRH unless it is given only for purposes of pituitary stimulation.

The mechanism of the central action of TRH remains obscure. As stated above, the hormone is widely distributed in brain, and this has been shown both by assay of brain regions (Jackson and Reichlin, 1974b; Winokur and Utiger, 1974) and by radioautography (Stumpf and Sar, 1973). Thus, the hormone could reasonably be expected to exert a variety of effects. In our laboratory preliminary work in the rat has suggested that after i.v. TRH the activity of cyclic adenosine monophosphate may

References p. 7–9

be increased in brain but not in peripheral tissues. However, an adequate assessment of this possibility must await the employment of ultra fast techniques of killing animals. We have not been able to identify an action of TRH on brain serotonin, dopamine, or norepinephrine, and Reigle *et al.* (1974) have similarly found negative results regarding catecholamines. Keller *et al.* (1974), on the other hand, have very recently found in the rat that shortly after i.p. TRH there is a 20% increase in brain 3-methoxy-4-hydroxyphenylglycol (MHPG), the chief brain metabolic product of norepinephrine. TRH also increased the rate of incorporation of radioactive tyrosine into norepinephrine. An increase in norepinephrine activity after TRH would dovetail nicely with the reported antidepressant effect of the compound, as a deficiency of such activity has been suggested as being related to depressive disorders (Prange, 1964; Schildkraut, 1965; Bunney and Davis, 1965). In a similar way, Stein and Wise (1971) have postulated a norepinephrine deficit as well as a dopamine excess as being related to schizophrenia. Thus, the results of Keller *et al.* (1974) establish a sufficient mechanistic explanation for the preliminary findings regarding TRH in both depression and schizophrenia.

We have not been astonished to find that the apparent benefits of TRH are not specific to a single diagnostic group. TRH is a hormone, not a drug. It probably influences a variety of functions, the alteration of which have behavioral consequences that can reasonably be regarded as improvement, or aggravation, in any diagnostic entity in which that function is involved. The effects of TRH are not diagnosis specific, but neither are behavioral deficits. Depression and schizophrenia, for example, can usually be readily distinguished, but they nevertheless share features in common. Motor activity is often disordered in both. Mood, which may be primarily affected in depression, may be disordered in schizophrenia even when not to the extent or quality that would require the diagnosis of schizo-affective disorder. Thought disorder is primary to schizophrenia but a product of thought disorder, namely delusional thinking, is not rare in depression, especially if one so regards the depressed patient's assertions of guilt and worthlessness. Expectations of diagnostic specificity for the actions of TRH are also lessened by the finding that the hormone produces a discernible mood elevation in normal subjects (Wilson *et al.*, 1973b). After observing patients and normals, and after self-experimentation, we have conceived the idea that TRH broadly increases the coping capacity of the organism.

Another aspect of TRH physiology also promises to provide substantial insight into disorders of brain functions. May and Donabedian (1973) have developed a radioimmunoassay for TRH and applied it to studies of rat urine. Although subject to enzymatic destruction in blood, the polypeptide rapidly enters urine and once there is exceedingly stable. Urinary TRH, of course, comes only from brain. Therefore clinical science may learn more about brain from urinary studies of TRH than from urinary studies, say, of MHPG, which originates mostly in peripheral tissues (Maas and Landis, 1968).

Laboratory studies of TRH have kept pace with clinical studies. With Plotnikoff's leadership, we showed that in mice the hormone would potentiate the behavioral activation produced by pargyline–DOPA (Plotnikoff *et al.*, 1972a). This occurs even when mice are hypophysectomized and when rats are thyroidectomized (Plotnikoff *et al.*, 1974). These findings, along with our traditional interest in the thyroid axis in depression, formed the motivation for our original trial of TRH in depression. For a time thereafter we were stymied as to how to study TRH in animal systems. Segal and Mandell (1974) showed that slow intracerebroventricular infusion of TRH increased activity in the free-moving rat. However, we found that acute intracisternal injections and acute peripheral administration had little effect. After large doses animals showed some salivation, chewing, piloerection, and increased activity, but these effects were not profound. The enormous i.v. dose of 10 mg/rat produced death through apparent gross adrenergic stimulation, as R. Guillemin (personal communication) had noted, but efforts to detect subtler effects, such as the work of Breese and Cooper in trying to demonstrate an effect for TRH on self-stimulation in rats with median forebrain bundle implantations, were unrewarding (unpublished data).

An approach to the problem was revealed by the observation that preinjection or postinjection of TRH antagonizes the sedative and hypothermic effects of pentobarbital (Prange *et al.*, 1974). We have since discovered that TRH also antagonizes the effects of ethanol, chloral hydrate, reserpine, and all of 6 other barbiturates tested, but not the analgesic effects of morphine (unpublished data). The antagonism of phenobarbital, a mostly unmetabolized drug, is profound; yet antagonism of pentobarbital does not depend upon an effect on drug metabolism, for a search for such an effect was negative (Breese, unpublished data). The antagonism of ethanol by TRH provided a nice contrast between TRH and amphetamine, which otherwise bear certain similarities. Amphetamine, Breese found, does not antagonize ethanol sedation; it prolongs it (Breese *et al.*, 1974).

It is worthwhile to describe some of the parameters of pentobarbital antagonism by TRH, for in later work we have used the phenomenon as a screening device for the central activity of other polypeptides. The phenomenon holds in hypophysectomized mice (Breese, unpublished data); it does not depend upon altered metabolism of pentobarbital (Breese, unpublished data); it is greater during the day than during the night (unpublished data); it is increased in the cold (unpublished data); it is decreased, but not lost, in the warm (unpublished data); it is unaltered by prior administration of L-tryptophan or L-DOPA (unpublished data). When pentobarbital-treated mice are given intracisternal norepinephrine, hypothermia is diminished or even reversed, but sedation is not greatly affected (Breese, unpublished data). This is reason to think that TRH has brain effects other than the promotion of brain norepinephrine activity (Keller *et al.*, 1974).

Cognizant of these observations, we have pretreated pentobarbital-injected mice with a number of compounds. It is convenient here to list those which were without effect: L-pyroglutamic acid, L-histidine, L-proline, L-leucine, L-threonine, L-proline amide, luteinizing hormone-releasing hormone (LHRH), melanocyte-stimulating hormone-release inhibiting factor (MIF) and Substance P. Pyroglutamic acid, histidine, and proline amide, of course, are the constituents of TRH. Two compounds have been found to have pentobarbital reversing potency comparable to that of TRH: 3-methyl-histidine TRH and pyrozolyl TRH (unpublished data). Other workers have described the TSH releasing potencies of these compounds as compared to the potency of TRH (Vale *et al.*, 1973b). 3-Methyl-histidine TRH is 800% as potent, pyrozolyl TRH is 5% as potent. Thus, there is clearly a dissociation between pituitary and non-pituitary brain activity. Our attention has been particularly attracted by the results from the study of diiodo TRH and deamidated TRH. The former tends to exaggerate slightly the effects of pentobarbital, while the latter does so with statistical significance (unpublished data). The mechanism for the empirical observations is unknown.

TRH potentiates the behavioral activation caused in mice by the injection of pargyline and 5-hydroxytryptophan (5-HTP) (N. P. Plotnikoff, personal communication).

Somatotropin-release inhibiting factor (SRIF, somatostatin)

This tetradecapeptide (Brazeau *et al.*, 1973) inhibits the release of both growth hormone (Siler *et al.*, 1973; Brazeau *et al.*, 1974) and TSH (Vale *et al.*, 1973a). As noted above, an increase of its activity could account for two widely confirmed findings in depression: diminished growth hormone response to insulin and L-DOPA, and diminished TSH response to TRH. Its behavioral effects when given alone are consistent with the notion that it may be overactive in depression. In the same experiment in which they studied TRH, Segal and Mandell (1974) also infused SRIF into the lateral ventricle of the rat. Animals thus treated showed significant reduction in spontaneous activity without appearing sedated. Siler *et al.* (1973) gave large i.v. doses to monkeys and noted anecdotally that the animals seemed "tranquilized".

SRIF is the only hormone we have found, apart from TRH, that is active in the pentobarbital sedation test. In this system SRIF has the slight but statistically significant effect of prolonging sedation and exaggerating hyperthermia (unpublished data). This is further evidence that SRIF and pentobarbital are set in opposition at the central level just as they are at the pituitary level. Time of day does not influence the effects of SRIF on pentobarbital responses. However, the effects of SRIF are entirely lost in both warm and cold environments (unpublished data).

We believe that SRIF should be examined in standard screening tests for putative tranquilizers and for anticonvulsants. We have mentioned the plausibility of testing the SRIF-injected animal as a pharmacologic model of depression.

Luteinizing hormone-releasing hormone (LHRH)

LHRH is a decapeptide that causes the release from the pituitary gland of follicle-stimulating hormone and of luteinizing hormone (Matsuo *et al.*, 1971). Moss and McCann (1973) and Pfaff (1973), working independently, produced elegant demonstrations of a central action of LHRH. Ovariectomized rats were given doses of estrogen too small to reinstate mating behavior. When LHRH was then given, these behaviors occurred with normal frequency. TRH had no effect in this system (Moss and McCann, 1973). LHRH was active even after hypophysectomy (Pfaff, 1973).

LHRH has no effect on pentobarbital response in rodents (unpublished data).

L-Prolyl-L-leucyl-L-glycine amide

This tripeptide is often designated as melanocyte-stimulating hormone-release inhibiting factor (MIF) because it opposes the release of melanocyte-stimulating hormone in certain assay systems (Kastin *et al.*, 1971; Celis *et al.*, 1971). It is active in the pargyline–DOPA test (Plotnikoff *et al.*, 1971) like TRH, but inactive in the pargyline–5-HTP test (Plotnikoff, personal communication) unlike TRH. MIF antagonizes the tremors caused by oxotremorine (Plotnikoff *et al.*, 1972b). It does not alter pentobarbital response in rodents (unpublished data).

MIF appears to possess a certain degree of anti-Parkinsonian activity (Kastin and Barbeau, 1972) and also to oppose L-DOPA-induced dyskinesia (Kastin and Barbeau, 1972). Ehrensing and Kastin (1974) have presented preliminary evidence to suggest that MIF may have antidepressant activity. In one of their patients the symptoms of tardive dyskinesia yielded to administration of this tripeptide.

SUMMARY

This communication has been intended as a synopsis of work in progress or only recently completed. We have proposed as many ideas as confirmed observations and this performance aptly characterizes the burgeoning field of behavioral effects of hypothalamic hormones. We submit that such a field exists, and even this notion was novel a year or so ago. It should not be astonishing that an area so new is rather amorphous. In trying to locate it on an intellectual map one starts by searching for bridges to established territories. Thus, we and others have looked, for example, for connections between polypeptides on the one hand and monoamine neurotransmitters, cyclic adenosine monophosphate, and the like, on the other. While such bridges exist — the monoaminergic influences on peptidergic neurons, for example — they are probably not the only nor necessarily the most important foci of polypeptide activity. One must think of cholinergic systems, of inhibitory influences, and indeed of the possibility that polypeptides may be not only modulators of neural transmission, an idea not yet demonstrated, but even themselves transmitters.

ACKNOWLEDGEMENTS

This work was supported in part by U.S.P.H.S. Career Scientist Award MH-22536 (A.J.P.) and U.S.P.H.S. Grant MH-15631.

REFERENCES

BOWERS, C. Y., SCHALLY, A. V., ENZMANN, F., BOLER, J. AND FOLKERS, K. (1970) Porcine thyrotropin releasing hormone is (pyro)glu-his-pro(NH₂). *Endocrinology*, **86**, 1143–1153.
BOWERS, C. Y., FRIESEN, H. G., HWANG, P., GUYDA, H. J. AND FOLKERS, K. (1971) Prolactin and thyrotropin release in man by synthetic pyro-glutamyl-histidyl-prolineamide. *Biochem. biophys. Res. Commun.*, **45**, 1033–1041.

BRAZEAU, P., VALE, W., BURGUS, R., LING, N., BUTCHER, M., RIVIER, J. AND GUILLEMIN, R. (1973) Hypothalamic polypeptide that inhibits the secretion of immunoreactive pituitary growth hormone. *Science*, **179**, 77–79.

BRAZEAU, P., RIVIER, J., VALE, W. AND GUILLEMIN, R. (1974) Inhibition of growth hormone secretion in the rat by synthetic somatostatin. *Endocrinology*, **94**, 184–187.

BREESE, G. R., COTT, J. M., COOPER, B. R., PRANGE, JR., A. J. AND LIPTON, M. A. (1974) Antagonism of ethanol narcosis by thyrotropin releasing hormone. *Life Sci.*, **14**, 1053–1063.

BUNNEY, JR., W. E. AND DAVIS, J. M. (1965) Norepinephrine in depressive reactions: A review. *Arch. gen. Psychiat. (Chic.)*, **13**, 483–494.

BURGUS, R., DUNN, T. F., DESIDERIO, D. AND GUILLEMIN, R. (1969) Molecular structure of the hypothalamic thyrotropin-releasing factor (TRF) of ovine origin; demonstration of the pyroglutamyl-histidylprolinamide sequence by mass spectrometry. *C.R. Acad. Sci. (Paris)*, Ser. D, **269**, 1870–1873.

CELIS, M. E., TALEISNIK, S. AND WALTER, R. (1971) Regulation of formation and proposed structure of the factor inhibiting the release of melanocyte-stimulating hormone. *Proc. nat. Acad. Sci. (Wash.)*, **68**, 1428–1433.

DENIKER, P., GINESTET, D., LOO, H., ZARIFIAN, E. AND COTTEREAU, M.-J. (1974) Preliminary study on the action of hypothalamic thyrostimuline (thyrotropin releasing hormone or TRH) in depressive states. *Ann. med. Psychol.*, **1**, 249–255.

EHRENSING, R. H. AND KASTIN, A. J. (1974) Melanocyte-stimulating hormone-release inhibiting hormone as an antidepressant: A pilot study. *Arch. gen. Psychiat. (Chic.)*, **30**, 63–65.

FLEISCHER, N., BURGUS, R., VALE, W., DUNN, T. AND GUILLEMIN, R. (1970) Preliminary observations on the effect of synthetic thyrotropin releasing factor on plasma thyrotropin levels in man. *J. clin. Endocr.*, **31**, 109–112.

JACKSON, I. M. D. AND REICHLIN, S. (1974a) Thyrotropin releasing hormone (TRH): Distribution in hypothalamic and extrahypothalamic brain tissues of mammalian and submammalian chordates. *Endocrinology*, **96**, 854–862.

JACKSON, I. M. D. AND REICHLIN, S. (1974b) Thyrotropin releasing hormone (TRH): Distribution in the brain, blood and urine of the rat. *Life Sci.*, **14**, 2247–2257.

KASTIN, A. J., SCHALLY, A. V. AND VIOSCA, S. (1971) Inhibition of MSH release in frogs by direct application of L-prolyl-L-leucylglycinamide to the pituitary. *Proc. Soc. exp. Biol. (N.Y.)*, **137**, 1437–1439.

KASTIN, A. J. AND BARBEAU, A. (1972) Preliminary clinical studies with L-prolyl-L-leucyl-glycine amide in Parkinson's disease. *Canad. Med. Ass. J.*, **107**, 1079–1081.

KASTIN, A. J., EHRENSING, R. H., SCHALCH, D. S. AND ANDERSON, M. S. (1972) Improvement in mental depression with decreased thyrotropin response after administration of thyrotropin-releasing hormone. *Lancet*, **ii**, 740–742.

KELLER, H. H., BARTHOLINI, G. AND PLETSCHER, A. (1974) Enhancement of cerebral noradrenaline turnover by thyrotropin-releasing hormone. *Nature (Lond.)*, **248**, 528–529.

MAAS, J. W. AND LANDIS, D. H. (1968) *In vivo* studies of the metabolism of norepinephrine in the central nervous system. *J. Pharmacol. exp. Ther.*, **163**, 147–162.

MATSUO, H., ARIMURA, A., NAIR, R. M. G. AND SCHALLY, A. V. (1971) Synthesis of the porcine LH- and FSH-releasing hormone by the solid-phase method. *Biochem. biophys. Res. Commun.*, **45**, 822–827.

MAY, P. AND DONABEDIAN, R. K. (1973) A sensitive radioimmunoassay for thyrotropin releasing hormone. *Clin. chim. Acta (Amst.)*, **46**, 371–376.

MOSS, R. L. AND McCANN, S. M. (1973) Induction of mating behavior in rats by luteinizing hormone-releasing factor. *Science*, **181**, 177–179.

MUELLER, P. S., HENINGER, G. R. AND McDONALD, R. K. (1972) Studies on glucose utilization and insulin sensitivity in affective disorders. In *Recent Advances in the Psychobiology of the Depressive Illnesses*, T. A. WILLIAMS AND M. M. KATZ (Eds.), N.I.M.H., Rockville, N.Y., pp. 235–248.

PFAFF, D. W. (1973) Luteinizing hormone-releasing factor potentiates lordosis behavior in hypophysectomized ovariectomized female rats. *Science*, **182**, 1148–1149.

PLOTNIKOFF, N. P., KASTIN, A. J., ANDERSON, M. S. AND SCHALLY, A. V. (1971) DOPA potentiation by a hypothalamic factor, MSH release-inhibiting hormone (MIF). *Life Sci.*, **10**, 1279–1283.

PLOTNIKOFF, N. P., PRANGE, JR., A. J., BREESE, G. R., ANDERSON, M. S. AND WILSON, I. C. (1972a) Thyrotropin releasing hormone: enhancement of DOPA activity by a hypothalamic hormone. *Science*, **178**, 417–418.

PLOTNIKOFF, N. P., KASTIN, A. J., ANDERSON, M. S. AND SCHALLY, A. V. (1972b) Oxotremorine antagonism by a hypothalamic hormone, melanocyte-stimulating hormone release-inhibiting factor (MIF) (36558). *Proc. Soc. exp. Biol. (N.Y.)*, **140**, 811–814.

PLOTNIKOFF, N. P., PRANGE, JR., A. J., BREESE, G. R., ANDERSON, M. S. AND WILSON, I. C. (1974) The effects of thyrotropin releasing hormone on DOPA response in normal, hypophysectomized, and thyroidectomized animals. In *The Thyroid Axis, Drugs, and Behavior*, A. J. PRANGE, JR. (Ed.), Raven Press, New York, N.Y., pp. 103–113.

PRANGE, JR., A. J. (1964) The pharmacology and biochemistry of depression. *Dis. nerv. Syst.*, **25**, 217–221.

PRANGE, JR., A. J. AND WILSON, I. C. (1972) Thyrotropin releasing hormone (TRH) for the immediate relief of depression: A preliminary report. *Psychopharmacologia (Berl.)*, **26**, suppl., 82.

PRANGE, JR., A. J., WILSON, I. C., LARA, P. P., ALLTOP, L. B. AND BREESE, G. R. (1972) Effects of thyrotropin-releasing hormone in depression. *Lancet*, **ii**, 999–1002.

PRANGE, JR., A. J., BREESE, G. R., COTT, J. M., MARTIN, B. R., COOPER, B. R., WILSON, I. C. AND PLOTNIKOFF, N. P. (1974) Thyrotropin releasing hormone: Antagonism of pentobarbital in rodents. *Life Sci.*, **14**, 447–455.

REIGLE, T. G., AVNI, J., PLATZ, P. A., SCHILDKRAUT, J. J. AND PLOTNIKOFF, N. P. (1974) Norepinephrine metabolism in the rat brain following acute and chronic administration of thyrotropin releasing hormone. *Psychopharmacologia (Berl.)*, **37**, 1–6.

SACHAR, E. J., FINKELSTEIN, J. AND HELLMAN, L. (1971) Growth hormone responses in depressive illness. I. Response to insulin tolerance test. *Arch. gen. Psychiat. (Chic.)*, **25**, 263–269.

SCHILDKRAUT, J. J. (1965) The catecholamine hypothesis of affective disorders: A review of supporting evidence. *Amer. J. Psychiat.*, **122**, 509–522.

SEGAL, D. S. AND MANDELL, A. J. (1974) Differential behavioral effects of hypothalamic polypeptides. In *The Thyroid Axis, Drugs, and Behavior*, A. J. PRANGE, JR. (Ed.), Raven Press, New York, N.Y., pp. 129–133.

SILER, T. M., VAN DEN BERG, G. AND YEN, S. S. C. (1973) Inhibition of growth hormone release in humans by somatostatin. *J. clin. Endocr.*, **37**, 632–634.

STEIN, L. AND WISE, C. D. (1971) Possible etiology of schizophrenia: Progressive damage to the noradrenergic reward system by 6-hydroxydopamine. *Science*, **171**, 1032–1039.

STUMPF, W. E. AND SAR, M. (1973) ^{3}H-TRH and ^{3}H-proline radioactivity localization in pituitary and hypothalamus. *Fed. Proc.*, **32**, 1.

TAKAHASHI, S., KONDO, H., YOSHIMURA, M. AND OCHI, Y. (1973) Antidepressant effect of thyrotropin-releasing hormone (TRH) and the plasma thyrotropin levels in depression. *Folia psychiat. neurol. jap.*, **27**, 305-314.

TAUROG, A., OLIVER, C., ESKAY, R. L., PORTER, J. C. AND MCKENZIE, J. M. (1974) The role of TRH in the neoteny of the Mexican axolotl *(Ambystoma mexicanum)*. *Gen. comp. Endocr.*, **24**, 267–279.

TAUROG, A., OLIVER, C. AND PORTER, J. C. (1974) Metamorphosis in Mexican axolotl treated with TSH, TRH or LATS. *Gen. comp. Endocr.*, in press.

TIWARY, C. M., FRIAS, J. L. AND ROSENBLOOM, A. L. (1972) Response to thyrotropin in depressed patients. *Lancet*, **ii**, 1086.

TIWARY, C. M., ROSENBLOOM, A. L., ROBERTSON, M. F. AND PARKER, J. C. (1973) Improved behavior of hyperkinetic children given thyrotropin-releasing hormone (TRH). *Fourth Int. Congr. Int. Soc. Psychoneuroendocrinol., Berkeley, September 10–11*.

VALE, W., BRAZEAU, P., RIVIER, C., RIVIER, J., GRANT, G., BURGUS, R. AND GUILLEMIN, R. (1973a) Inhibitory hypophysiotropic activities of hypothalamic somatostatin. *Fed Proc.*, **32**, 211.

VALE, W., GRANT, G. AND GUILLEMIN, R. (1973b) Chemistry of the hypothalamic releasing factors — studies on structure–function relationships. In *Frontiers in Neuroendocrinology*, W. F. GANONG AND L. MARTINI (Eds.), Oxford University Press, New York, N.Y., pp. 375–413.

VAN DER VIS-MELSEN, M. J. E. AND WIENER, J. D. (1972) Improvement in mental depression with decreased thyrotropin response after administration of thyrotropin-releasing hormone. *Lancet*, **ii**, 1415.

WILSON, I. C., LARA, P. P. AND PRANGE, JR., A. J. (1973a) Thyrotropin-releasing hormone in schizophrenia. *Lancet*, **ii**, 43–44.

WILSON, I. C., PRANGE, JR., A. J., LARA, P. P., ALLTOP, L. B., STIKELEATHER, R. A. AND LIPTON, M. A. (1973b) TRH (lopremone): Psychobiological responses of normal women. I. Subjective experiences. *Arch. gen. Psychiat. (Chic.)*, **29**, 15–21.

WINOKUR, A. AND UTIGER, R. D. (1974) Thyrotropin-releasing hormone: regional distribution in rat brain. *Science*, **185**, 265–267.

Prolyl-Leucyl-Glycine Amide (PLG) and Thyrotropin-Releasing Hormone (TRH): DOPA Potentiation and Biogenic Amine Studies

NICHOLAS P. PLOTNIKOFF

Experimental Therapy Division, Abbott Laboratories, North Chicago, Ill. (U.S.A.)

INTRODUCTION

The finding by our group that thyrotropin-releasing hormone (TRH) is active in the pargyline–3,4-dihydroxy-phenylalanine (DOPA) mouse activation test formed in part the motive for trials of the hormone as a remedy for depression (Plotnikoff *et al.*, 1972). Prange and Wilson showed that TRH has a fast onset of antidepressant activity (Prange and Wilson, 1972; Prange *et al.*, 1972). This finding was confirmed by Kastin *et al.* (1972) and Van der Vis-Melsen and Wiener (1972). Thus, the value of this pharmacological test for identifying substances that have clinical antidepressant activity was further confirmed.

With these clinical findings at hand, it became a matter of interest to examine the activity of TRH in more detail on the behavioral response of DOPA and to examine the activity of related substances in this test. In the course of this work, it was rational to include in addition to the DOPA test, an animal test that relates to cerebral indoleamines because these substances have also been implicated in the pathogenesis of depression (Coppen, 1967; Glassman, 1969; Lapin and Oxenkrug, 1969). The final phase of the present work was to examine the influence of TRH on levels of cerebral biogenic amine concentrations in brain.

Earlier studies by Plotnikoff *et al.* (1971, 1972, 1973) indicated that prolyl-leucyl-glycine amide (PLG, often designated as melanocyte-stimulating hormone release-inhibiting factor (MIF)) potentiated behavioral effects of DOPA both in intact as well as hypophysectomized mice when administered by the intraperitoneal (i.p.) route; PLG also antagonized the central and peripheral effects of oxotremorine and deserpidine in mice. The present report examines the effects of PLG on DOPA potentiation and brain biogenic amine levels in rats and mice following acute and repeated doses.

MATERIALS AND METHODS

Behavioral tests of the potentiation of the effects of DOPA and pargyline were conducted in the Everett DOPA potentiation test as previously reported (Plotnikoff

References p. 22–23

et al., 1971). The critical variable in the DOPA test is the dose of pargyline (from 40 to 50 mg/kg) depending on age and strain of rodent employed. In addition, DL-DOPA (200 mg/kg, i.p.) gives more sustained behavioral effects than L-DOPA. This consists of observations of increases in irritability reactions, spontaneous motor activity caused by the test drug and squealing in animals treated with the test drug, DOPA and pargyline. The times after administration of PLG at which the behavioral ratings were made are indicated in the tables. The Swiss albino mice used in these behavioral studies and ablated animals were obtained from the Charles River Laboratories and the Attech Laboratories, Madison, Wisc. Both Long–Evans (Simonsen Labs.) and Sprague–Dawley rats (Charles River Labs.) were also used in testing DOPA potentiation (Everett, 1966).

The levels of dopamine (DA), norepinephrine (NE), homovanillic acid (HVA), and serotonin in the brain were determined by techniques previously reported from this laboratory (Everett and Borcherding, 1970; Everett and Yellin, 1971; Minard and Grant, 1972). For the experiments in which catecholamine levels were measured in the brains of mice, IRC male mice (17–22 g) were given PLG for either 1 or 5 days and decapitated 1 hr after the last i.p. injection. DA and HVA were also measured in male Long–Evans rats (200 g) decapitated 3–4 hr after a single i.p. injection of PLG or 1 hr after 5 successive days of a single i.p. administration of PLG.

RESULTS

Behavioral studies

No loss of activity or formation of tolerance to the behavioral potentiation of DOPA by TRH (Table I). Thus, in a wide dose range (0.05–8 mg/kg), TRH was found to be active in the Everett DOPA potentiation test when administered daily for 5 days.

TABLE I

EFFECTS OF TRH ON DOPA RESPONSE IN PARGYLINE-TREATED MICE AFTER SINGLE AND MULTIPLE DOSE ADMINISTRATION

The TRH was administered 1 hr prior to DOPA. In the case of chronic treatment, mice were treated for 5 days and tested 1 hr after the last dose. The degree of potentiation was: 1, slight; 2, moderate; 3, marked. Control mice received pargyline (40 mg/kg) and DOPA (100 mg/kg) which showed only slight effects. Each row indicates an experiment.

	Oral	*Chronic (5 days)*
Control	1	1
0.1	1	3
0.2	1	3
0.4	2	3
0.8	3	3
1.6	—	3

TABLE II

DOPA POTENTIATION IN MICE 1 AND 4 HR AFTER ORAL ADMINISTRATION OF PLG

Mice	Dose (mg/kg, p.o.)	Behavioral rating***	
		At 1 hr	At 4 hr
Normal	Controls	1	1
Intact	0.125*	1	1 (intact)
	0.25	3	1
	0.5	3	2
	1	3	2 2 (pinealectomy)
	2	3	3 3
	4	3	3 3
	8	3	3 3
	16	3	3 3
Hypophysectomized	0.05**	1	1
	0.1	1	1
	0.2	2	1
	0.4	3	3
	0.8	3	3
	1.6	3	3
	4	3	3
	8	3	3
	16	2	2
	Controls	1	1

* Six to 9 mice per dose at 1 hr and 20–36 mice per dose at 4 hr.
** Four to 8 mice per dose.
*** Behavioral rating: 1 = slight; 2 = moderate; and 3 = marked potentiation of DOPA–pargyline.

Indeed, there appeared to be an accumulative effect resulting in greater potency on the fifth day.

Marked potentiation of the behavioral effects of DOPA was observed in mice when PGL was administered by the oral route. Even low oral doses of PLG were found to be active in the DOPA test 1 and 4 hr after administration. Five days of treatment (Table II) were also effective.

Ablation studies

Table III shows that intraperitoneal administration of TRH is effective in females. It also shows that activity of TRH is not lost in ovariectomized mice. By comparison with Table I, it can be seen that there is a tendency for TRH to be more potent in female than in male mice in the pargyline–DOPA test. By these criteria it is more potent in normal female than ovariectomized mice as well.

In a series of ablation studies, TRH was found to be active in the DOPA test in adrenalectomized, thymectomized, unilaterally nephrectomized, splenectomized, parathyroidectomized, castrated, and pinealectomized mice (Table IV) (Hollander

TABLE III

EFFECT OF TRH IN INTACT AND OVARIECTOMIZED FEMALE MICE*

TRH (mg/kg, i.p. route)	Behavioral rating			
(A) Intact female mice				
0.05	2	1		
0.1	3	2		
0.2	3	2		
0.4	3	3		
0.8	3	3		
1.6	3	3		
(B) Ovariectomized mice				
0.05	1	1	1	
0.1	1	1	1	
0.2	1	2	1	2
0.4	2	2	2	2
0.8	3	3	2	3
1.6	3	3	3	3

* Animals were treated and rated as in Table I. TRH was administered 1 hr before DOPA. Rows of numbers indicate different experiments.

TABLE IV

DOPA POTENTIATION BY TRH IN ABLATED MICE

Surgical procedure	Dose (mg/kg, i.p. route)	Behavioral rating at 1 hr
None (intact)	0.05	1
	0.1	1
	0.2	2
	0.4	3
	0.8	3
Adrenalectomy	0.05	1
	0.1	2
	0.2	2
	0.4	3
	0.8	3
Thymectomy	0.05	1
	0.1	2
	0.2	2
	0.4	3
	0.8	3
Nephrectomy (unilateral)	0.05	1
	0.1	1
	0.2	2
	0.4	3
	0.8	3

(be continued on next page)

TABLE IV *(continued)*

Surgical procedure	Dose (mg/kg, i.p. route)	Behavioral rating at 1 hr
Splenectomy	0.05	1
	0.1	1
	0.2	2
	0.4	3
	0.8	3
Parathyroidectomy	0.05	2
	0.1	3
	0.2	3
	0.4	3
	0.8	3
Castration	0.05	1
	0.1	2
	0.2	3
	0.4	3
	0.8	3
Pinealectomy	0.1	2
	0.2	3
	0.4	3
	0.8	2

TABLE V

DOPA POTENTIATION BY PLG IN ABLATED MICE

Surgical procedure	Dose (mg/kg, i.p.)	Behavioral rating at 1 hr
None (intact)	0.025*	1
	0.05	1
	0.1	2
	0.2	3
	0.4	3
	0.8	3
	1.6	3
Adrenalectomy	0.05*	1
	0.1	1
	0.2	2
	0.4	2
	0.8	3
	1.6	3

(be continued on next page)

* Twelve mice per dose.

TABLE V *(continued)*

Surgical procedure	Dose (mg/kg, i.p.)	Behavioral rating at 1 hr	
		Controls (intact female)	
Ovariectomy**	0.05*	1	1
	0.1	1	1
	0.2	2	2
	0.4	3	2
	0.8	3	3
	1.6	3	3
Splenectomy	0.05*	1	
	0.1	1	
	0.2	2	
	0.4	3	
	0.8	3	
	1.6	3	
Parathyroidectomy	0.05*	1	
	0.1	2	
	0.2	3	
	0.4	3	
	0.8	3	
	1.6	3	
Castration	0.05*	1	
	0.1	2	
	0.2	3	
	0.4	3	
	0.8	3	
	1.6	3	
Nephrectomy (unilateral)	0.05*	1	
	0.1	2	
	0.2	3	
	0.4	3	
	0.8	3	
	1.6	3	
Thymectomy	0.05*	1	
	0.1	2	
	0.2	2	
	0.4	3	
	0.8	3	
	1.6	3	

* Eight mice per dose.
** All other mice were males.

et al., 1972; Prange *et al.*, 1973). Of great interest was the finding that TRH appeared to be more active in parathyroidectomized, castrated and pinealectomized mice.

In a series of (ablation) studies, PLG was found to be active in the DOPA test in adrenalectomized, ovariectomized, splenectomized, parathyroidectomized, castrated, unilaterally nephrectomized and thymectomized mice (Table V). In addition, PLG

TABLE VI

DOPA POTENTIATION IN RATS AFTER PLG

Dose (mg/kg, i.p.)	Behavioral rating (at 4 hr)	
	Intact	Thyroidectomized
Males		
0.05*	1	1
0.1	1	1
0.2	2	2
0.4	3	3
0.8	3	3
Females		
0.05**	1	1
0.1	1	1
0.2	1	1
0.4	2	2
0.8	3	2
1.6	3	3

* Eight rats per dose.
** Four rats per dose.

was effective in hypophysectomized as well as pinealectomized mice in the same test at similar doses (Table II).

Behavioral potentiation of DOPA was also observed with PLG in rats. This was found both in intact and thyroidectomized males as well as in intact and ovariectomized female rats (Table VI).

TRH plus imipramine

In the present body of work, the pargyline–DOPA test was used for a final time to

TABLE VII

POTENTIATION OF BEHAVIORAL EFFECTS OF DOPA IN MICE BY TRH AND IMIPRAMINE

Imipramine dose	Behavioral rating	
	Imipramine alone	Imipramine plus TRH (0.1 mg/kg, i.p.)*
0.5 mg/kg (oral)	1	1
1	1	2
2	1	2
2.5	1	3
5	1	3
10	2	3
20	2	3

* This dose of TRH alone causes only 1 + (slight) activation, which is the same as the control value.

References p. 22–23

TABLE VIII

EFFECTS OF TRH ON THE MOUSE 5-HTP POTENTIATION TEST

The doses of TRH were administered 1 hr prior to DL-5-hydroxytryptophan (HTP) (100 mg/kg). All mice received pargyline (40 mg/kg) 2 hr before TRH.

TRH alone (i.p. route)		Imipramine alone (oral route)		Imipramine plus TRH*	
mg/kg	Behavior (1)	mg/kg	Behavior	mg/kg	Behavior
0.1	1	10	1	10	1
0.2	2	20	1	20	1
0.4	2	40	1	40	1
0.8	3	80	2	80	3

* Dose of TRH was 0.1 mg/kg which produced a 1 + behavioral rating.

discern whether TRH would amplify the well-known effects of imipramine in this test model. Table VII confirmed once again the activity of TRH and the activity of imipramine. Furthermore, it shows that the activities of the two substances potentiate or at least add to each other's effects. This would commend to the clinical investigator a trial of TRH as a potentiator of imipramine and such a trial finds precedent in the extensive work of Prange *et al.* (1969) who have used triiodo-thyronine as an adjunct to treatment with imipramine.

Serotonin potentiation by TRH

Table VIII shows that TRH is active in the serotonin potentiation test. However, when TRH and imipramine were given together, no potentiation was observed.

α-Methyl-p-tyrosine and TRH

Pretreatment of mice with α-methyl-*p*-tyrosine markedly reduced the activity of TRH in the DOPA potentiation test but did *not* abolish it (Table IX).

The effects of TRH and PLG on brain biogenic amines

The above work strongly suggested an interaction between TRH and brain biogenic amines. For this reason it was of interest to examine the effects of TRH treatment on the levels of these substances. Groups of male Swiss–Webster mice were treated with various doses of i.p. TRH for 5 days or with controlled injection. Table X shows that none of the doses employed had reliable effect on brain dopamine, norepinephrine, or serotonin. It can be seen that the behaviorally active doses of TRH were without effect on brain amines (Prange *et al.*, 1972).

Neurochemical studies in normal intact mice did not reveal any significant alteration

TABLE IX

EFFECT OF α-METHYL-p-TYROSINE ON TRH IN THE DOPA POTENTIATION TEST

Pretreatment with α-methyl-p-tyrosine (300 mg/kg, i.p., 4 hr).

TRH (mg/kg, i.p.)	Behavioral rating at 1 hr
0.4	1
0.8	2
1.6	3

TABLE X

EFFECT OF TRH ON THE BRAIN BIOGENIC AMINES IN MICE

Animals were treated with various doses of TRH for 5 days and killed 1 hr after the last dose of TRH.

Controls	Dopamine (µg/g)	Norepinephrine (µg/g)	Serotonin (µg/g)
Oral route	0.91 ± 0.02	0.59 ± 0.01	0.55 ± 0.02
TRH (mg/kg)			
0.5	0.96 ± 0.02	0.61 ± 0.01	0.56 ± 0.05
1.0	0.94 ± 0.03	0.57 ± 0.02	0.52 ± 0.01
2.0	0.91 ± 0.01	0.55 ± 0.01	0.55 ± 0.02
4.0	1.01 ± 0.02	0.55 ± 0.01	0.51 ± 0.02
8.0	0.93 ± 0.01	0.55 ± 0.01	0.54 ± 0.01

of brain levels of biogenic amines after a single or after 5 daily injections of PLG (Tables XI and XII).

As can be seen upon examination of the results presented in Table XIII, PLG did not increase the level of DA in rat brain even at this high dose of 100 mg/kg. Nor did it increase the levels of HVA, the presence of which might be an indirect indication

TABLE XI

BRAIN BIOGENIC AMINE LEVELS IN MICE AFTER A SINGLE INJECTION OF PLG

Dose (mg/kg, i.p.)	Number of mice	Dopamine**	Mean ± S.E. (µg/g)*	
			Norepinephrine	Serotonin
0 (controls)	3	1.06 ± 0.03	0.50 ± 0.01	0.62 ± 0.01
10	3	1.16 ± 0.04	0.49 ± 0.01	0.57 ± 0.02
20	3	1.11 ± 0.01	0.47 ± 0.01	0.57 ± 0.01
40	3	1.12 ± 0.05	0.49 ± 0.01	0.59 ± 0.01
80	3	1.11 ± 0.05	0.44 ± 0.03	0.54 ± 0.01

* One hour after treatment.
** Levels measured according to Everett and Borcherding (1970).

References p. 22–23

TABLE XII

BRAIN BIOGENIC AMINE LEVELS IN MICE AFTER DAILY INJECTION OF PLG FOR 5 DAYS

PLG (mg/kg, i.p.)	Number of mice	Dopamine**	Mean ± S.E. (µg/g)*	
			Norepinephrine	Serotonin
0 (controls)	3	0.65 ± 0.01	0.49 ± 0.00	0.33 ± 0.01
5	4	0.67 ± 0.00	0.51 ± 0.00	0.31 ± 0.01
10	4	0.67 ± 0.00	0.51 ± 0.00	0.31 ± 0.00
20	4	0.65 ± 0.00	0.51 ± 0.00	0.30 ± 0.00

* One hour after last injection.
** Levels measured according to Minard and Grant (1972).

TABLE XIII

BRAIN BIOGENIC AMINE LEVELS IN RATS AFTER 1 AND 5 DAILY INJECTIONS OF PLG

Dopamine level was measured according to Minard and Grant (1972). Homovanillic acid was measured on column effluents with method of Murphy *et al.* (1969).

Tissue	Dose PLG (mg/kg, i.p.)	No. of days injected	DA	HVA
Whole brain	0	—	0.60 ± 0.03 (5)*	—
	100	1	0.64 ± 0.02 (4)	—
Caudate nucleus	0	—	10.6 ± 0.30 (5)	1.49 ± 0.07 (5)
	100	1	10.5 ± 0.39 (5)	1.52 ± 0.13 (5)
Caudate nucleus	0	—	10.3 ± 0.30 (8)	1.32 ± 0.06 (7)
	100	5	11.3 ± 0.41 (8)	1.14 ± 0.06 (8)

* Mean ± S.E. (number of animals in parentheses).

of the turnover of DA. None of the paired values (Table VIII) were significantly different from each other at the 0.05 level of probability (Murphy *et al.*, 1969).

DISCUSSION

It can readily be seen that the 4 hormones of the hypothalamic–pituitary–thyroid axis are active in the pargyline–DOPA test in mice. So far as has been discerned, TRH is active in both sexes. In female mice, the actions of TRH were not dependent upon the presence of the ovary. Furthermore, the activity of TRH depends neither upon the pituitary gland, nor on the thyroid gland.

The present studies indicate that removal of the adrenals, thymus, one kidney, spleen, parathyroid, testes, ovaries, or pineal gland did not prevent the activity of TRH in the dopamine potentiation test. However, the potency of TRH was reduced in ovariectomized, but increased in castrated, parathyroidectomized, or pinealecto-mized mice. Thus, there appears to be endocrine interaction with TRH from these glands.

The studies described here also indicate that removal of the adrenals, ovaries, testes, spleen, thyroid, parathyroid, kidney, or thymus does not alter the actions of PLG in the test system. Although these organs might not have been expected to be involved in the actions of PLG, the pituitary could have been. Oral administration of PLG to hypophysectomized mice again demonstrated that the pituitary gland is not required for the actions of PLG in the DOPA potentiation test. The effectiveness of PLG in mice in which these organs have been ablated further supports our concept of the extra-endocrine effects of PLG.

Present findings are consistent with those of Breese et al. (1974) that TRH does not elevate brain levels of dopamine, norepinephrine and serotonin. It should be pointed out, however, that brain levels of dopamine are 50% higher in TRH-treated mice than in control mice, 20 min after DOPA administration in the Everett test. Dopaminergic receptors are probably affected since our studies showed that α-methyl-p-tyrosine reduced the effects of TRH.

Since the test system used in this study involves DOPA, it was reasonable to examine brain levels of biogenic amines after administration of PLG. Mice did not show any significant alteration in the total brain content of dopamine, norepinephrine, or serotonin after either a single injection or 5 daily injections of PLG. Similarly, dopamine content of the rat brain was not altered by PLG. The caudate nucleus, an area of the brain particularly rich in catecholamines, was specifically examined for changes in content of DA or HVA after either 1 or 5 daily injections of PLG, but no changes were found.

Thus, if TRH and PLG affect dopaminergic systems, they may do so by a direct action which does not involve alterations in levels of dopamine (Lahti et al., 1972). Such speculations must be considered with the reservations that total brain content of some catecholamines does not necessarily reflect uptake or turnover rates, or even alterations in small areas of the brain. Further studies are required to determine whether TRH and PLG may be acting as neurotransmitters in the systems in which we have shown them to have extra-endocrine effects (Kastin and Barbeau, 1973; Prange et al., 1974).

SUMMARY

The central nervous system activity of TRH (thyrotropin-releasing hormone) and MIF (melanocyte-stimulating hormone-release inhibiting factor, prolyl-leucyl-glycine amide (PLG)) was discovered by means of the Everett brain dopamine potentiation test for antidepressant activity and the Everett oxotremorine antagonism test for antiparkinson activity. When either TRH or MIF was administered over 5 days the original level of activity was maintained in the dopamine potentiation test. No evidence of tolerance was observed. A clear separation of central effects from periph-

eral endocrine effects was demonstrated for both TRH and MIF in hypophysectomized animals. The central effects of TRH or MSH release from the pituitary. Furthermore, ablation of the adrenals, ovaries, testes, pineal, spleen, parathyroid, one kidney,
or thymus, did not disrupt the behavioral potentiation of dopamine by TRH or MIF.
Biogenic amine brain levels in mice and rats were not altered by TRH or MIF.

REFERENCES

BREESE, G. R., COOPER, B. R., PRANGE, JR., A. J., COTT, J. M. AND LIPTON, M. A. (1974) Interactions
    of thyrotropin-releasing hormone with centrally acting drugs. In *The Thyroid Axis, Drugs and
    Behavior*, A. J. PRANGE, JR. (Ed.), Raven Press, New York, N.Y., pp. 115–127.
COPPEN, A. (1967) The biochemistry of affective disorders. *Brit. J. Psychiat.*, **113**, 1237–1264.
EVERETT, G. M. (1966) The DOPA response potentiation test and its use in screening for antidepressant
    drugs. In *Excerpta Medica International Congress Series No. 122*, Excerpta Medica, Amsterdam,
    pp. 164–167.
EVERETT, G. M. AND YELLIN, T. O. (1971) Effect of 4-chlorophenoxyamphetamine (A-6587), D-
    amphetamine and 4-chloroamphetamine of biogenic amines and behavior in mice. *Res. Commun.
    Chem. Path. Pharm.*, **2**, 407–410.
EVERETT, G. M. AND BORCHERDING, J. W. (1970) L-Dopa effect on concentrations of dopamine,
    norepinephrine and serotonin in brains of mice. *Science*, **168**, 849.
GLASSMAN, A. (1969) Indoleamines and affective disorders. *Psychosom. Med.*, **31**, 107–114.
HOLLANDER, C. S., MITSUMA, T., SHENKMAN, L., WOOLF, P. AND GERSHENGORN, M. C. (1972)
    Thyrotropin-releasing hormone: evidence for thyroid response to intravenous injection in man.
    Science, **175**, 209–210.
KASTIN, A. B., EHRENSING, R. N., SCHALCH, D. S. AND ANDERSON, M. S. (1972) Improvement in
    mental depression with decreased thyrotroping response after administration of thyrotropin-
    releasing hormone. *Lancet*, **ii**, 740–742.
KASTIN, A. J. AND BARBEAU, A. (1973) Preliminary clinical studies with L-prolyl-L-leucyl-glycine
    amide in Parkinson's disease. *J. Canad. Med. Ass.*, **107**, 1079–1081.
LAPIN, I. P. AND OXENKRUG, G. F. (1969) Intensification of the central serotonergic process as a
    possible determinant of the thymoleptic effect. *Lancet*, **ii**, 132–136.
LAHTI, R. A., MCALLISTER, B. AND WOZNIAK, J. (1972) Apomorphine antagonism of the elevation
    of homovanillic acid induced by antipsychotic drugs. *Life Sci.*, **11**, 605–609.
MINARD, F. N. AND GRANT, D. S. (1972) A convenient method for the chromatographic analyses of
    norepinephrine, dopamine and serotonin. *Biochem. Med.*, **6**, 46–52.
MURPHY, G. F., ROBINSON, D. AND SHARMAN, D. F. (1969) The effect of tropolone on the formation
    of 3,4-dihydroxyphenylacetic acid and 4-hydroxy-3-methoxphenyl-acetic acid in the brain of the
    mouse. *Brit. J. Pharmacol.*, **36**, 107–110.
PLOTNIKOFF, N. P., KASTIN, A. J., ANDERSON, M. S. AND SCHALLY, A. V. (1971) DOPA potentiation
    by a hypothalamic factor, MSH release-inhibiting hormone (MIF). *Life Sci.*, **10**, 1279–1283.
PLOTNIKOFF, N. P., KASTIN, A. J., ANDERSON, M. S. AND SCHALLY, A. V. (1973) Deserpidine antag-
    onism by a tripeptide, L-prolyl-L-leucylglycinamide. *Neuroendocrinology*, **11**, 67–71.
PLOTNIKOFF, N. P., PRANGE, JR., A. J., BREESE, G. R., ANDERSON, M. S. AND WILSON, Y. C. (1972)
    Thyrotropin releasing hormone: enhancement of DOPA activity by a hypothalamic hormone.
    Science, **178**, 417–418.
PRANGE, JR., A. J. (1973) The use of drugs in depression: its theoretical and practical basis. *Psychiat.
    Ann.*, **13**, 56–75.
PRANGE, A. J., SISK, J. L., WILSON, I. C., MORRIS, C. E., HALL, C. D. AND CARMAN, J. S. (1974)
    Balance, permission, and discrimination among amines: a theoretical consideration of L-tryptophan
    in disorders of movement and affect. In *Serotonin and Behavior*, J. D. BARCHAS AND E. USDIN
    (Eds.), Academic Press, New York, N.Y.
PRANGE, JR., A. J. AND WILSON, I. C. (1972) Thyrotropin releasing hormone (TRH) for the immediate
    relief of depression: a preliminary report. *Psychopharmacologia*, Suppl., **26**, 82.
PRANGE, JR., A. J., WILSON, I. C., LARA, P. P., ALLTOP, L. B. AND BREESE, G. R. (1972) Effects of
    thyrotropin-releasing hormone in depression. *Lancet*, **ii**, 999–1002.

Prange, Jr., A. J., Wilson, I. C., Lara, P. P., Wilber, J. F., Breese, G. R., Alltop, L. B. and Lipton, M. A. (1973) Thyrotropin releasing hormone: psychobiological responses of normal women. II. Pituitary–thyroid responses. *Arch. gen. Psychiat.*, **29**, 15–21.

Prange, Jr., A. J., Wilson, I. C., Rabon, A. M. and Lipton, M. A. (1969) Enhancement of imipramin antidepressant activity by thyroid hormone. *Amer. J. Psychiat.*, **126**, 457–469.

Van der Vis-Melsen, M. J. E. and Wiener, J. D. (1972) Improvement in mental depression with decreased thyrotropin response after administration of thyrotropin-releasing hormone. *Lancet*, **ii**, 1415.

Studies on Pituitary Hormones and Releasing Hormones in Depression and Sexual Impotence

O. BENKERT

Psychiatrische Klinik der Universität München, Nussbaumstrasse 7, 8 Munich 2 (G.F.R.)

INTRODUCTION

Studies over the last few years on releasing hormones signify a novel starting-point in biological psychiatry. Besides the question whether releasing hormones have therapeutical effects or not in psychiatric disorders, the influence of pituitary hormones on psychiatric disorders can now be extensively studied, which has been facilitated by developing radioimmunoassays. In the following experiments some of these questions in respect to research of depression and sexual impotence will be discussed.

First we raised the question, whether just as in animal experiments the influence of biogenic amines on the hypothalamic–pituitary axis could be demonstrated on the human, too. This was studied by measuring the plasma concentration of some pituitary hormones in healthy subjects after giving precursors of catecholamines and serotonin and *p*-chlorophenylalanine (PCPA), the inhibitor of the biosyntheses of serotonin.

(I) Effect of L-DOPA, DL-5-HTP and L-PCPA on pituitary hormones in healthy subjects

(A) L-DOPA (3,4-dihydroxyphenylalanine)

In several studies on man it has been shown that *growth-hormone* (GH) secretion could be stimulated by L-DOPA (Boyd *et al.*, 1970; Kansal *et al.*, 1972; Perlow *et al.*, 1972; Souvatzoglou *et al.*, 1973; Sachar, 1975).

On the other hand it was observed in some of these studies that GH response to oral and intravenous L-DOPA is variable. We were interested to see whether different dosages of L-DOPA in combination with the decarboxylase inhibitor, Ro4-4602, were able to increase the GH secretion more than L-DOPA alone, since it has been demonstrated that L-DOPA in combination with Ro4-4602 leads to a higher increase of dopamine concentration in the brain than L-DOPA alone (Butcher and Engel, 1969; Henning and Rubenson, 1970; Bartholini *et al.*, 1971; Maj *et al.*, 1971; Benkert *et al.*, 1973a).

All 5 subjects tested demonstrated an adequate increase of the plasma GH levels after adequate insulin-induced hypoglycemia (Table I). The mean maximal response

TABLE I

PLASMA LEVELS OF GROWTH HORMONE (ng/ml) FOLLOWING L-DOPA, L-DOPA + Ro4-4602, DL-5-HTP + Ro4-4602 AND INSULIN

Time (min)	L-DOPA 25.0 mg	Ro4-4602 pretreatment					Insulin (0.15 U/kg body wt.)
		L-DOPA				DL-5-HTP 150.0 mg	
		12.5 mg	25.0 mg	50.0 mg	75.0 mg		
−15	2.1	1.9	2.2	2.5	1.7	1.8	3.0
0	2.0	2.1	2.0	2.2	1.6	1.8	3.2
10	1.9	2.4	2.2	1.1	1.2	1.6	
20	1.8	2.9	1.4	2.5	1.3	1.5	
30	1.9	4.9	1.8	2.0	1.4	1.2	4.7
40	2.5	5.5	2.3	2.1	1.9	1.4	22.7
60	2.7	4.6	2.4	1.6	2.0	1.9	35.1
75	1.6	3.3	1.9	1.8	2.0	1.5	
90	1.8	4.3	1.7	1.1	1.6	1.9	45.3
105	1.6	2.2	1.3	1.3	2.5	1.2	
120	1.6	2.9	1.9	1.8	1.3	2.1	
135	2.0	1.1	2.4	3.9	1.5	1.7	
150	1.9	1.3	1.9	5.5	1.6	2.7	
165	2.5	2.4	1.2	4.4	1.9	2.4	
180	2.7	3.3	2.1	3.1	1.9	1.6	
195		2.9	2.6	2.1	2.4	1.5	
210		2.6	1.6	2.6	4.2	2.3	
225		2.1	1.9	2.5	4.1	2.0	
240		3.2	1.5	2.2	2.7	1.9	
	n = 5 $\bar{x}$ = 2.0 s = 0.36	n = 4 $\bar{x}$ = 2.9 s = 1.18	n = 3 $\bar{x}$ = 1.9 s = 0.39	n = 4 $\bar{x}$ = 2.4 s = 1.12	n = 4 $\bar{x}$ = 2.1 s = 0.85	n = 4 $\bar{x}$ = 1.8 s = 0.39	n = 5 $\bar{x}$ = 19.0 s = 20.9

was 45.3 ± 9.9 ng GH/ml ± S.E.M. The same subjects received 25 mg L-DOPA and only two subjects showed a slight increase of plasma GH levels, the mean remaining below 7.7 ng/ml. L-DOPA, after pretreatment with the decarboxylase inhibitor (for 5 days, 3 × 125 mg Ro4-4602), caused only a slight increase of the GH plasma level in 3 subjects. Although one subject showed an increase 40 min after 12.5 mg L-DOPA to a maximum of 16.4 ng/ml, and two other subjects showed a late GH rise after 50 mg and 75 mg respectively, the mean GH increase of all subjects was not statistically significant at any of the L-DOPA levels (Table I).

It must be mentioned that only male subjects were studied and that the GH increase is more pronounced and more consistent among females than among males (Merimee et al., 1967). This could be one explanation for missing a statistically significant GH increase in our experiments. Also, in our studies L-DOPA was administered intravenously, in contrast to the oral application in most of the above mentioned studies.

In 4 subjects, plasma levels of *luteinizing hormone* (LH) were measured over a period of 4 hr in 15-min intervals after L-DOPA alone or in combination with Ro4-4602 (see dosages in Table I). All subjects showed the typical episodic LH secretion.

This pattern of episodic LH secretion was not significantly influenced by L-DOPA in various dosages, with or without Ro4-4602 pretreatment.

The inability to influence the pattern of LH secretion in men by administration of L-DOPA has been shown previously (Boyd *et al.*, 1970; Eddy *et al.*, 1971; Perlow *et al.*, 1972; Souvatzoglou *et al.*, 1973) and is confirmed and extended by these findings, inasmuch that also very *high* doses of L-DOPA in combination with Ro4-4602 have no influence on the LH serum pattern.

(B) DL-5-HTP (5-hydroxytryptophan)

All subjects who received DL-5-HTP were pretreated with Ro4-4602 in the same manner as those described above. Two subjects were injected with 75 mg DL-5-HTP, 2 subjects with 100 mg DL-5-HTP and 4 subjects with 150 mg DL-5-HTP. Blood collections were again sampled from 15 min before until 4 hr after the injection of DL-5-HTP.

In contrast to Imura *et al.* (1973) who found stimulation of GH secretion after 5-HTP, we did not see any influence of the serotonin precursor on GH secretion (Table I).

The effect of DL-5-HTP on LH-secretion in men has not been investigated. Although animal work suggested that serotonin might inhibit LH secretion (O'Steen, 1964; Kordon *et al.*, 1968) we did not find any influence of DL-5-HTP given at doses of 75, 100, and 150 mg intravenously after decarboxylase inhibitor pretreatment. The possible discrepancy between men and animals might be due to species specific control of gonadotropin secretion.

The findings that LH and GH blood levels are not, or not regularly, influenced by the administration of precursors of biogenic amines, which are known to cross the blood–brain barrier and lead to accumulation of dopamine and serotonin in the brain, demonstrate that the measurements of these hormones will not serve as an indicator for the brain concentration of biogenic amines, as could have been anticipated by the results of earlier investigations (Benkert *et al.*, 1973b).

(C) L-PCPA (para-chlorophenylalanine)

We then attempted to find out if the inhibition of the biosynthesis of serotonin could have an influence on the secretion of the pituitary hormones and several steroid hormones. Contradictory results have been reported on the effect of PCPA on gonadotropins, ovulation and testicular function in animals (Donoso *et al.*, 1971; Brown and Fawke, 1972; Kordon and Glowinski, 1972; Bliss *et al.*, 1972; Gawienowski *et al.*, 1973).

In 6 healthy male subjects the effect of L-PCPA (1.5 g/day over a period of 12 days) on the plasma levels of the following hormones was measured: LH, follicle-stimulating hormone (FSH), GH, thyrotropin (TSH), testosterone, estrone, estradiol, 17-α-hydroxyprogesterone and cortisol. LH and FSH were measured before and after L-PCPA treatment over a period of 4 hr at 15-min intervals between 9 a.m. and 1 p.m. The other hormones were measured under the same conditions but only in hourly intervals. 5-Hydroxyindole-acetic acid (5-HIAA) in the urine decreased significantly

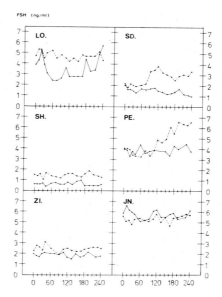

Fig. 1. Effect of ʟ-PCPA on plasma FSH in healthy male subjects. Plasma FSH was measured in 6 subjects over 240 min at 15-min intervals before (solid line) and after (dotted line) intake of 1.5 g ʟ-PCPA daily for 12 days.

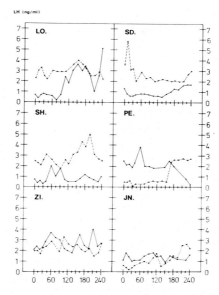

Fig. 2. Effect of ʟ-PCPA on plasma LH in healthy male subjects. Plasma LH was measured in 6 subjects over 240 min in 15-min intervals before (solid line) and after (dotted line) intake of 1.5 g ʟ-PCPA daily for 12 days.

($P < 0.025$) from 6.06 ± 2.8 µg/ml to 1.75 ± 0.96 µg/ml after L-PCPA treatment. A slight but not significant increase in FSH plasma level is seen in 5 subjects after L-PCPA when compared to the basic levels; but the individual values are still within the normal range (Fig. 1). No influence of L-PCPA could be recorded for LH (Fig. 2), for testosterone, nor for the other hormones mentioned above. These results will be reported in more detail elsewhere, including the assay procedures (Benkert *et al.*, to be published).

These results demonstrate that inhibition of the biosynthesis of serotonin with the above mentioned dosages of L-PCPA has no influence on pituitary hormones or steroid hormones in male subjects. Thus there is no effect on the pituitary–gonadal axis — an effect which might have been assumed in explaining the effect of PCPA on male sexual behavior.

(II) LH plasma concentration in manic and depressive patients

The report of a correlation between GH release and the initial phase of slow-wave sleep (ref. in Rubin, 1975), the report of the possible changes of the GH response in respect to the insulin tolerance test in depressive illness (Sachar, 1975), the report of a short but rapid antidepressive effect of thyrotropin-releasing hormone (TRH) (Prange, 1975) and the reports about the neurotropic effects of TRH in animal experiments (Plotnikoff, 1975) have stimulated us to explore the possibility of

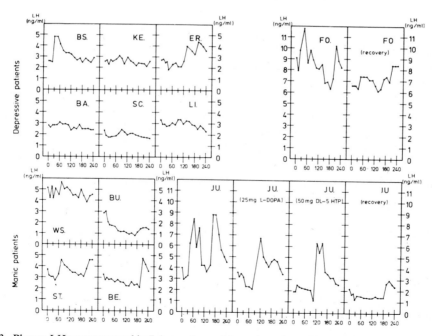

Fig. 3. Plasma LH was measured in 7 depressive and 5 manic patients for 240 min at 15-min intervals. Additionally, LH was measured in patient "FO" during recovery and in patient "JU" during the manic status, after stimulation with 25 mg L-DOPA and 50 mg DL-5-HTP and during the recovery.

References p. 34–36

disturbances in the secretion of another gonadotropin (LH) in the manic-depressive illness. LH plasma levels were measured in 7 monopolar endogenously depressed male patients and 5 manic male patients of whom 1 patient ("JU", Fig. 3) had a bipolar endogenous depression (2 manic and 1 depressive phases). None of the patients had been pretreated with antidepressants nor minor tranquilizers for 2 weeks before, and neuroleptics for 6 weeks before the day of LH determination. Plasma samples had been taken every 15 min over a period of 4 hr starting at 9 a.m., with the exception of 2 manic patients, starting in the evening. Six depressive and 4 manic patients had LH plasma levels within the normal range. The high LH level of the depressed patient "FO" was unprecedented in our male samples without endocrinological diseases. After recovery the high LH spikes disappeared. A similar case is the manic patient "JU". His LH plasma levels were very high in the manic status and within the normal range during recovery, when the high spikes also disappeared. In the manic status we tried to stimulate LH in intervals of 2 days with DL-5-HTP and L-DOPA in this patient; however, the LH plasma level showed no significant differences to the basic LH level in the manic status (Fig. 3).

We think that these findings might further hint at an endocrine dysfunction in *some* endogenously depressed patients in the manic or depressive status, demonstrated by an increased LH plasma level. Certainly this statement is to be made under the above mentioned conditions without considering the whole 24-hr rhythm.

(III) Effect of releasing hormones in depressive patients

(A) TRH, LHRH and placebo in a doubleblind-crossover study

The report of a short but rapid antidepressive effect of TRH, first described by Prange, has been followed by several single case and doubleblind studies either substantiating or refuting these claims (Kastin *et al.*, 1972; Van der Vis-Melsen and Wiener, 1972; Itil, 1973; Cassano *et al.*, 1973; Dimitrikoudi *et al.*, 1974; Ehrensing *et al.*, 1974; Maggini *et al.*, 1974; van den Burg *et al.*, 1975). It was therefore the aim of this study to determine whether the reported antidepressive effects previously observed were specific to TRH, or whether similar results could be produced by another hypothalamic factor, luteinizing hormone-releasing hormone (LHRH) or placebo. Thus we carried out a doubleblind-crossover study with 12 female endogenously depressed patients, 9 monopolar and 3 bipolar.

The patients were treated in a randomized order with a single injection of 600 μg TRH, 500 μg LHRH and placebo and rated for changes in their depression scores over a 6-day period. The patients were assessed over an 8-day period using both the Hamilton Depressions-Scale and a self-rating scale 3 times per day at 9 a.m., 1 p.m. and 5 p.m. and the 100 mm line at hourly intervals from 7 a.m. to 6 p.m. Previous to the wash-out period the patients could be pretreated with antidepressants or minor tranquilizers. No significant differences were seen among the various treatments (Figs. 4 and 5). Nevertheless, in 11 patients sudden transient or longer lasting improvements were observed. These improvements were described on the basis of the rater's global observation together with the patients' own reports and differed from the usual daily variations. These sudden improvements were reported 6 times with LHRH, 4 times with TRH and 3 times with placebo. The question arises whether or not the antidepressive effects of TRH, reported earlier in the literature, were of a similar nature; if they were, we suppose that such sudden improvements are usual in depressed patients independent of medication.

(B) Imipramine plus TRH or placebo in a doubleblind study

The reported neurotropic effects of TRH in animals especially in the combination with the tricyclic antidepressant drug, imipramine (Plotnikoff, 1975), raised the question whether the combination of TRH plus imipramine could shorten the latency and improve the antidepressive effect of imipramine. It could be demonstrated in several experiments that TRH given orally has the same physiological effect as TRH given i.v. (Benkert et al., to be published). Therefore, 10 female and 10 male depressed patients received, in addition to an imipramine basic therapy (3×50 mg/day oral), TRH (2×40 mg/day oral) or placebo for 14 days in a doubleblind technique. Again the Hamilton Depressions-Scale and a self-rating scale were used. But there was neither a difference in the degree nor in the time of the beginning of the antidepressive effect after 14 days of TRH and placebo for the female or the male group. Similar results concerning the combination of TRH plus amytriptyline were reported by Coppen (personal communication).

These results clearly support the suggestion that TRH has no therapeutic anti-depressive effect.

(IV) Effect of releasing hormones in sexual impotent patients

(A) TRH in a doubleblind-crossover study

TRH was given to sexually impotent patients for a therapeutic purpose. This was done on the one hand to stimulate hypothalamic centers, which might be possible because of the neurotropic effect of TRH (Plotnikoff, 1975). On the other hand the thyroid-stimulating effect of TRH was required.

TRH was given orally to 12 impotent patients in a dose of 40 mg/daily for 4 weeks in a doubleblind-crossover technique compared with placebo. The 12 patients were selected in a randomized order to receive placebo in the first 4 weeks and then TRH for 4 weeks or vice versa. The patients had to state their daily sexual feelings and behavior in a questionnaire.

The calculation of the daily questionnaires and the subjective evaluation by the doctor proved that TRH gave no more of a therapeutic effect than placebo.

(B) LHRH in a doubleblind study

Recently, animal experiments have given evidence that LHRH may play a role in the induction of mating behavior (Moss and McCann, 1973) and facilitate lordosis responses in female rats (Pfaff, 1973).

LHRH has been given as a nasal spray in a doubleblind study to 6 sexually impotent

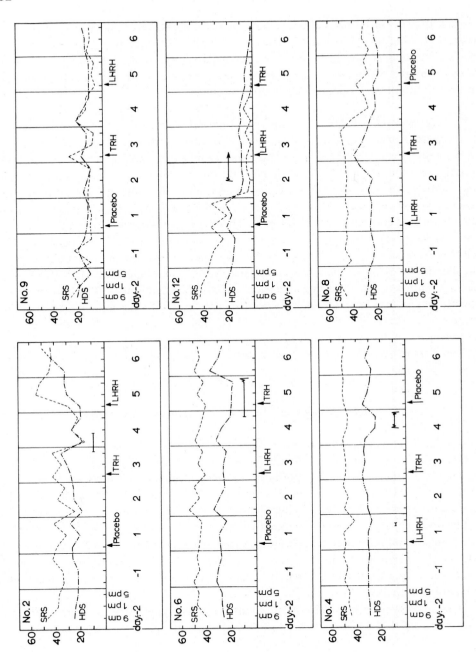

Fig. 4.

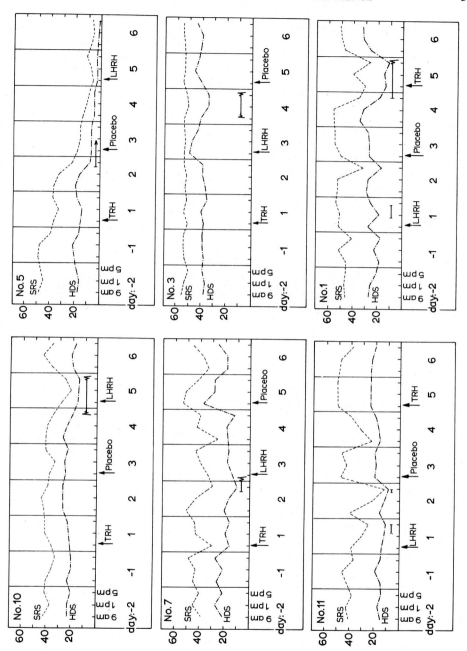

Figs. 4 and 5. Diagrams of the changes occurring during the 6-day therapy in 12 female depressed patients. Placebo, TRH (600 μg) and LHRH (500 μg) were injected intravenously at 9.15 a.m. Patients with corresponding dose-schedules were compared in the diagram (*i.e.* No. 2 and No. 9: 1, placebo; 2, TRH; 3, LHRH). Day −2, −1: wash-out period. On the first day of the wash-out period all patients also received a placebo infusion intravenously. SRS: Self-rating scale (v. Zerssen), HDS: Hamilton Depressions-Scale. Lines with squared-off ends: sudden improvements within the specified time limits. Lines with spiky ends: sudden improvements approximately within the specified time limits.

References p. 34–36

patients. All received placebo spray for 2 weeks, thereafter 3 patients received LHRH spray (1 mg/day) for 4 weeks, and the other 3 patients received placebo spray for 4 weeks. At the end of the trial a 2-week placebo spray treatment followed for all patients. After the trial the patients had to fill out the questionnaires for a further 2 months. Two placebo patients observed no effect; 1 patient reported an improvement under placebo which lasted only until the end of the treatment. One of the patients taking LHRH showed a good increase in penile erection after the beginning of the LHRH period; the effect was uninterrupted after discontinuing the spray. The second patient in the LHRH group had a strong increase in penile erection *after* changing from LHRH to placebo spray. The third patient in the LHRH group reported an unpleasant sensibility in the penis and in the testes and experienced emission of sperms during urination until the end of the placebo period. But *after* discontinuation of LHRH he observed an increase of penile erection during intercourse, uninterrupted in the drug-free period until the end of the sixth week.

Because only 6 patients have been treated to date, a final result cannot be given. However, in comparison to other drug studies in impotent patients using TRH, L-DOPA, PCPA and antiserotonergic substances, the results with LHRH in sexually impotent patients, especially after discontinuation of treatment, must be noted.

SUMMARY

L-DOPA, DL-5-HTP and L-PCPA have no statistically significant effect on LH and GH plasma levels. Further, L-PCPA has no effect on FSH, TSH, testosterone or other steroid hormones in male subjects.

An indication of the existence of an endocrine dysfunction in some endogenously depressed patients is demonstrated by a high LH plasma level in the manic and depressive status and the disappearance of the high LH spikes during recovery in 2 of 12 male patients.

No significant therapeutic differences were seen between TRH, LHRH and placebo in endogenously depressed patients. Transient improvements were subjectively observed under all drugs. The combination of imipramine plus TRH has no better and no quicker an effect than imipramine plus placebo in depressed patients.

TRH has no more of a therapeutic effect than placebo in sexually impotent patients. The effect of LHRH seems to be more promising in these patients.

REFERENCES

BARTHOLINI, G., CONSTANTINIDIS, R., TISSOT, R. AND PLETSCHER, A. (1971) Formation of mono-amines from various acids in the brain after inhibition of extracerebral decarboxylase. *Biochem. Pharmacol.*, **20**, 1243–1247.

BENKERT, O., GLUBA, H. AND MATUSSEK, N. (1973a) Dopamine, noradrenaline and 5-hydroxytrypt-amine in relation to motor activity, fighting and mounting behaviour. *Neuropharmacology*, **12**, 177–186.

BENKERT, O., LAAKMANN, G., SOUVATZOGLOU, A. AND VON WERDER, K. (1973b) Missing indicator function of growth hormone and luteinizing hormone blood levels for dopamine and serotonin concentration in the human brain. *J. Neural Transm.*, **34**, 291–299.

BLISS, E. L., FRISCHAT, A. AND SAMUELS, L. (1972) Brain and testicular function. *Life Sci.*, **11**, 231–238.

BOYD, A. E., LEBOVITZ, H. E. AND PFEIFFER, J. B. (1970) Stimulation of human growth hormone secretion by L-DOPA. *New Engl. J. Med.*, **283**, 1425–1429.

BROWN, P. S. AND FAWKE, L. (1972) Effects of reserpine, *p*-chlorophenylalanine, *α*-methyltyrosine, thymoxamine or methallibure on pituitary FSH in male rats. *J. Reprod. Fertil.*, **28**, 167–175.

BURG, W. VAN DEN, VAN PRAAG, H. M., BOS, E. R. H., VAN ZANTEN, A. K., PIERS, D. A. AND DOORENBOS, H. (1975) TRH as a possible quick-acting but short-lasting antidepressant. In *Hormones, Homeostasis and the Brain, Progr. Brain Res.*, Vol. 42, W. H. GISPEN, TJ. B. VAN WIMERSMA GREIDANUS, B. BOHUS AND D. DE WIED (Eds.), Elsevier, Amsterdam, pp. 68–69.

BUTCHER, L. L. AND ENGEL, J. (1969) Behavioral and biochemical effects of L-DOPA after peripheral decarboxylase inhibition. *Brain Research*, **15**, 233–242.

CASSANO, G. B., CASTROGIOVANNI, P., CARRARA, S., MARTINO, E., LOI, A. M., AMBROSINO, N., PINCHERA, A. E BASCHIERI, L. (1973) Effetti del TRH in soggetti con dinsrome depressiva. *G. Endocrinol. Pisana*.

DIMITRIKOUDI, M., HANSON-NORTY, E. AND JENNER, F. A. (1974) TRH in psychoses. *Lancet*, i, 456.

DONOSO, A. O., BISHOP, W., FAWCETT, C. P., KRULICH, L. AND McCANN, S. M. (1971) Effects of drugs that modify brain monoamine concentrations on plasma gonadotropin and prolactin levels in the rat. *Endocrinology*, **89**, 774–784.

EDDY, R. L., JONES, A. L., CHAKMAKJIAN, Z. H. AND SILVERTHORNE, M. C. (1971) Effect of levodopa (L-DOPA) on human hypophyseal trophic hormone release. *J. clin. Endocr.*, **33**, 709–712.

EHRENSING, R. H., KASTIN, A. J., SCHALCH, D. S., FRIESEN, H. G., VARGAS, J. R. AND SCHALLY A. V. (1974) Affective state and thyrotropin and prolactin responses after repeated injections of thyrotropin-releasing hormone in depressed patients. *Amer. J. Psychiat.*, **131**, 714–718.

GAWIENOWSKI, A. M., MERKER, J. W. AND DAMON, R. A. (1973) Alteration of sexual behaviour and sex accessory glands by *p*-chlorophenylalanine and testosterone. *Life Sci.*, **12**, 307–315.

HENNING, M. AND RUBENSON, A. (1970) Central hypotensive effect of L-3,4-dihydroxyphenylalanine in the rat. *J. Pharm. Pharmacol.*, **22**, 553–560.

IMURA, H., NAKAI, Y. AND YOSHIMI, T. (1973) Effect of 5-hydroxytryptophan (5-HTP) on growth hormone and ACTH release in man. *J. clin. Endocr.*, **36**, 204–206.

ITIL, T. M. (1973) *Summary of Clinical, Psychopharmacological and Neurophysical Studies, ECDEU 11 Progress Report*, NIMH, Washington, D.C.

KANSAL, P. C., BUSE, J., TALBERT, O. R. AND BUSE, M. G. (1972) The effect of L-DOPA on plasma growth hormone, insulin and thyroxin. *J. clin. Endocr.*, **34**, 99–105.

KASTIN, A. J., EHRENSING, R. H., SCHALCH, D. S. AND ANDERSON, M. S. (1972) Improvement in mental depression with decrease thyrotropin response after administration of thyrotropin-releasing hormone. *Lancet*, ii, 740–742.

KORDON, C., JAVOY, F., VASSENT, G. AND GLOWINSKI, J. (1968) Blockade of superovulation in the immature rat by increased brain serotonin. *Europ. J. Pharmacol.*, **4**, 169–174.

KORDON, C. AND GLOWINSKI, J. (1972) Role of hypothalamic monoaminergic neurones in the gonadotrophin release-regulating mechanisms. *Neuropharmacology*, **11**, 153–162.

MAGGINI, C., GUAZZELLI, M., MAURI, M., CARRARA, S., FORNARO, P., MARTINO, E., MACCHIA, E. AND BASCHIERI, L. (1974) Sleep, clinical and endocrine studies in depressive patients treated with thyrotropin releasing hormone. Presented to the *2nd European Congress on Sleep Research, Rome*.

MAJ, J., GRABOWSKA, M. AND MOGILNICKA, E. (1971) The effect of L-DOPA on brain catecholamines and motility in rats. *Psychopharmacologia (Berl.)*, **22**, 162–171.

MERIMEE, T. J., RABINOWITZ, D., RIGGS, L., BURGESS, J. A., RIMOIN, D. L. AND McKUSICK, V. A. (1967) Plasma growth hormone after arginine infusion. *New Engl. J. Med.*, **23**, 434–439.

MOSS, R. L. AND McCANN, S. M. (1973) Induction of mating behaviour in rats by luteinizing hormone-releasing factor. *Science*, **181**, 177–179.

O'STEEN, W. K. (1964) Serotonin suppression of luteinization in gonadotropin-treated, immature rats. *Endocrinology*, **74**, 885–888.

PERLOW, M. J., SASSIN, J. F., BOYAR, R., HELLMANN, L. AND WEITZMANN, E. D. (1972) Release of human growth hormone, follicle stimulating hormone, and luteinizing hormone in response to L-dihydroxyphenylalanine (L-DOPA) in normal man. *Dis. nerv. Syst.*, **33**, 804–810.

PFAFF, D. W. (1973) Luteinizing hormone-releasing factor potentiates lordosis behaviour in hypophysectomized ovariectomized female rats. *Science*, **182**, 1148–1149.

PLOTNIKOFF, N. P. (1975) Prolyl-leucyl-glycine amide (PLG) and thyrotropin-releasing hormone (TRH): DOPA potentiation and biogenic amine studies. In *Hormones, Homeostasis and the Brain, Progr. Brain Res.*, *Vol. 42*, W. H. GISPEN, TJ. B. VAN WIMERSMA GREIDANUS, B. BOHUS AND D. DE WIED (Eds.), Elsevier, Amsterdam, pp. 11–23.

PRANGE, JR., A. J., WILSON, I. C., BREESE, G. R. AND LIPTON, M. A. (1975) Behavioral effects of hypothalamic releasing hormones in animals and men. In *Hormones, Homeostasis and the Brain, Progr. Brain Res.*, *Vol. 42*, W. H. GISPEN, TJ. B. VAN WIMERSMA GREIDANUS, B. BOHUS AND D. DE WIED (Eds.), Elsevier, Amsterdam, pp. 1–10.

RUBIN, R. T. (1975) Sleep-endocrinology studies in man. In *Hormones, Homeostasis and the Brain, Progr. Brain Res.*, *Vol. 42*, W. H. GISPEN, TJ. B. VAN WIMERSMA GREIDANUS, B. BOHUS AND D. DE WIED (Eds.), Elsevier, Amsterdam, pp. 73–80.

SACHAR, E. J. (1975) Twenty-four-hour cortisol secretory patterns in depressed and manic patients. In *Hormones, Homeostasis and the Brain, Progr. Brain Res.*, *Vol. 42*, W. H. GISPEN, TJ. B. VAN WIMERSMA GREIDANUS, B. BOHUS AND D. DE WIED (Eds.), Elsevier, Amsterdam, pp. 81–91.

SOUVATZOGLOU, A. K., VON WERDER, K. AND BOTTERMANN, P. (1973) The effect of intravenous L-DOPA on growth hormone and luteinizing hormone levels in man. *Acta endocr. (Kbh.)*, **73**, 259–265.

VAN DER VIS-MELSEN, M. J. E. AND WIENER, J. D. (1972) Improvement in mental depression with decreased thyrotropin response after administration of thyrotropin-releasing hormone. *Lancet*, **ii**, 1415.

Releasing Hormones and Sexual Behavior

ROBERT L. MOSS, S. M. McCANN AND C. A. DUDLEY

Department of Physiology, University of Texas Health Science Center at Dallas, Southwestern Medical School, Dallas, Texas 75235 (U.S.A.)

INTRODUCTION

It has been known for many years that mating in the female rat is dependent on the ovarian steroids, estrogen and progesterone (Beach, 1947). Removal of the ovaries results in the complete cessation of copulatory behavior. The heat response, in ovariectomized females, can be initiated by exogenous treatment with daily doses of estrogen over a period of days (Davidson *et al.*, 1968; Pfaff, 1970), or with relatively small doses of estrogen followed by progesterone (Boling and Blandau, 1939). In the regular 4-day cyclic rat, the secretion of ovarian steroids and subsequent mating behavior is controlled by the gonadotropins from the anterior pituitary (Young *et al.*, 1941), which, in turn, are under hypothalamic regulation (McCann and Porter, 1969).

Hypothalamic control over anterior pituitary function is thought to be mediated by the action of hypophyseotropic hormones, *i.e.* the releasing and inhibiting factors (McCann *et al.*, 1973; Motta *et al.*, 1973). Research on the subject of releasing factors has focused principally on the elucidation of (1) their chemical structure, (2) the neural and pharmacological determinants of their "release mechanism", and (3) their involvement in the secretion of anterior pituitary hormones. An extensive literature exists in these areas, and we will make no attempt to review it here. (For a current review, see Greep and Porter, 1973.) Instead, we would like to focus on a less well-studied area, and discuss the role which luteinizing hormone-releasing hormone (LHRH) may play in the regulation of overt sexual behavior.

At first glance, the possibility of an interaction between LHRH and sexual receptivity appears quite unlikely. Yet, upon further analysis, the temporal relationship that exists in the female rat between the release of ovarian hormones, releasing factors, pituitary gonadotropins and the onset of sexual receptivity becomes apparent. In most species that show spontaneous ovulatory cycles, the period of behavioral estrus coincides with the ovulatory period; that is, a period of sexual receptivity ensues shortly following the time of preovulatory luteinizing hormone (LH) release. For instance, it is thought that in the proestrous rat, ovarian estrogen acts on the hypothalamus to initiate release of LHRH which, in turn, results in a preovulatory discharge of LH from the anterior pituitary (Everett, 1964; Ramirez and McCann, 1964; McCann and Porter, 1969). Shortly after the peak of plasma LH, ovarian progesterone is secreted and this is followed by the onset of heat (Blandau *et al.*, 1941; Beach, 1948; Schwartz, 1969; Feder *et al.*, 1971). Thus, the hypothalamus controls anterior pituitary functions by means of releasing factors and the anterior pituitary in turn controls estrogen secretion by the ovary through gonadotropins. Heat has been thought to be ultimately induced by the ovarian hormones.

Of interest is the possibility that the specific hypothalamic tissue which regulates LH secretion may also mediate sexual receptivity. LHRH is found in a band of tissue extending from the medial preoptic area through the ventral aspect of the hypothalamus to the median eminence–arcuate region from which LHRH is presumably released into the portal capillaries (Crighton *et al.*, 1970; Krulich *et al.*, 1971; Quijada *et al.*, 1971; Barry *et al.*, 1973a and b). On the other hand, the primary region concerned with mating behavior in the female rat appears to be the preoptic–anterior hypothalamic complex. Although this hypothalamic tissue is certainly involved in sexual receptivity (Brookhart *et al.*, 1940; Dey *et al.*, 1942; Law and Meager, 1958; Lisk, 1962; Singer, 1968; Powers and Valenstein, 1972; Moss *et al.*, 1974), the exact functional role of neurons in this area remains to be specified.

These aforementioned findings have initiated a query as to the effect of LHRH and gonadotropins on the induction of mating behavior in the rat and have afforded a new dimension in the elucidation of the hypothalamic–pituitary–gonadal behavioral interaction. As a first step toward answering this question, the series of studies described in this paper were carried out in the senior author's laboratory.

GENERAL METHOD

The experiments were carried out on sexually experienced Sprague–Dawley female (N = 109) and male (N = 24) rats of the Simonsen Laboratories, Gilroy, Calif. Each animal was housed in an individual cage, maintained on a modified day–night lighting cycle of 14 hr light and 10 hr darkness (lights going off at 2 p.m.) (Moss and Cooper, 1973), and given Purina Rat Chow and water *ad libitum*.

All surgical procedures, *i.e.* ovariectomies (OVX) and/or adrenalectomies (ADX) in the female rat as well as castration (CASX) in the male rat, were performed under ether anesthesia. The mating protocol was begun by placing the experimental animal in a mating arena with a known sexually active partner according to the method previously described (Moss, 1971; Moss and McCann, 1973). The mating session was started when the male mounted the female rat and was terminated at the end of 15 min. All hormones were injected subcutaneously (s.c.) prior to the mating session.

Luteinizing hormone-releasing hormone activates lordosis behavior

Recently, we have examined the possible role of the gonadotropins and releasing factors in the facilitation of lordosis behavior in the female rat. The procedures have been described in previous publications (Moss and McCann, 1973; Moss, 1974). All ovariectomized rats were injected with estrone (E, 0.25 mg) alone or E followed 42 hr

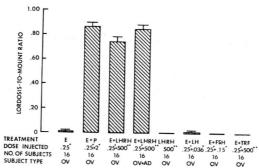

Fig. 1. Effect of gonadotropins, ovarian hormones and releasing factors on lordosis behavior in the female rat. * = mg; ** = ng; E = estrone; P = progesterone; OV = ovariectomy; AD = adrenalectomy.

later by progesterone (P, 2 mg) or 48–50 hr later by either LHRH (500 ng), LH (24 μg/100 g), FSH (50 μg/100 g; follicle stimulating hormone) or TRH (500 ng; thyrotropin-releasing hormone).

Hormone-primed female rats were tested for lordosis with a vigorous stud male (expressed as the lordosis-to-mount ratio; L/M) approximately 50–52 hr after the E injection. Lordosis was scored when the back was arched and the head raised during a mount alone, mount with intromission or with intromission and ejaculation.

The initial study demonstrated that LHRH in sufficient doses can facilitate lordosis in the E-primed OVX female rat (Moss and McCann, 1973). Ovariectomized females treated with E alone or E in combination with either LH, FSH or TRH displayed little or no lordosis behavior in response to male sexual contact. On the other hand, animals primed with E in combination with either P or LHRH exhibited sexual behavior typified by a high L/M. Further experiments confirmed as well as extended the aforementioned findings. As expected, E-primed, LHRH-treated OVX animals exhibited lordosis behavior following ADX. This finding suggests that adrenal progesterone is not involved in the LHRH facilitation of lordosis behavior. A summary of these data is presented in Fig. 1. To determine whether the response to LHRH was specific, we tested another releasing factor, TRH. This one seemed particu-

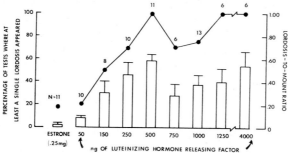

Fig. 2. Dose–response relationship between doses of LHRH and induction of lordosis behavior. Open bars give lordosis-to-mount ratio; solid dots give percentage of animals displaying at least one lordosis; vertical bars give standard error of the mean.

References p. 44–46

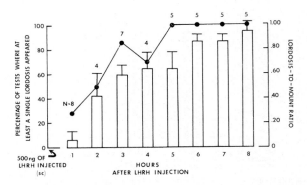

Fig. 3. Time-course for the initiation of the LHRH-facilitated lordosis response. Open bars give lordosis-to-mount ratio; solid dots give percentage of animals displaying at least one lordosis; vertical bars give standard error of the mean.

larly appropriate since it is localized in the bed nucleus of the stria terminalis (Quijada *et al.*, 1971), a region near the LHRH-containing and sexual behavior centers. Lordosis behavior was observed in only one of 50 tests with TRH.

We next concentrated our efforts on the minimal dose of LHRH needed to initiate lordosis in the E-primed OVX female rat. The results of this experiment are summarized in Fig. 2. In the initial experiments, 500 ng of LHRH was used to induce lordosis behavior, whereas a dose 10-fold smaller (50 ng of LHRH) resulted in only 20% of the animals displaying at least a single lordosis. There was no significant difference in the number of animals displaying a single lordosis while under the influence of E alone or E in combination with 50 ng of LHRH. When the LHRH dose level was increased from 50 to 150 to 500 ng, the percentage of animals displaying at least a single lordotic response increased from 20% to 50% to 95%. In terms of lordosis behavior, some animals responded to 50 ng of LHRH (L/M = 0.08), but the majority of the animals displayed consistent lordosis behavior (L/M = 0.45) only after an injection of 250 ng of LHRH. Thus, the percentage of animals showing at least one lordosis increased with progressive doses (50–150–250–500 ng) of LHRH. Under the present experimental conditions, the minimal effective dose of LHRH needed to produce a significant change in female sexual behavior is 150 ng.

The data illustrated in Fig. 3 depict the time-course of the LHRH response. Approximately 2 hr after LHRH injection (500 ng), about 50% of the E, LHRH-primed OVX animals displayed at least a single lordosis response, but the best and most consistent behavior occurred 3–4 hr post-injection (L/M = 0.60; 75–80% of animals showed at least a single lordosis). The LHRH-induced behavior persisted for 8 hr and then decreased rapidly, which is also characteristic of the receptive period seen in the E, P-primed animal.

In general, during a high peak of sexual arousal, E, P-primed female rats display characteristic sexual behaviors including a stiff-legged hopping gait, darting behavior and rapid vibratory movements of the ears. In the present experiment, the majority of E, LHRH-primed animals displayed some hopping and darting behavior but at the same time, displayed resistive behavior characteristic of a non-receptive female. The significance of this finding has not yet been determined.

In the next series of experiments, the effect of LHRH on the onset and duration of the sexual receptivity period in the normal 4-day cyclic female rat was studied. In the proestrous female, 500 ng of LHRH administered 6, 4 and 2 hr prior to the normal "onset" of the "heat" period did not advance the onset of sexual receptivity. In the same manner, LHRH injected 6, 4 and 2 hr prior to the termination of the heat period had no effect in prolonging receptivity. In addition, the behavior patterns observed during mating in the proestrous animal were not modified by LHRH administered during the heat period.

Activation of male sexual behavior by luteinizing hormone-releasing hormone

The medial preoptic area and medial forebrain bundle have been implicated as being an integral part of neural systems mediating male sexual behavior in the rat (Caggiula and Hoebel, 1966; Heimer and Larsson, 1967; Giantonio *et al.*, 1970; Hitt *et al.*, 1970; Malsbury, 1971; Harvey and Lints, 1971). In the case of the medial preoptic area, lesions in this area have been shown to disrupt male sexual behavior while electrical stimulation has been shown to facilitate ejaculation. Since LHRH has been localized to the medial preoptic area, it was of considerable interest to explore the effect of LHRH on male sexual behavior.

Sexually experienced intact and hormone-primed CASX male rats were injected with LHRH or saline and tested in the mating arena with a sexually active E, P-primed female rat. During the mating test the occurrence of mounts (M) with thrusting but no intromission, mounts with intromission (I) and ejaculation (E) as well as the time to achieve the first M, I and E was recorded. All CASX males were treated with either 25 or 10 μg of testosterone proprionate (TP) alone or TP in combination with LHRH (500 ng or saline), while the intact males were treated only with saline or LHRH.

In the first series of experiments, we investigated the effect of LHRH on sexual behavior in the intact male rat. All intact males were sexually experienced and tested under two conditions, namely, under the influence of saline and LHRH. The data were analyzed by a paired comparison test. LHRH or saline was injected s.c. into male rats, 2 hr prior to the mating test. There was no significant difference in the number of Ms, Is or L/M ratios observed during the 15-min testing period between the saline- and LHRH-treated animals. On the other hand, LHRH significantly reduced ($P < 0.05$) the time to first I and E as compared to times obtained in saline-treated animals (Fig. 4). These findings appear to be comparable to the data obtained in the OVX E, LHRH-primed female rat.

At this point, it was thought that a proper comparison would better be made with OVX E, LHRH-primed females if the males were CASX and treated with TP. After demonstrating good sexual behavior, the males were castrated and treated with TP (at a dose too low to initiate good behavior) and were then injected with either saline or 500 ng of LHRH. The TP injections were begun 48 hr after surgery at a dose level

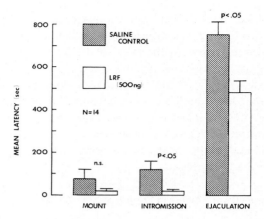

Fig. 4. Paired comparison of mean latency to first mount, first intromission and first ejaculation under saline and LHRH treatments.

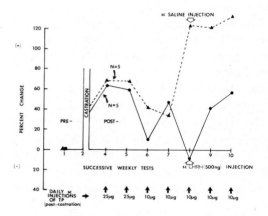

Fig. 5. Post-castration comparison of percent change in time to ejaculation under testosterone proprionate (TP) in combination with either a single injection of LHRH (solid lines) or saline (dashed lines). All substances were injected subcutaneously (s.c.).

of 25 μg/day for 2 weeks and were continued at 10 μg/day for the duration of the experiment. Analysis by *t*-test revealed no significant differences between the saline- and LHRH-treated animals in the number of Ms, Is and Es or in the time to achieve the first M and I. A single injection of LHRH (500 ng) to the experimental group produced a significant decrease in the time to achieve ejaculation, while a single injection of saline to the control group had no effect. No other significant differences in the data recorded were observed (Fig. 5). Thus, LHRH facilitated ejaculation in the TP-primed CASX male rat. It should be noted here that CASX male rats treated with saline in combination with LHRH (no TP injected) displayed little or no copulatory behavior.

DISCUSSION

The administration of synthetic LHRH in this investigation has demonstrated that LHRH exerts (1) a facilitatory effect on the occurrence of the lordosis response, and (2) a stimulatory action on the ejaculatory response. After an injection of LHRH, OVX female rats pretreated with E in doses too low to initiate behavior, displayed lordosis patterns that differed little from those produced by progesterone. The LHRH-facilitated behavior was shown to be specific, in that only a few females exhibited the lordosis pattern in response to E alone or E in combination with LH, FSH or TRH. In addition to supporting our original findings (Moss and McCann, 1973), we were able to demonstrate that the LHRH-facilitated lordosis behavior is independent of adrenal progesterone. Thus, this effect is apparently not mediated by pituitary or adrenal hormones. Confirmation of our original findings has been reported in the estradiol-primed hypophysectomized, OVX female rat (Pfaff, 1973). Here again, this provides further evidence for the view that the effect is caused by LHRH itself rather than by the gonadotropins liberated by the neurohormone.

Similar findings to that obtained in the E, LHRH-primed OVX female rat were observed in the male rat. Injections of LHRH in the intact and TP-primed CASX male rat decreased the time required to achieve ejaculation. It should be noted here that LHRH did not have a significant effect on sexual behavior in the intact cyclic female rat, *i.e.* injections of LHRH in proestrous animals did not advance or prolong the sexual receptivity period.

Thus, the results indicate that another hormone, namely LHRH, in addition to E and P in the female and to TP in the male, can induce mating behavior in the rat. Under the conditions of these experiments, LHRH alone did not lead to mating behavior in CASX males or OVX females. This suggests that E-priming in the OVX females and TP-priming in the CASX males is a necessary condition to obtain a high level of copulatory behavior.

The results presented here provide a physiological explanation for the anatomical overlapping of the centers regulating mating behavior and producing LHRH. Axons or collaterals from LHRH-producing neurons may project to neurons concerned with arousal levels during mating behavior. The localization of estrogen concentrating as well as LHRH neurons in the medial preoptic area provides a further anatomical basis for this concept (Pfaff, 1968; Pfaff and Keiner, 1973; McCann *et al.*, 1975). Thus, LHRH may function not only to trigger an ovulatory discharge of LH, but also to induce mating by activating the preoptic–anterior hypothalamic complex. It may act in conjunction with gonadal steroids to bring about mating behavior several hours following the preovulatory discharge of LH which is also presumably evoked by release of LHRH. Our ability to induce copulatory behavior with LHRH in the OVX, E-primed rat and to facilitate mating in CASX males given suboptimal doses of TP is certainly consistent with this concept. The time lag between the injection of LRF on the one hand, and the induction of mating behavior on the other, suggests that this is not a simple monosynaptic mechanism, but may involve an intermediate step, such as the activation of protein synthesis in the postsynaptic neurons of the mating center.

SUMMARY

The role of luteinizing hormone-releasing hormone (LHRH) in activating mating behavior was examined in estrone (E)-primed ovariectomized (OVX) and normal proestrous female rats (4-day cycles) as well as in testosterone proprionate (TP)-primed castrated and intact male rats. Subcutaneous administration of synthetic LHRH in E-primed OVX as well as OVX-adrenalectomized female rats facilitated the appearance of lordosis behavior. No consistent lordotic behavior was observed in response to LHRH alone, E alone or E in combination with luteinizing hormone (LH), follicle-stimulating hormone (FSH) or thyrotropin-releasing hormone (TRH). In the proestrous female, LHRH administered prior to the ovulatory surge of LH or post-ovulation did not advance, induce nor prolong sexual receptivity in any of the animals studied. In the sexually active intact male rat as well as in the TP-primed castrated male rat, LHRH enhanced mating behavior. Subcutaneous administration of LHRH in intact male rats resulted in a significant decrease in the time to the first intromission and to subsequent ejaculation, while in the TP-primed castrated male only a significant decrease in the time to ejaculation was observed. No mating behavior was observed in castrated rats treated with LHRH alone. It is suggested that LHRH plays a role in the facilitation of sexual behavior.

ACKNOWLEDGEMENTS

The authors are indebted to Dr. S. N. Preston of Parke-Davis Company for the estrone and progesterone; Dr. R. Deghenghi of Ayerst Ltd. for the luteinizing hormone-releasing hormone; Dr. J. Dorn of Abbott Laboratories for the thyrotropin-releasing hormone and the Endocrinology Study Section, National Institutes of Health for the luteinizing hormone and the follicle-stimulating hormone. The authors also thank Susie Zavislan for assistance in the preparation of the manuscript.

This investigation has been supported by Research Grant USPHS NS10434-END, awarded to Dr. Moss.

REFERENCES

BARRY, J., DUBOIS, M. P. AND POULAIN, P. (1973a) LRF producing cells of the mammalian hypothalamus. *Z. Zellforsch.*, **146**, 351–366.
BARRY, J., DUBOIS, M. P., POULAIN, P. ET LEONARDELLI, J. (1973b) Charactérisation et topographie des neurones hypothalamiques immunoréactifs avec des anti-corps anti-LRF de synthèse. *C. R. Acad. Sci. (Paris)*, **276**, 3191–3193.
BEACH, F. A. (1947) A review of physiological and psychological studies of sexual behavior in mammals. *Physiol. Rev.*, **27**, 240–307.

BEACH, F. A. (1948) *Hormones and Behavior*, Hoeber, New York, N.Y., pp. 1–368.

BLANDAU, R. J., BOLING, R. J. AND YOUNG, W. C. (1941) The length of heat in the albino rat as determined by the copulatory response. *Anat. Rec.*, **79**, 453–463.

BOLING, J. L. AND BLANDAU, R. J. (1939) The estrogen–progesterone induction of mating responses in the spayed female rat. *Endocrinology*, **25**, 359–364.

BROOKHART, J. M., DEY, F. L. AND RANSON, S. W. (1940) Failure of ovarian hormones to cause mating reactions in spayed guinea pigs with hypothalamic lesions. *Proc. Soc. exp. Biol. (N.Y.)*, **44**, 61–64.

CAGGIULA, A. R. AND HOEBEL, B. G. (1966) "Copulation-reward site" in the posterior hypothalamus. *Science*, **153**, 1284–1285.

CRIGHTON, D. B., SCHNEIDER, H. P. G. AND McCANN, S. M. (1970) Localization of LH-releasing factor in the hypothalamus and neurohypophysis as determined by *in vivo* assay. *Endocrinology*, **87**, 323–329.

DAVIDSON, J. M., SMITH, E. R., RODGERS, C. H. AND BLOCK, G. J. (1968) Stimulation of female sex behavior in adrenalectomized rats with estrogen alone. *Endocrinology*, **82**, 193–195.

DEY, F. L., LEININGER, C. R. AND RANSON, S. W. (1942) The effects of hypothalamic lesions on mating behavior in female guinea pigs. *Endocrinology*, **30**, 323–326.

EVERETT, J. W. (1964) Central neural control of reproductive functions of the adenohypophysis. *Physiol. Rev.*, **44**, 373–431.

FEDER, H. H., BROWN-GRANT, K. AND CORKER, C. S. (1971) Pre-ovulatory progesterone, the adrenal cortex and the "critical period" for luteinizing hormone release in rats. *J. Endocrinol.*, **50**, 29–39.

GIANTONIO, G. W., LUND, N. L. AND GERALL, A. A. (1970) Effect of diencephalic and rhinencephalic lesions on the male rat's sexual behavior. *J. comp. physiol. Psychol.*, **73**, 38–46.

GREEP, R. O. AND PORTER, J. E. (Eds.) (1973) Hypothalamic control of fertility. *J. Reprod. Fertil.*, **Suppl. 20**, 1–170.

HARVEY, J. A. AND LINTS, C. E. (1971) Lesions in the medial forebrain bundle: Relationship between pain sensitivity and telencephalic content of serotonin. *J. comp. physiol. Psychol.*, **74**, 28–36.

HEIMER, L. AND LARSSON, K. (1967) Impairment of mating behavior in male rats following lesions in the preoptic–anterior hypothalamic continuum. *Brain Res.*, **3**, 248–263.

HITT, L. C., HENDRICKS, S. E., GINSBERG, S. I. AND LEWIS, J. H. (1970) Disruption of male, but not female, sexual behavior in rats by medial forebrain bundle lesions. *J. comp. physiol. Psychol.*, **73**, 377–384.

KRULICH, L., QUIJADA, M., ILLNER, P. AND McCANN, S. M. (1971) The distribution of hypothalamic hypophysiotropic factors in the hypothalamus of the rat. *Proc. XXV Int. Congr. Physiol. Sci.*, **9**, 326.

LAW, T. AND MEAGER, W. (1958) Hypothalamic lesions and sexual behavior in the female rat. *Science*, **128**, 1626–1627.

LISK, R. D. (1962) Diencephalic placement of estradiol and sexual receptivity in the female rat. *Amer. J. Physiol.*, **203**, 493–496.

MALSBURY, C. W. (1971) Facilitation of male rat copulatory behavior by electrical stimulation of the medial preoptic area. *Physiol. Behav.*, **7**, 797–805.

McCANN, S. M. AND PORTER, J. C. (1969) Hypothalamic pituitary stimulating and inhibiting hormones. *Physiol. Rev.*, **49**, 240–284.

McCANN, S. M., KRULICH, L., COOPER, K. J., KALRA, P. S., KALRA, S. P., LIBRERTUN, C., NEGRO-VILAR, A., ORAIS, R., RONNEKLEIV, O. AND FAWCETT, C. P. (1973) Hypothalamic control of gonadotrophin and prolactin secretion, implications for fertility control. In *Proc. First Int. Planned Parenthood Fed. Biol. Workshop* (*J. Reprod. Fertil.*, Suppl. 20), R. O. GREEP AND J. E. PORTER (Eds.), Blackwell Scientific Publications, Osney Mead, Oxford, pp. 43–60.

McCANN, S. M., KRULICH, L., QUIJADA, M., WHEATON, J. AND MOSS, R. L. (1975) Gonadotropin-releasing factors: sites of production, secretion and action in the brain. In *Anatomical Neuroendocrinology, Proc. Conference on Neurobiology of CNS-Hormones*, W. E. STUMPF AND L. D. GRANT (Eds.), Karger, Basel, in press.

MOSS, R. L. (1971) Modifications of copulatory behavior in the female rat following olfactory bulb removal. *J. comp. physiol. Psychol.*, **74**, 374–382.

MOSS, R. L. (1974) Relationship between central regulation of gonadotropins and mating behavior in female rats. In *Reproductive Behavior*, W. A. SADLER (Ed.), Plenum, New York, pp. 55–76.

MOSS, R. L. AND COOPER, K. J. (1973) Temporal relationship of spontaneous and coitus-induced release of luteinizing hormone in the normal cyclic rat. *Endocrinology*, **92**, 1748–1753.

Moss, R. L. and McCann, S. M. (1973) Induction of mating behavior in rats by luteinizing hormone-releasing factor. *Science*, **181**, 177–179.

Moss, R. L., Paloutzian, R. F. and Law, O. T. (1974) Electrical stimulation of forebrain structures and its effect on copulatory as well as stimulus-bound behavior in ovariectomized hormone-primed rats. *Physiol. Behav.*, **12**, 997–1004.

Motta, M., Piva, F. and Martini, L. (1973) New findings on the central control of gonadotrophin secretion. In *Proceedings of the First International Planned Parenthood Federation Biological Workshop (J. Reprod. Fertil.*, Suppl. 20), R. O. Greep and J. E. Porter (Eds.), Blackwell Scientific Publications, Osney Mead, Oxford, pp. 27–42.

Pfaff, D. W. (1968) Uptake of estradiol-17β-H^3 in the female rat brain. An autoradiographic study. *Endocrinology*, **82**, 1149–1155.

Pfaff, D. W. (1970) Mating behavior of hypophysectomized rats. *J. comp. physiol. Psychol.*, **72**, 45–50.

Pfaff, D. W. (1973) Luteinizing hormone-releasing factor potentiates lordosis behavior in hypophysectomized ovariectomized female rats. *Science*, **182**, 1148–1149.

Pfaff, D. W. and Keiner, M. (1973) Atlas of estradiol-concentrating cells in the central nervous system. *J. comp. Neurol.*, **151**, 121–159.

Powers, B. and Valenstein, E. S. (1972) Sexual receptivity: Facilitation by medial preoptic lesions in female rats. *Science*, **175**, 1003–1005.

Quijada, M., Krulich, L., Fawcett, C. P., Sundberg, D. K. and McCann, S. M. (1971) Localization of TSH-releasing factor (TRF), LH-RF and FSH-RF in rat hypothalamus. *Fed. Proc.*, **30**, 2.

Ramirez, V. D. and McCann, S. M. (1964) Fluctuations in plasma luteinizing hormone concentrations during the estrous cycle of the rat. *Endocrinology*, **74**, 814–816.

Schwartz, N. B. (1969) A model for the regulation of ovulation in the rat. *Rec. Progr. Hormone Res.*, **25**, 1–55.

Singer, J. J. (1968) Hypothalamic control of male and female sexual behavior in female rats. *J. comp. physiol. Psychol.*, **69**, 738–742.

Young, C. W., Boling, J. L. and Blandau, R. J. (1941) The vaginal smear picture, sexual receptivity and time of ovulation in the albino rat. *Anat. Rec.*, **80**, 37–45.

Interaction of the Tripeptide Pyroglutamyl-Histidyl-Proline Amide (Thyrotropin-Releasing Hormone) with Brain Norepinephrine Metabolism: Evidence for an Extrahypophyseal Action of TRH on Central Nervous System Function

JON M. STOLK AND BRUCE C. NISULA

*Departments of Psychiatry and Pharmacology, Dartmouth Medical School, Hanover, N. H. 03755
and Reproduction Research Branch, National Institute of Child Health and Human Development,
National Institutes of Health, Bethesda, Md. 20014 (U.S.A.)*

INTRODUCTION

A rapidly expanding body of information has implicated several polypeptides as potent regulators of anterior pituitary function. These compounds are thought to be synthesized within specialized nerve cells in the hypothalamus, and exert their effects by being released into the hypothalamo-hypophyseal portal system and either stimulating or inhibiting the release of a particular tropic hormone by specific anterior pituitary cells. Parenteral administration of small quantities of these polypeptides has a profound effect on anterior pituitary function, a finding in concert with their postulated role as endogenous regulators of hypophyseal hormone metabolism. Thus, microgram quantities of the tripeptide pyroglutamyl-histidyl-proline amide (thyrotropin-releasing hormone, TRH) given to man result in a rapid stimulation of thyrotropin secretion followed by a more prolonged increase in circulating thyroid hormone concentration (Fleischer *et al.*, 1970; Hollander *et al.*, 1972).

However, while the anterior pituitary is extremely sensitive to the injection of the polypeptides a number of extrahypophyseal actions have recently been documented, indicating that these peptides may play a significant role in the central nervous system independent of the pituitary. Luteinizing hormone-releasing hormone (LHRH) has been shown to potentiate lordosis behavior in hypophysectomized, ovariectomized female rats (Pfaff, 1973). Similarly, melanocyte-stimulating hormone release-inhibiting factor (MIF) potentiated the behavioral effects of L-DOPA (3,4-dihydroxyphenyl-alanine) in pargyline-treated hypophysectomized rats (Plotnikoff *et al.*, 1971). TRH has the same activity as MIF in the DOPA–pargyline test system (Plotnikoff *et al.*, 1972); in addition, the intravenous injection of TRH results in the prompt emergence from ether anesthesia in rats (unpublished observations), an effect occurring so rapidly (within 10 sec) that mediation by the pituitary–thyroid axis is most unlikely. Finally, two groups have reported rapid ameliorations of symptomatology following TRH administration to psychiatric patients suffering from depression (Kastin *et al.*,

References p. 55–56

1972; Prange *et al.*, 1972). In view of the suspected associations between a wide variety of animal and human behaviors with brain catecholamines (see Barchas *et al.*, 1972), the indications cited above led us to study potential direct interactions between TRF and brain catecholamine containing neuronal systems.

Effects of TRH on brain catecholamine metabolism

Our initial study was directed at exploring potential effects of TRH on *in vivo* brain catecholamine metabolism. We chose to employ a procedure, recently developed in our laboratory, for estimating the conversion of intracisternally injected [³H]dopamine to [³H]norepinephrine by the enzyme dopamine-β-hydroxylase (DβH; EC 1.14.2.1) in rat brain (Stolk, 1973 and 1975; Stolk and Hanlon, 1973). Male Sprague–Dawley rats were given an intravenous injection of 1 mg/kg synthetic TRH (Gross *et al.*, 1973) in a 0.9 % saline–1 % bovine serum albumin vehicle; control rats received the vehicle alone. All rats were injected intracisternally with 1.36 ng [1-³H]dopamine 10 min later. Labeled catecholamine levels in 3 brain regions were measured by column chromatography–liquid scintillation spectrometry 45 min after the intracisternal injection.

Accumulation of [³H]norepinephrine was not affected by TRH treatment in either the cortex or the diencephalon, as shown in Fig. 1. However, [³H]norepinephrine levels were reduced significantly after TRH in the medulla–pons (Fig. 1A). A subsequent study in which 5 μg/kg triiodothyronine (T$_3$) was injected intraperitoneally 30 min before the intracisternal administration of 1.52 ng [1-³H]dopamine revealed no significant effect of the T$_3$ on [³H]norepinephrine accumulation in any brain region. Thus, the effect of TRH on conversion of [³H]dopamine to [³H]norepinephrine in medulla–pons is not mediated by stimulation of hormone secretion from the thyroid.

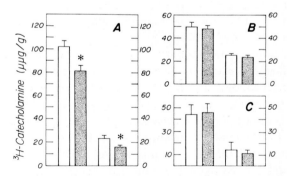

Fig. 1. *In vivo* DβH activity in medulla–pons (panel A), cortex (panel B) and diencephalon (panel C) following treatment with intravenous saline (open bars) or with 1 mg/kg TRH (stippled bars). The two bars nearest the left side of each panel represent the mean [³H]norepinephrine levels ± S.E.M. found in controls or TRH-treated subjects 45 min after the intracisternal injection of 1.36 ng [³H]-dopamine; the two bars nearest the right side of each panel represent the mean [³H]dopamine levels remaining in brain at the time of sacrifice. The intravenous administration of saline or TRH preceded intracisternal dopamine injections by 30 min. An asterisk denotes a significant difference ($P < 0.05$) from the appropriate control value.

The *in vivo* effects of TRH on brain catecholamine metabolism described above could be attributed to: (1) an inhibition of [³H]dopamine transport into neurons capable of converting the labeled substrate to [³H]norepinephrine; (2) an inhibition of the enzyme DβH converting dopamine to norepinephrine; or (3) accelerated release and/or catabolism of the [³H]norepinephrine formed from precursor. Although accumulation of labeled dopamine is reduced by TRH in medulla–pons tissue at the time of sacrifice (Fig. 1A), no such effect is observed in the other brain regions tested. Inhibition of [³H]dopamine entry into DβH containing neurons is, therefore, considered unlikely. Further, Breese *et al.* (1974) were unable to detect effects of TRH on norepinephrine release or degradation, making this an unlikely possible mechanism resulting in reduced [³H]norepinephrine content. These data, therefore, suggested that TRH was affecting the conversion of labeled dopamine to norepinephrine.

A direct action of TRH on DβH activity was investigated using an *in vitro* system for estimating enzyme activity. DβH activity was measured by the coupled enzyme procedure developed by Molinoff *et al.* (1971); an appropriate substrate is converted to a β-hydroxylated amine by DβH, and the latter product is methylated enzymatically to a radioactive compound using the enzyme phenylethanolamine-N-methyltransferase (PNMT; EC 2.1.1.28) and labeled S-adenosyl-L-methionine as the methyl donor. Two DβH sources were tested: (1) a preparation of the bovine adrenal enzyme partially purified by ammonium sulfate fractionation and Sephadex G-200 chromatography, and (2) a crude homogenate of rat adrenal gland. TRH concentration in the incubation mixture ranged from about 10^{-9} to 10^{-5} M; these concentrations of TRH were without effect on the second (PNMT) step of the enzyme assay. The results are summarized in Table I.

TABLE I

EFFECT OF PYROGLUTAMYL-HISTIDYL-PROLINE AMIDE (TRH) ON PARTIALLY PURIFIED DOPAMINE-β-HYDROXYLASE (DβH) ACTIVITY AND ON ACTIVITY CONTAINED IN A CRUDE ADRENAL GLAND HOMOGENATE

*[TRH]** *(CM)*	*Partially purified DβH***	*Crude adrenal homogenate****
	Mean counts/min/assay tube	
0	4075	3161
10^{-9}	3022	—
10^{-8}	2463	2160
10^{-7}	2342	—
10^{-6}	2089	1554
10^{-5}	1423	—

* Synthetic pyroglutamyl-histidyl-proline amide dissolved in 0.9% saline containing 0.5% bovine serum albumin. The saline–albumin solution without added TRH was used in control (0 TRH) tubes.
** Partially purified DβH was obtained from fresh bovine adrenal medullae. Tissue was homogenized in 0.32 M sucrose, subjected to ammonium sulfate fractionation and Sephadex G-200 chromatography. Ten microliters of the partially purified enzyme preparation (protein content: 9 mg/ml) were used in each assay tube.
*** Rat adrenal glands were homogenized in 100 vol. of 5 mM Tris buffer (pH 7.5) containing 0.1% Triton X; 100 μl of supernatant were used in each assay tube.

References p. 55–56

Addition of TRH to the incubation medium resulted in a significant reduction of enzyme activity using both DβH sources. Reduction of DβH activity by 50% was observed at about 10^{-6} M TRH; even very low concentrations of TRH (10^{-9} M) caused a significant reduction in DβH activity. These data, while they cannot explain the regional specificity of the TRH-induced reduction in conversion of [³H]dopamine to [³H]norepinephrine *in vivo*, indicate that the tripeptide probably affects DβH activity directly; moreover, the effect of TRH on *in vivo* norepinephrine metabolism occurs in a brain region distinct from that reported to be related with stimulation of thyrotropin release (Martin and Reichlin, 1970). Our findings suggest that TRH has a direct effect on brain norepinephrine metabolism that is independent of the pituitary–thyroid axis, observations that are consistent with the postulate that TRH has central nervous system activity unrelated to the anterior pituitary and possibly associated with catecholaminergic mechanisms. This thesis was explored further by studying the effect of procedures resulting in altered TRH levels in brain.

Effects of altered thyroid function on brain catecholamine metabolism

According to the predicted relationship between TRH, thyrotropin (TSH) and circulating thyroid hormones one would anticipate an inverse relationship between thyroid status and hypothalamo-hypophyseal activity. In accord with the relationship predicted by the latter negative feedback loop we began to study alterations of *in vivo* catecholamine metabolism associated with induced modifications in pituitary–thyroid status.

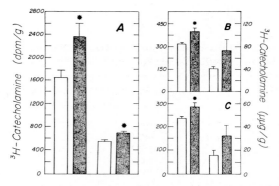

Fig. 2. Effect of radiothyroidectomy on formation of [³H]catecholamines from L-[3,5-³H]tyrosine in hindbrain tissue (medulla–pons plus cerebellum; panel A) or from *in vivo* DβH measurements in medulla–pons (panel B) or in cerebellum (panel C). The two bars nearest the left side of each panel represent the mean [³H]norepinephrine content ± S.E.M. in controls (open bars) or in thyroidectomized rats (stippled bars); the two bars nearest the right side of each panel represent mean [³H]dopamine levels in the same subjects. The catecholamine precursor for the data in panel A was 125 μCi L-[3,5-³H]tyrosine (1 Ci/mmole; Amersham–Searle) injected intravenously 1 hr before sacrifice. The dose of [³H]dopamine for the *in vivo* DβH study (panels B and C) was 3.43 ng (10 Ci/mmole; New England Nuclear) injected intracisternally 45 min before sacrifice. An asterisk denotes a significant difference ($P < 0.05$) compared to the appropriate control value. See legend of Table II for the radiothyroidectomy protocol details.

Male Sprague–Dawley rats were rendered hypothyroid by radioiodide treatment; 250 μCi [^{131}I] as sodium iodide was injected intraperitoneally 1 week after rats were placed on a low-iodine test diet. This schedule was shown by Maloof *et al.* (1952) to cause essentially complete destruction of functioning thyroid tissue. Objective parameters of hypothyroidism, including weight gain and circulating TSH levels, verified the efficacy of thyroid radioablation. Initial estimates of catecholamine metabolism were obtained by measuring the accumulation of labeled dopamine and/or norepinephrine in several tissues after the intravenous injection of L-[3,5-^{3}H]-tyrosine. Levels of [^{3}H]dopamine and [^{3}H]norepinephrine were elevated in all tissues tested, confirming the initial observations of Lipton *et al.* (1968) and Prange *et al.* (1970). [^{3}H]Norepinephrine levels in heart and spleen were increased markedly

TABLE II

EFFECT OF RADIOTHYROIDECTOMY ON FORMATION OF [^{3}H]NOREPINEPHRINE FROM L-[3,5-^{3}H]TYROSINE
IN RAT HEART AND SPLEEN TISSUE

Male Sprague–Dawley rats were placed on a low-iodine diet (Remington) for 2 weeks prior to receiving an i.p. injection of saline (Control) or 250 μCi [^{131}I]sodium iodide (New England Nuclear); both groups remained on the low-iodine diet for an additional week, after which they were given regular rat chow. Four weeks after saline or radioiodide treatment, rats received an i.v. injection of 125 μCi L-[3,5-^{3}H]tyrosine (1 Ci/mmole; Amersham-Searle) and were sacrificed 1 hr later.

Organ	Measure	Enzyme activity (mean $\pm$ S.E.M.; $n = 6$)	
		Control	Thyroidectomy
Heart	Weight (mg)	1000 $\pm$ 30	743 $\pm$ 16*
	Organ:body weight (mg:g)	2.99 $\pm$ 0.06	2.51 $\pm$ 0.05*
	[^{3}H]Norepinephrine (disint./min/g)	564 $\pm$ 42	2010 $\pm$ 172*
Spleen	Weight (mg)	842 $\pm$ 53	458 $\pm$ 32*
	Organ:body weight (mg:g)	2.28 $\pm$ 0.10	1.55 $\pm$ 0.12*
	[^{3}H]Norepinephrine (disint./min/g)	838 $\pm$ 99	2978 $\pm$ 415*

* Significantly different ($P < 0.05$) from control values.

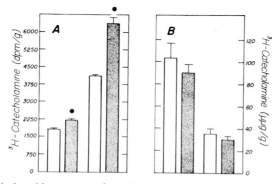

Fig. 3. Effect of radiothyroidectomy on formation of [^{3}H]catecholamines from L-[3,5-^{3}H]tyrosine (panel A) or from *in vivo* DβH measurements (panel B) in rat forebrain. See Fig. 2 legend for further experimental details.

References p. 55–56

21 days after radioiodide treatment (Table II); similar observations applied to hind-brain (medulla, pons and cerebellum; Fig. 2A). Interestingly, [^{3}H]dopamine accumulation from tyrosine was affected primarily in forebrain tissue where norepinephrine levels changed but slightly (Fig. 3A).

Estimates of *in vivo* DβH activity were ascertained in hypothyroid rats using the procedure described above in the TRH studies (Fig. 1). Radiothyroidectomized rats revealed a prominent increase in [^{3}H]norepinephrine formed from an intracisternal injection of 3.43 ng [^{3}H]dopamine in both medulla–pons and cerebellum (Fig. 2B and C, respectively); this observation is in close agreement with results obtained in the labeled tyrosine study (see Fig. 2A). Accumulation of [^{3}H]norepinephrine from [^{3}H]dopamine was not affected in the telencephalon (Fig. 3B); it will be recalled that norepinephrine formation from labeled tyrosine increased only slightly in this brain region (Fig. 3A), again revealing close concordance between the *in vivo* [^{3}H]-dopamine and L-[3,5-^{3}H]tyrosine studies.

These data indicate clearly that thyroidectomy results in a regionally specific increase in norepinephrine formation. Emlen *et al.* (1972) previously reported that hypothyroidism results in increased levels of tyrosine hydroxylase activity measured *in vitro* in the basal ganglia, a finding that is supported by our observation of enhanced [^{3}H]dopamine accumulation from L-[3,5-^{3}H]tyrosine in forebrain (Fig. 3A). However, this observation on tyrosine hydroxylase cannot account for the (1) disproportionately small increase in forebrain norepinephrine production from labeled tyrosine (Fig. 3A), and (2) the disproportionately small increase in hindbrain [^{3}H]dopamine formation from labeled tyrosine (Fig. 2A). We interpret these data to indicate that the effect of radiothyroidectomy on tyrosine hydroxylase is localized to the nigro-neostriatal dopamine tract. Measures of *in vitro* DβH activity reveal that thyroid ablation results in a slight decrease in medulla–pons enzyme activity compared to controls (Table III); other brain regions did not reveal any change in *in vitro* DβH activity. Thus, the observed increases in norepinephrine accumulation *in vivo* in both medulla–pons and cerebellum (Fig. 2) are not due to increases in the amount of synthetic enzymes present, and since *in vitro* DβH activity in medulla–pons is decreased

TABLE III

EFFECT OF RADIOTHYROIDECTOMY ON *in vitro* DOPAMINE-β-HYDROXYLASE ACTIVITY IN RAT BRAIN REGIONS

Brain region	Enzyme activity (mean $\pm$ S.E.M.)	
	Control*	Thyroidectomy**
Medulla–pons	220 $\pm$ 6	174 $\pm$ 6***
Hypothalamus	138 $\pm$ 14	152 $\pm$ 13
Cerebral cortex	94 $\pm$ 8	98 $\pm$ 16
Cerebellum	58 $\pm$ 8	61 $\pm$ 7

* See legend of Table II for details of radiothyroidectomy protocol.
** Enzyme activity is expressed as units, where 1 unit equals 1 nmole product formed/20 min/g of brain tissue.
*** Significantly different ($P < 0.05$) from control value.

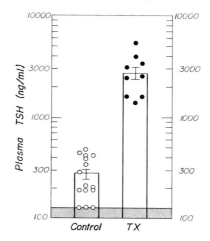

Fig. 4. Effect of radiothyroidectomy (TX) on plasma thyrotropin (TSH) level. The levels of TSH were determined by radioimmunoassay using a standard reference preparation (NIAMD-Rat TSH-RP-1). Mean TSH content, in ng/ml, $\pm$ S.E.M. for the individual animals shown on the graph are plotted on a log scale. Details of the radiothyroidectomy protocol are described in legend of Table II.

in thyroidectomized rats (Table III), the specific activity of existing DβH *in vivo* must be increased.

The fact that TRH affects catecholamine mechanisms in the same brain regions as thyroidectomy may be more than coincidental. Contrary to expectations based upon a negative feedback loop, thyroidectomy does not result in an increased concentration of TRH in brain; in fact, TRH levels are *decreased* significantly in hypothyroidism (Bassiri and Utiger, 1974; Jackson *et al.*, 1974a). Since T$_3$ treatment is without effect on *in vivo* DβH activity, and since the accumulation of [^{3}H]norepinephrine from intra-cisternal [^{3}H]dopamine or intravenous L-[3,5-^{3}H]tyrosine increases in radiothyroid-ectomized rats despite marked elevation of circulating TSH levels (Fig. 4), the evidence points very strongly toward a direct effect of TRH itself on brain norepinephrine metabolism. Our data are consistent with the view that TRH levels vary inversely with norepinephrine production in rat hindbrain, and that the tripeptide could be influencing DβH activity directly (Table I) to cause this change.

Prospectus for an extrahypophyseal role of TRH in central nervous system function

Recent evidence by Jackson *et al.* (1974b) demonstrates unequivocally that TRH is distributed throughout the brain and is not confined to the hypothalamus–adeno-hypophysis; additionally, the tripeptide is found in the brains of a wide variety of vertebrates, including primitive species lacking an anterior pituitary. Jackson *et al.* (1974b) concluded on the basis of the latter studies that pyroglutamyl-histidyl-proline amide plays an important role in brain function unrelated to pituitary–thyroid regulation. While the extreme sensitivity of the adenohypophysis to the tripeptide cannot be denied, the role of the compound in regulation of the thyrotroph has recently come under close critical scrutiny. First of all, TSH is not the only tropic hormone released upon parenteral administration of the tripeptide, since circulating prolactin levels increase markedly following pyroglutamyl-histidyl-proline amide treatment (Burgus *et al.*, 1970; Jacobs *et al.*, 1971). Secondly, prolactin is equally sensitive to the releasing effects of the tripeptides as is TSH, even though both tropic hormones are known to be regulated independently physiologically (Jacobs *et al.*, 1973; Snyder *et al.*, 1973). Finally, pyroglutamyl-histidyl-proline amide levels in the hypothalamus vary directly with thyroid function, not inversely as predicted by the negative feedback loop theory of pituitary–thyroid regulation (Bassiri and Utiger, 1974; Jackson *et al.*, 1974a). These findings, along with observations summarized in the Introduction, have provoked inquiries into an extrahypophyseal role for pyroglutamyl-histidyl-proline amide.

Appropriate models for non-hypophyseal effects of polypeptides can be found in the metabolism and action of the posterior pituitary hormones, oxytocin and vasopressin. Both are synthesized within brain neurons and have their primary sites of action far removed from the neurohypophysis. With respect to pyroglutamyl-histidyl-proline amide, the existence of significant quantities of the tripeptide and the presence of active mechanisms for metabolizing the compound in many brain regions outside of the hypothalamus argues for extrahypophyseal activity. Jackson *et al.* (1974b) even have demonstrated that non-thyroidal, extrahypophyseal stimuli can cause marked effects on pyroglutamyl-histidyl-proline amide levels in extrahypothalamic brain regions; tripeptide levels in frog pineal, but not those in the hypothalamus, are sensitive to alterations in environmental lighting.

Our data offer suggestive evidence for a neuroregulatory function of pyroglutamyl-histidyl-proline amide on brain norepinephrine metabolism. The results presented are not inconsistent with the idea that the tripeptide regulates the activity of DβH within noradrenergic neurons in the brain stem. Thus, pyroglutamyl-histidyl-proline amide has a direct inhibitory effect on enzyme activity when administered acutely (Fig. 1; Table I), and tonic reduction in brain levels of the peptide results in relaxation of inhibition exerted on existing DβH protein (Fig. 3). This hypothesis, while it encompasses the known extrahypothalamic distribution of pyroglutamyl-histidyl-proline amide and its metabolic actions on catecholamine function both *in vivo* and *in vitro*, does not explain several facets of the data presented above. For instance, why hindbrain DβH activity *in vivo* is affected specifically remains an open question. Additionally, the mechanisms regarding the tripeptide's penetration through the blood–brain barrier, its uptake into neurons, its intraneuronal storage, its accessibility to vesicles containing DβH, and its release from neurons need to be examined in detail to evaluate the legitimacy of the hypothesis presented. Several of the latter aspects are currently being pursued actively in our laboratory, and only after the potential neuroregulatory role of the tripeptide has been subjected to the same critical scrutiny as the initially proposed hypophyseal role of TRH, can this more general function in brain be entertained seriously.

SUMMARY

The ability of the tripeptide pyroglutamyl-histidyl-proline amide (thyrotropin-releasing hormone) to modify the final step in norepinephrine biosynthesis was assessed *in vivo* and *in vitro*. One mg/kg of the tripeptide significantly reduced accumulation of norepinephrine formed from intracisternally injected [^{3}H]dopamine, an action observed in brain stem but not in other brain regions. Pyroglutamyl-histidyl-proline amide also was an effective *in vitro* inhibitor of dopamine-β-hydroxylase activity. Assessment of norepinephrine formation *in vivo* in hypothyroid rats, where levels of endogenous pyroglutamyl-histidyl-proline amide are low, revealed a marked increase compared to control (euthyroid) rats; these effects, again, were confined to hindbrain regions. These results support an extrahypothalamo-hypophyseal action of the tripeptide, and suggest a potential role for pyroglutamyl-histidyl-proline amide in regulating norepinephrine biosynthesis in some brain regions.

ACKNOWLEDGEMENTS

The participation of Ms. Madelyn Stolk, Ms. Maralyn Kaufman and Mr. Dee Van Riper in the conduct of this research is gratefully acknowledged.

We would like to thank the National Institute of Arthritis, Metabolism and Digestive Diseases (NIAMDD) Rat Pituitary Hormone Distribution Program for the TSH radioimmunoassay reagents.

Research in this paper was supported by USPHS Grants MH 21090, MH 24625 and MH 25601.

REFERENCES

BARCHAS, J. D., CIARANELLO, R. D., STOLK, J. M., BRODIE, H. K. H. AND HAMBURG, D. A. (1972) Biogenic amines and behavior. In *Hormones and Behavior*, S. LEVINE (Ed.), Academic Press, New York, N.Y., pp. 235–329.

BASSIRI, R. M. AND UTIGER, R. D. (1974) Thyrotropin-releasing hormone in the hypothalamus of the rats. *Endocrinology*, **94**, 188–197.

BREESE, G. R., PRANGE, A. J. AND LIPTON, M. A. (1974) Pharmacological studies of thyroid–imipramine interaction in animals. In *The Thyroid Axis, Drugs and Behavior*, A. J. PRANGE, JR. (Ed.), Raven Press, New York, N.Y., pp. 29–48.

BURGUS, R., DUNN, T. F., DESIDERIO, D., WARD, D. N., VALE, W. AND GUILLEMIN, R. (1970) Characterization of ovine hypothalamic hypophysiotropic TSH-releasing factor. *Nature (Lond.)*, **226**, 321–325.

EMLEN, W., SEGAL, D. S. AND MANDELL, A. J. (1972) Thyroid state: effects on pre- and postsynaptic central noradrenergic mechanisms. *Science*, **175**, 79–82.

FLEISCHER, N., BURGUS, R., VALE, W., DUNN, T. F. AND GUILLEMIN, R. (1970) Preliminary observations on the effect of synthetic thyrotropin releasing factor on plasma thyrotropin levels in man. *J. clin. Endocr.*, **31**, 109–112.

GROSS, E., NODA, K. AND NISULA, B. (1973) Solid phase synthesis of peptides with carboxyl-terminal amides — thyrotropin-releasing factor (TRF). *Angew. Chem. int. Edit.*, **12**, 664–665.

HOLLANDER, C. S., MITSUMA, T., SHENKMAN, L., WOOLF, P. AND GERSHSENGORN, M. C. (1972)

Thyrotropin-releasing hormone: evidence for thyroid response to intravenous injection in man. *Science*, **175**, 209–210.

JACKSON, I. M. D., GAGEL, R., PAPAPETROU, P. AND REICHLIN, S. (1974a) Pituitary, hypothalamic and urinary thyrotropin releasing hormone (TRH) concentration in altered thyroid states of rat and man. *Clin. Res.*, **22**, 342A.

JACKSON, I. M. D., SAPERSTEIN, R. AND REICHLIN, S. (1974b) Thyrotropin-releasing hormone (TRH): distribution in hypothalamic and extrahypothalamic brain tissues of mammalian and submammalian chordates. *Fifty-sixth Annual Meeting of the Endocrine Society, 1974, Atlanta, Georgia*, Abstract No. 23.

JACOBS, L. S., SNYDER, P. J., UTIGER, R. D. AND DAUGHADAY, W. H. (1973) Prolactin response to thyrotropin-releasing hormone in normal subjects. *J. clin. Endocr.*, **36**, 1069–1073.

JACOBS, L. S., SNYDER, P. J., WILBUR, J. F., UTIGER, R. D. AND DAUGHADAY, W. H. (1971) Increased serum prolactin after administration of synthetic thyrotropin releasing hormone (TRH) in man. *J. clin. Endocr.*, **33**, 996–998.

KASTIN, A. J., EHRENSING, R. H., SCHALCH, D. S. AND ANDERSON, M. S. (1972) Improvement in mental depression with decreased thyrotropin response after administration of thyrotropin-releasing hormone. *Lancet*, **ii**, 740–742.

LIPTON, M. A., PRANGE, JR., A. J., DAIRMAN, W. AND UDENFRIEND, S. (1968) Increased rate of nor-epinephrine biosynthesis in hypothyroid rats. *Fed. Proc.*, **27**, 399.

MALOOF, F., DOBYNS, B. M. AND VICKERY, A. L. (1952) The effects of various doses of radioactive iodine on the function and structure of the thyroid of the rat. *Endocrinology*, **50**, 612–638.

MARTIN, J. B. AND REICHLIN, S. (1970) Thyrotropin secretion in rats after hypothalamic electrical stimulation or injection of synthetic TSH-releasing factor. *Science*, **168**, 1366–1368.

MOLINOFF, P. B., WEINSHILBOUM, R. AND AXELROD, J. (1971) A sensitive enzymatic assay for dopamine-β-hydroxylase. *J. Pharmacol. exp. Ther.*, **178**, 425–431.

PFAFF, D. W. (1973) Luteinizing hormone-releasing factor potentiates lordosis behavior in hypo-physectomized ovariectomized female rats. *Science*, **182**, 1148–1149.

PLOTNIKOFF, N. P., KASTIN, A. J., ANDERSON, M. S. AND SCHALLY, A. T. (1971) DOPA potentiation by a hypothalamic factor, MSH release-inhibiting hormone (MIF). *Life Sci.*, **10**, 1279–1283.

PLOTNIKOFF, N. P., PRANGE, JR., A. J., BREESE, G. R., ANDERSON, M. S. AND WILSON, I. C. (1972) Thyrotropin releasing hormone: enhancement of dopa activity by a hypothalamic hormone. *Science*, **178**, 417–418.

PRANGE, JR., A. J., MEEK, J. L. AND LIPTON, M. A. (1970) Catecholamines: diminished rate of synthesis in rat brain and heart after thyroxine treatment. *Life Sci.*, **9**, 901–907.

PRANGE, JR., A. J., WILSON, I. C., LARA, P. P., ALLTOP, L. B. AND BREESE, G. R. (1972) Effects of thyrotropin-releasing hormone in depression. *Lancet*, **ii**, 999–1002.

SNYDER, P. J., JACOBS, L. S., UTIGER, R. D. AND DAUGHADAY, W. H. (1973) Thyroid hormone inhibition of the prolactin response to thyrotropin-releasing hormone. *J. clin. Invest.*, **52**, 2324–2329.

STOLK, J. M. (1973) Estimation of *in vivo* dopamine-β-hydroxylase activity in rat brain. *J. Pharmacol. exp. Ther.*, **186**, 230–240.

STOLK, J. M. (1975) Evidence for reversible inhibition of brain dopamine-β-hydroxylase activity *in vivo* by amphetamine analogues. *J. Neurochem.*, **24**, 135–142.

STOLK, J. M. AND HANLON, D. P. (1973) Inhibition of brain dopamine-β-hydroxylase activity by methimazole. *Life Sci.*, **12**, 417–423.

Vasopressin as a Neurotransmitter in the Central Nervous System: Some Evidence from the Supraoptic Neurosecretory System

J. D. VINCENT AND E. ARNAULD

Laboratoire de Neurophysiologie, Université de Bordeaux II, 24 rue Paul Broca, 33000 Bordeaux (France)

There is some evidence to suggest that the neurohormones might be considered as central synaptic transmitters. These polypeptides are synthesized by neurons whose location in the brain is well established (the magnocellular system for antidiuretic hormone and oxytocin) or still uncertain (the parvocellular system for pituitary releasing factors). It is generally thought that the neurosecretory cells do not form specialized junctions with other neurons, but secrete their products exclusively into the blood stream; however, Barry (1954, 1958) and more recently Sterba (1973) have suggested that "extrapituitary neurosecretory pathways" may exist in the central nervous system and have proposed the existence of "neurosecretory synapses". Furthermore, polypeptide hormones have numerous effects on the brain (for review, see de Wied, 1974).

A major difficulty in validating these hypotheses arises from the lack of a morphologically and functionally defined set of neurons in which the capacity of a neurohormone to act as a neurotransmitter may be tested. In this report we should like to propose the supraoptic neurosecretory system as a model. We have previously suggested (Vincent and Hayward, 1970) that the excitation–inhibition sequence produced in the supraoptic nucleus cells upon osmotic stimulation may result from a system of recurrent collaterals forming direct or indirect inhibitory connections with the neurosecretory cells. According to the Dale's principle *(one neuron–one transmitter)*, Nicoll and Barker (1971) have proposed that the neurosecretory product itself might serve a synaptic function and mediate this recurrent inhibition. The existence of a recurrent inhibition (RI) in the supraoptic neurosecretory system (NSO) and the possible role of vasopressin as a neurotransmitter will be discussed.

The recurrent inhibition in the supraoptic neurosecretory system

The results of our electrophysiological studies in the unanesthetized monkey on the response of hypothalamic neurons to intracarotid osmotic stimuli (Hayward and Vincent, 1970) led us to present a schematic interpretation of the possible cellular connections in the osmoreceptor supraoptic nuclear complex (Fig. 1). We proposed

References p. 65–66

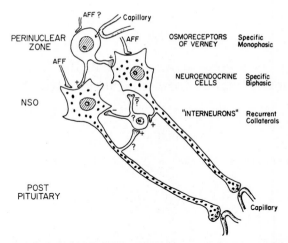

Fig. 1. Schematic interpretation of the possible cellular connections in the osmoreceptor–supraoptic nuclear complex of the monkey (Vincent and Hayward, 1970). AFF = afferent; NSO = supraoptic neurosecretory system.

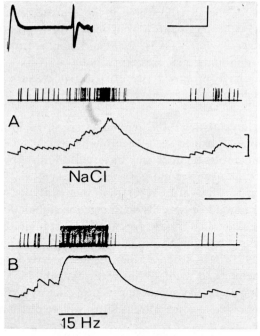

Fig. 2. Responses of an antidromically identified NSO cell to osmotic and antidromic stimuli. In the upper part of the figure, superimposition of 10 antidromic potentials at a fixed latency (time calibration is 10 msec, amplitude 0.5 mV). A and B show the response of the unit to stimulation; the upper line corresponds to the pulse output from a pulse height discriminator triggered by action potentials in the window; the lower line is the analog output proportional to the rate of unit discharge; time calibration, 5 sec; amplitude, 10 spikes/sec. A: biphasic response of the unit to an i.c. osmotic stimulus (hypertonic sodium chloride solution 0.45 *M*, 1 ml). B: inhibitory response to a train of antidromic stimuli (12 V, 15 Hz, 5 sec).

that the "osmoreceptors" are distinct neurons lying in the perinuclear zone of the NSO and responding "specifically" to an osmotic stimulus with a monophasic discharge; we further suggested that the supraoptic neuroendocrine cells respond to an osmotic stimulus with an initial acceleration in firing, due to synaptic driving by the osmoreceptors, followed quickly by an inhibitory phase, possibly due to recurrent activation of inhibitory interneurons or as a result of direct action on these neuroendocrine cells with a slow inhibitory post-synaptic potential. The neurosecretory nature of these "biphasic" cells (Fig. 2) is confirmed by their antidromic activation from the posterior pituitary (Vincent et al., 1972).

Although recurrent collaterals from neurosecretory axons have been seen in Golgi preparations (Christ, 1966), there is no good anatomical proof that such a system exists in the NSO, though the possibility is supported by much electrophysiological evidence.

By intracellular recordings of preoptic neurosecretory cells in the goldfish, Kandel (1964) was able to demonstrate a depression of firing after stimulation of the posterior pituitary, accompanied by a hyperpolarization of the membrane potential (antidromic IPSP). Several papers have now appeared describing recurrent inhibition in

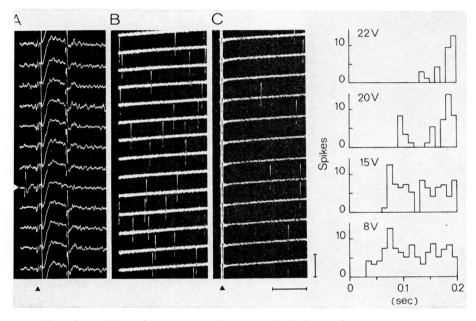

Fig. 3. Effect of stimulation of the posterior pituitary on the discharge of a supraoptic neurosecretory cell. Stimuli were applied at a rate of 1/sec with a strength of 20 V and a duration of 0.6 msec. Threshold for antidromic invasion was 9.5 V. A: responses to single shocks; the arrow marks a spontaneously occurring spike responsible for cancellation of the antidromic action potential. B: spontaneous random discharges occurring in the absence of electrical stimulation. C: cessation of spontaneous discharge, following a response to antidromic stimulus. Calibrations are 0.2 mV, 25 msec for A; and 75 msec for B and C. On the right: column poststimulus time histograms after 8, 15, 20, 22 V stimuli. Note that the reduction of the probability of firing exists for a subthreshold value of the stimulus (8 V) and increases with the intensity of the stimulus (number of stimuli, 200 for each histogram).

References p. 65–66

TABLE I

PATTERNS AND RATES OF FIRING OF HYPOTHALAMIC SUPRAOPTIC NEURONS AS A FUNCTION OF PLASMA OSMOLARITY DURING WATER DEPRIVATION

S.D., standard deviation; in brackets, percentages.

Plasma osmolarity (mOsM/kg)	Number of neurons studied	Pattern of firing			Firing rate (spikes/sec)		Recurrent inhibition
		Irregular	Phasic	Continuous	Mean	S.D. of mean	
299	16	14 (88)	2 (12)	—	1.01	0.79	15 (94)
300–309	6	3 (50)	3 (50)	—	1.84	0.55	5 (83)
310–319	12	2 (17)	8 (66)	2 (17)	2.41	1.29	7 (58)
320–329	2	—	1 (50)	1 (50)	4.07*	2.87*	1
330–339	12	—	5 (42)	7 (58)	5.28	4.11	5 (42)
340	23	—	7 (30)	16 (70)	7.19	4.24	7 (30)

* individual values.

the NSO system after posterior pituitary or stalk stimulation in different mammalian species (Kelly and Dreifuss, 1970; Koizumi and Yamashita, 1971; Barker *et al.*, 1971; Negoro and Holland, 1972).

Evidence for RI in the primate is given by our observation in the unanesthetized monkey of a long inhibition period (30–110 msec) following the antidromic invasion of the cell. By a train of repetitive antidromic stimulation, it is possible to produce inhibition similar to that which follows orthodromic activation of a cell by an osmotic stimulus (Fig. 2A and B); in both cases, the duration of the inhibition is proportional to the magnitude of the preceding activation. By using poststimulus histogram analysis (computed by PDP 8E), RI can be demonstrated in 37 of 42 antidromically identified neurons of the NSO. Fig. 3 shows that the length of the period of reduced probability of discharge increases with the strength of the stimulus. Moreover, RI can be produced by a stimulus that is subthreshold for activation of the somatic antidromic spike. This observation and also the duration of the inhibition (the absolute refractory period of antidromic activation determined by repetitive stimulation never exceeds 5 msec) excludes the possibility of a direct influence of the antidromic action potential on the membrane.

On the other hand we observed in the normally hydrated monkey (Arnauld *et al.*, 1974) that 12% of the spontaneously active neuroendocrine cells discharged phasically by alternating periods of excitation and inhibition. Following withdrawal of drinking water, the proportion of these intermittently firing neurons increased markedly with increasing plasma osmolarity and hormonal release (Table I). This finding suggests that phasically active neurons of the NSO are those engaged in neurohypophyseal hormone secretion. This contention gains support from our previous finding that acute stimulation of the neurosecretory cell by intracarotid osmotic stimulation leads to a biphasic change in membrane excitability characterized by the excitation–inhibition sequence. Finally, it is tempting to speculate that the recurrent inhibition phenomenon contributes to the oscillatory pattern of firing which is reflected in the pattern of release of the neurohormonal product.

Identity of the synaptic transmitter mediating RI: antidiuretic hormone as a possible neurotransmitter

Since electrophysiological evidence exists to support the view that the NSO neuro-secretory cells possess synaptic ability, they must either release the hormone at synapses or elaborate a separate transmitter substance. The latter possibility is based on electron microscopic evidence of small "synaptoid vesicles" beside the large neurosecretory granules; but the physiological significance of these vesicles is not clear and it is possible that they may only represent a different stage in the elaboration of neurosecretion.

By using a pharmacological approach and microelectrophoretic injections of the suspected transmitter substances, Nicoll and Barker (1971) eliminated acetylcholine, noradrenaline, glycine and gamma-aminobutyric acid as mediators of RI. On the other hand the view that the neurosecretory product itself might mediate the inhibition

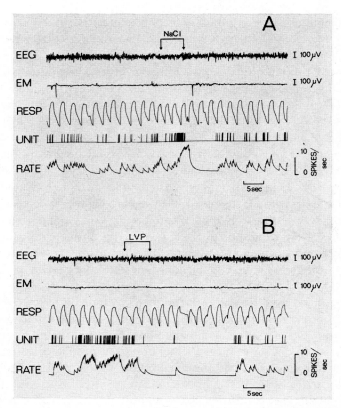

Fig. 4. Response of a neurosecretory cell A: to intracarotid injection of hypertonic sodium chloride solution (0.45 M, 1 ml), B: to an intracarotid injection of lysine vasopressin (LVP) (5 × 10⁻⁹ M, 1 ml). Labels: EEG, biparietal electrocorticogram; EM, eye movements; RESP, respiration; UNIT and RATE, pulse output and integration of the unit discharge.

was supported by the observation of a clearcut inhibition of firing following the administration of lysine vasopressin (LVP) to the NSO cells by microelectrophoresis.

To confirm this hypothesis, we have tested the effect of an *intracarotid (i.c.) injection of LVP* on the firing rate neurosecretory neurons identified by their responses to osmotic and antidromic stimulations. Six monkeys were prepared using our techniques of chronic single unit recording, i.c. injection and polygraphic recording of behavioral parameters of the conscious monkeys (Hayward and Vincent, 1970). In 3 animals urine was collected from a sterile indwelling bladder catheter. The renal action of LVP was verified by free water clearance studies in two animals. During some experimental sessions, the urine flow was held constant by intravenous infusion of mannitol. In one animal blood pressure was measured by an electronic sphygmo-manometer (RACIA 315 M).

Of the 33 cells analyzed, 26 responded to the i.c. injections of LVP (Sandoz, 5 × 10⁻⁹ M, isotonic saline solution, 1 ml injected over a period of 5–10 sec) with a rapid decrease of their firing rate, and sometimes a total inhibition and generally returned

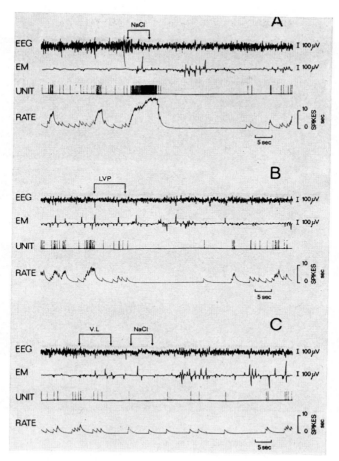

Fig. 5. A and B: legends as in Fig. 4. C shows the refractory period to an osmotic stimulus after an i.c. injection of lysine vasopressin.

to the baseline within 20–50 sec with or without a rebound effect (Fig. 4). This response was not observed in 19 randomly encountered hypothalamic cells. Repeated identical LVP injections produced reproducible inhibitory effects. Osmotic stimulation during the inhibitory period following LVP injection produced no response (Fig. 5). An i.v. injection of a 4 times more concentrated LVP solution caused no change in the NSO unit firing. Elevation in arterial blood pressure, comparable to that produced by the LVP injection, following i.v. injection of phenylephrine hydrochloride (1 mg/kg), failed to produce any comparable depression in NSO unit firing. No correlation was shown between NSO firing rate and changes in renal outflow, as clearly demonstrated in the monkey under mannitol infusion. Finally there is good evidence that LVP can cross the brain–blood barrier (de Wied, 1969). Taken together, these findings support the view that LVP has a direct action on the hypothalamo-neurohypophyseal system.

Our experiments on water-deprived monkeys may also favor our hypothesis. Five monkeys were subjected to water deprivation up to 7 days followed by a 4-day

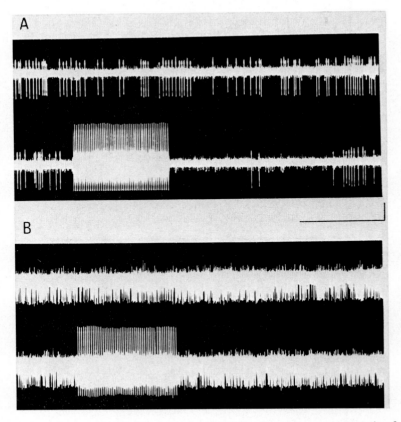

Fig. 6. A: spontaneous discharge of a neurosecretory NSO cell and response to a train of repetitive antidromic stimuli (10 Hz, 12 V, 0.5 msec) in a normally hydrated monkey; note the clearcut inhibition after the stimulation. B: neurosecretory NSO cell in a dehydrated monkey; note the continuous firing and the absence of inhibition after a train of repetitive antidromic stimuli. Calibrations: 5 sec, 0.1 mV.

rehydration period. Four to 8 neurons were recorded daily (Table I). The mean firing frequency of supraoptic neurons increased with the observed rise in plasma osmotic pressure. Initially, as reported above, an increasing proportion of cells displayed a phasic pattern of discharge with bursts of activity followed by silent periods. In a majority of cells, clearcut RI was observed. After the fifth day of water deprivation, most of the cells (70%) discharged continuously at a high rate, and RI was no longer present (Fig. 6). The mean firing frequency returned to control values after 2 days of rehydration. On the fourth day, the cells were either silent or firing very slowly. RI could again be demonstrated when a sufficient level of spontaneous firing existed. Since it has been shown that prolonged dehydration causes a severe depletion of neurosecretory material in the nerve terminals, the disappearance of RI and of the phasic pattern is consistent with the view that RI is related to the presence of neurosecretory material at the neuron terminals. Nevertheless the general increase in the NSO excitability may be sufficient to explain our observations.

On the other hand, we have recently reported (Dreifuss *et al.*, 1973) evidence which did not support our tentative hypothesis in that RI is still present in neurons of the NSO of rats which are homozygous for hypothalamic diabetes insipidus (Brattleboro strain) and have an absolute deficiency of vasopressin synthesis. This result does not exclude the possibility that a vasopressin-like substance possessing neuromediating activity, but lacking any hormonal function, exists in neurons.

Finally, we have recently observed in the unanesthetized rabbit (unpublished observations) that RI is present in some neurons, the axons of which terminate in the median eminence. These preliminary results are insufficient to support the widespread occurrence of RI but may give an illustration of the so-called ultra-short feedback mechanism proposed for the parvocellular neurosecretory system by Motta *et al.* (1970).

SUMMARY

It has been suggested that the excitation–inhibition sequence produced in the supra-optic neurosecretory neurons of the unanesthetized monkeys after osmotic stimulation may result from recurrent inhibition (RI) mediated by neurosecretory axon collaterals. Electrophysiological evidence for RI was given by the observation of a period of reduced firing following antidromic invasion of the cell. According to Dale's law of "one neuron–one transmitter" it has been proposed that the neurosecretory product might also serve a synaptic function and mediate the RI. The i.c. administration of lysine vasopressin depressed the spontaneous firing of neurosecretory cells and their response to osmotic stimulation. These changes were apparently unrelated to variations in renal outflow or systemic blood pressure. Disappearance of RI was observed after 5 days of water deprivation when a total depletion of vasopressin in the system is expected to occur. The only observation inconsistent with a neurotransmitter role for vasopressin in mediating RI is that RI persists in Brattleboro rats which apparently lack vasopressin.

ACKNOWLEDGEMENTS

The authors' gratitude is due to Dr A. Findlay who kindly read this manuscript and offered valuable editorial advice and to Dr B. Dufy and Dr B. Bioulac, for their cooperation. Mr R. Miguelez prepared the figures, Mrs Bonhomme-Caillaud, Mr G. Labayle and Mr F. Rodriguez provided valuable technical assistance.

This work was supported by "La Fondation pour la Recherche Médicale Française", I.N.S.E.R.M. (A.T.P. 3) and C.N.R.S. (E.R.A. 493).

REFERENCES

ARNAULD, E., VINCENT, J. D. AND DREIFUSS, J. J. (1974) Changes in the firing patterns of hypothalamic supraoptic neurones during water deprivation in monkeys. *Science*, **185**, 535–537.

BARKER, J. L., CRAYTON, J. W. AND NICOLL, R. A. (1971) Antidromic and orthodromic responses of paraventricular and supraoptic neurosecretory cells. *Brain Res.*, **33**, 353–366.

BARRY, J. (1954) Neurocrinie et synapses neurosecrétoires. *Arch. Anat. micr. Morph. exp.*, **43**, 310–320.

BARRY, J. (1958) Les voies neurosecrétoires extra-hypophysaires et le problème de l'action nerveuse centrale des hormones post-hypophysaires. *J. méd. Lyon*, **935**, 1065–1074.

CHRIST, J. F. (1966) Nerve supply, blood supply and cytology of the neurohypophysis. In *The Pituitary Gland, Vol. 3*, G. W. HARRIS AND B. T. DONOVAN (Eds.), University of California Press, Berkeley, Calif., pp. 62–130.

DREIFUSS, J. J., NORDMANN, J. AND VINCENT, J. D. (1973) Recurrent inhibition of supraoptic neurosecretory cells in homozygous Brattleboro rats. *J. Physiol. (Lond.)*, **237**, 25–27P.

HAYWARD, J. N. AND VINCENT, J. D. (1970) Osmosensitive single neurones in the hypothalamus of unanaesthetized monkeys. *J. Physiol. (Lond.)*, **210**, 947–972.

KANDEL, E. R. (1964) Electrical properties of hypothalamic neuroendocrine cells. *J. gen. Physiol.*, **47**, 691–717.

KELLY, J. S. AND DREIFUSS, J. J. (1970) Antidromic inhibition of identified rat supraoptic neurons. *Brain Res.*, **22**, 406–409.

KOIZUMI, K. and YAMASHITA, H. (1971) Studies of antidromically identified neurosecretory cells of the hypothalamus by intracellular and extracellular recordings. *J. Physiol. (Lond.)*, **221**, 683–705.

MOTTA, M., PIVA, F. AND MARTINI, P. (1970) The hypothalamus as the center of endocrine feedback mechanisms. In *The Hypothalamus*, L. MARTINI, M. MOTTA AND F. FRASCHINI (Eds.), Academic Press, New York, N.Y., pp. 463–489.

NEGORO, H. AND HOLLAND, H. C. (1972) Inhibition of unit activity in the hypothalamic paraventricular nucleus following antidromic activation. *Brain Res.*, **42**, 385–402.

NICOLL, R. A. AND BARKER, J. L. (1971) The pharmacology of recurrent inhibition in the supraoptic neurosecretory system. *Brain Res.*, **35**, 501–511.

STERBA, G. (1973) Ascending neurosecretory pathways of peptidergic type. In *VI International Symposium on Neurosecretion*, Abstracts, London, p. 3.

VINCENT, J. D. AND HAYWARD, J. N. (1970) Activity of single cells in the osmoreceptor–supraoptic nuclear complex in the hypothalamus of the waking rhesus monkey. *Brain Res.*, **23**, 105–108.

VINCENT, J. D., ARNAULD, E. AND NICOLESCU-CATARGI, A. (1972) Osmoreceptors and neurosecretory cells in the supraoptic complex of the unanesthetized monkey. *Brain Res.*, **45**, 278–281.

WIED, D. DE (1969) Effects of peptide hormones on behavior. In *Frontiers in Neuroendocrinology*, W. F. GANONG AND L. MARTINI (Eds.), Oxford University Press, New York, N.Y., pp. 97–140.

WIED, D. DE (1974) Pituitary–adrenal system, hormones and behavior. In *The neurosciences Third Study Program*, F. O. SCHMITT AND F. G. WORDEN (Eds.), MIT Press, Cambridge, Mass., pp. 653–666.

Free Communications

Ultrashort feedback effects of releasing hormones

M. Hyyppä, S. Justo, M. Motta and L. Martini — *Departments of Endocrinology and Pharmacology, University of Milan, Milan (Italy)*

Previous experiments had indicated that the subcutaneous administration of crude hypothalamic extracts containing FSH-RH and devoided of any FSH and sex steroid contamination may bring about a significant reduction of FSH-RH stores in the hypothalamus of castrated, hypophysectomized rats. These experiments suggested the possibility that the brain might contain receptors sensitive to circulating levels of FSH-RH, and that FSH-RH might directly regulate its own production via an "ultra-short" feedback effect[1]. Similar experiments have now been repeated using synthetic LH-RH and its effects have been evaluated on hypothalamic LH-RH stores of castrated, hypophysectomized male rats. LH-RH contained in the hypothalamus has been evaluated injecting hypothalamic extracts into the carotid artery of castrated estrogen-pretreated female rats and measuring the rise of radioimmunoassayable LH in their serum. It has been found that castration and hypophysectomy are followed by a significant increase of LH-RH in the hypothalamus. Subcutaneous or intracarotid treatments with repeated doses of synthetic LH-RH are able to bring back to normal the elevated levels of hypothalamic LH-RH in castrated, hypophysectomized animals. These data further support the view that releasing hormones have direct effects on the brain and speak in favor of the existence of "ultrashort" feedback mechanisms controlling gonadotropin secretion.

Supported by Ford Foundation Grant.

1 Hyyppä, M., Motta, M. and Martini, L., *Neuroendocrinology*, 7 (1971) 227–235.

Modification of *in vitro* neurotransmitter release from rat brain slices by hypophyseotropic factors

A. H. Mulder and P. G. Smelik — *Department of Pharmacology, Medical Faculty, Free University, Amsterdam (The Netherlands)*

Some of the hypothalamic peptides which are involved in regulation of pituitary function have been reported to exert behavioral effects[3]. These peptides may act by modifying some of the processes involved in central neurotransmission. In particular, effects on catecholamines have been reported[1,2].

We have investigated the effect of hypophysectomy and of melanocyte-stimulating hormone-release inhibiting factor (MIF) and thyrotropin-releasing hormone (TRH) on depolarization-induced release of several central neurotransmitter substances from tissue slices of rat striatum and hypothalamus after labeling *in vitro* with the radio-active neurotransmitters.

After hypophysectomy, release of dopamine (DA) from striatal slices was markedly increased. Release of acetylcholine was also augmented. In contrast, hypophysectomy appeared to result in a significant inhibition of noradrenaline (NA) release from hypothalamic slices. Effects on other neurotransmitters were only small.

MIF considerably enhanced the release of DA and 5-HT from striatal slices whereas it decreased release of NA and 5-HT from hypothalamic tissue. TRH only slightly increased release of DA and 5-HT from striatum, but was as effective as MIF in inhibiting release of NA and 5-HT from hypothalamus.

Our data suggest that there may be some specificity in the action of MIF and TRH, in that not all neurotransmitters are affected to the same extent. Another significant finding is, that the action of these peptides is stimulatory in the striatum, but inhibitory in the hypothalamus.

1 FRIEDMAN, E., *et al.*, *Science*, 182 (1973) 831.
2 KELLER, H. H., *et al.*, *Nature (Lond.)*, 248 (1974) 528.
3 PRANGE, A. J., *et al.*, In *Frontiers in Catecholamine Research*, E. USDIN AND S. H. SNYDER (Eds.), Pergamon Press, Oxford, 1973, pp. 1149–1155.

TRH as a possible quick-acting but short-lasting antidepressant

W. VAN DEN BURG, H. M. VAN PRAAG, E. R. H. BOS, A. K. VAN ZANTEN, D. A. PIERS AND H. DOORENBOS — *Department of Biological Psychiatry, Isotope Laboratory, Department of Internal Medicine, Division of Endocrinology, Medical Faculty, University of Groningen, Groningen (The Netherlands)*

Recently Prange *et al.*[1] reported that TRH has an antidepressant effect. Their evidence suggested that it is a very quick-acting albeit short-lasting therapeutic agent. Most patients showed a lowered plasma TSH-response after TRH injection.

This report is the result of a more extensive investigation, attempting to replicate Prange's findings.

Method. A group of 10 patients with an endogenous depressive syndrome was injected on 4 consecutive days with placebo and TRH (500 μg, i.v.) alternately, either in the order TRH–placebo–TRH–placebo, or *vice versa* (double reversal design). Blood samples were taken at various points of time. Several behavior measures were used. The double-blind inquiry centered around 3 questions: (1) are the rapid improvements reported by Prange reproducible? (2) is there a longer-lasting beneficial effect? (3) is there a lowered TSH-response in depressive patients after TRH administration?

Results. Question 1: taking only the first 2 days into consideration, a very slight quick-acting antidepressive effect seems likely, although this did not emerge clearly.

Thereafter no effect was observable. *Question 2:* no overall beneficial effect could be observed. *Question 3:* the TSH response indeed appears to be lowered in depressives. Serum thyroxine and resin uptake were normal, indicating normal thyroid function.

1 PRANGE, A. J., JR., *Lancet*, II (1972) 999–1002.

Action of releasing factors on unit activity in the forebrain

R. G. DYER AND R. E. J. DYBALL — *ARC Institute of Animal Physiology, Babraham, Cambridge CB2 4AT (Great Britain)*

Single unit activity was recorded from the cerebral cortex and rostral hypothalamus in urethane anesthetized rats. Recordings were made from the central barrel of multi-barrelled micropipettes. The outer barrels were filled with 1.0 M sodium glutamate, 0.01 M oxytocin, 0.01 M LHRH, 0.03 M TRH and 2 M sodium chloride. A drug was considered to influence the activity of a cell if changes in firing rate, in excess of 20% of the resting rate, were induced by application of ejecting currents (5–30 nA) to the drug containing barrels. Responses which could not be reproduced were excluded.

In the cerebral cortex TRH, LHRH and oxytocin were without effect (N = 12).

In the rostral hypothalamus 24 cells were tested successfully. Glutamate caused excitation (N = 10) or was without effect (N = 2). Oxytocin was always without effect (N = 8). LRH inhibited the discharge of 4 cells out of 12 and TRH had a similar effect upon 7 cells out of 17. One cell was excited by TRH. Several units responded to one releasing factor and were uninfluenced by the other.

The results demonstrate that releasing factors directly influence the electrical activity of the hypothalamus.

Session II

HORMONES AND SLEEP

Chairmen: E. D. WEITZMAN (Bronx, N.Y.)
E. J. SACHAR (Bronx, N.Y.)

Sleep-Endocrinology Studies in Man

ROBERT T. RUBIN

Department of Psychiatry, U.C.L.A. School of Medicine, Harbor General Hospital Campus, Torrance, Calif. 90509 (U.S.A.)

It is now well established that a major controlling factor in endocrine regulation is the central nervous system (CNS) (Reichlin, 1974). The secretion rate of an anterior pituitary hormone such as ACTH (corticotropin) depends on a balance between CNS driving (so-called "open-loop" mechanisms) and negative feedback to the pituitary and brain by glucocorticoids from the adrenal cortex (so-called "closed-loop" mechanisms). The importance of CNS driving mechanisms in ACTH regulation may be inferred from (1) its pulsatile, episodic release pattern (Gallagher *et al.*, 1973), (2) its prominent circadian rhythm (De Lacerda *et al.*, 1973) which is abolished by hypothalamic deafferentation (Halász, 1969), (3) its alterability by stimulation of suprahypothalamic brain centers such as the amygdala and hippocampus (Rubin *et al.*, 1966), and its exquisite sensitivity to many different kinds of psychological stress (Rubin and Mandell, 1966; Mason, 1971).

A major body of data contributing to the recognition of the importance of CNS open-loop mechanisms in normal endocrine functioning has come from studies of the neuroendocrinology of sleep (Rubin *et al.*, 1973a; Sassin, 1974; Rubin *et al.*, 1974a; Takahashi, 1974), most of which have been published only in the last 6 years. The phenomenon of sleep is a superb paradigm for the study of CNS open-loop mechanisms in humans for several reasons. First, in adult humans sleep is normally monotonic; *i.e.*, we normally sleep only once in each 24-hr period. Therefore, sleep *versus* waking provides a good contrast for examining circadian rhythms in endocrine function. (For the elucidation of circadian rhythms, hormone release patterns must be determined not only during the hours of sleep, but throughout the entire 24-hr period, as has been done in many studies.)

Second, during the time of sleep there are large qualitative shifts of CNS activity, *e.g.* slow-wave (stage 3–4) or deep sleep *versus* rapid eye movement (REM) or dreaming sleep. These shifts are regular, being part of a basic rest–activity cycle that is detectable throughout the 24 hr (Kleitman, 1969), and thus they provide an ultradian CNS rhythm for the modulation of endocrine activity. In adults there is normally a gradient during the sleep period, with stage 3–4 sleep being concentrated into the early hours, whereas REM episodes are concentrated into the later hours of sleep. This time differential is an important consideration in sleep neuroendocrinology, and the bottom of Fig. 1 presents it graphically.

References p. 78–80

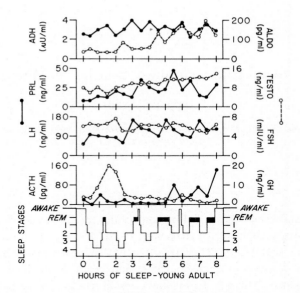

Fig. 1. Composite representation of the typical secretion patterns (plasma levels) of 8 hormones during a normal 8-hr sleep period in a young adult man. REM = rapid eye movement sleep; ACTH = adrenocorticotropic hormone; GH = growth hormone; LH = luteinizing hormone; FSH = follicle-stimulating hormone; PRL = prolactin; TESTO = testosterone; ADH = antidiuretic hormone; ALDO = aldosterone. Hormones named on left side of figure depicted by dots and solid line; those named on right side depicted by open circles and dashed line.

Third, the biogenic amine neurotransmitters — serotonin, dopamine, norepinephrine — and also acetylcholine appear to play a prominent role in the CNS regulation of anterior pituitary hormone secretion, via the hypothalamic releasing and inhibiting factors (Schally *et al.*, 1973; De Wied and De Jong, 1974). These neurotransmitters also appear to be involved in the triggering and maintenance of sleep stages (Jouvet, 1972). In the cat, in which most neurochemical sleep research has been done, many experiments suggest that slow-wave sleep is triggered by serotoninergic neurons in the median raphe nuclei of the brain stem, and REM sleep is primed by a serotoninergic mechanism. The maintenance of REM sleep depends on pontine noradrenergic and cholinergic mechanisms located in the region of the locus coeruleus (Morgane and Stern, 1972). These neurochemical data from cats are, however, at some odds with human neuropharmacologic studies of sleep, which suggest that increasing brain catecholamine levels decreases REM sleep, and conversely, lowering catecholamines increases REM (Wyatt, 1972). Thus, only limited inferences about the role of specific neurotransmitters in human sleep staging may be drawn from animal work.

The 6 anterior pituitary hormones (ACTH, GH (growth hormone), LH (luteinizing hormone), FSH (follicle-stimulating hormone), prolactin, TSH (thyrotropin)) have received the greatest attention for several reasons, including the obvious anatomical and functional proximity of the pituitary to the CNS, the 40-year-old concept of stress activation of the pituitary–adrenal cortical axis and its long-recognized prominent circadian rhythm, and the recent development of specific and sensitive radio-immunoassay techniques for the measurement of each of these hormones. Other hormones also are receiving considerable interest as newer measurement techniques are devised, such as the target gland hormones, cortisol, testosterone, estradiol, progesterone and 17-hydroxy-progesterone; the posterior pituitary hormone, vaso-pressin; components of other endocrine axes such as the renin–angiotensin–aldosterone system; and hormones thought to have little CNS modulation, such as parathormone.

Each of the 6 anterior pituitary hormones has now been shown to be released in a pulsatile, episodic manner, and each has its own unique secretion pattern during sleep and the 24-hr sleep–wake cycle in adult humans. We have considered many of the pertinent studies in earlier reviews (Rubin *et al.*, 1973a; Rubin *et al.*, 1974a), and here only the highlights will be mentioned. Fig. 1 shows a composite of 5 of the anterior pituitary hormones, ACTH, GH, LH, FSH, and prolactin, as well as testosterone, antidiuretic hormone and aldosterone, in a young adult.

ACTH has a prominent circadian rhythm, with lowest blood levels in the early hours of the sleep period, and then a rapid increase in levels in the latter few hours of sleep, reaching a maximum about the time of awakening. Once established, this rhythm appears to have considerable inertia, persisting when sleep is forced into a 3-hr ultradian cycle (Weitzman *et al.*, 1974) and taking several weeks to readjust when the sleep–wake cycle is reversed. The individual secretory episodes of ACTH do not correlate well with REM sleep episodes, but they do occur most frequently during the hours when REM sleep is maximal.

GH, in contrast to ACTH, is released soon after sleep onset and is closely linked to slow-wave sleep. Factors which alter GH secretion during waking hours have much less effect on the slow-wave sleep-related release of GH. In contrast to the inertia of the ACTH rhythm following the alteration of sleep, GH immediately responds to a shifted sleep schedule, being released at the new time of onset of slow-wave sleep. The metabolic importance of this sleep-GH release is not known. Normally, it occurs at the time when ACTH and glucocorticoid levels are at their lowest. GH promotes protein synthesis in conjunction with other anabolic hormones, whereas the gluco-corticoids are catabolic toward proteins; thus the timing of the slow-wave sleep-related GH release may permit unopposed facilitation of protein synthesis in the brain and other organs, perhaps playing a role in memory consolidation and learning.

Studies of sleep-GH release in other animals indicate that man and chair-restrained baboons are the only primates that show a single large GH peak; this phenomenon is not present in rhesus monkeys or in dogs (Takahashi, 1974). This difference may be on the basis of the monophasic, circadian pattern of sleep in man and baboons compared to other animals.

The gonadotropins, LH and FSH, show very little circadian rhythm in adult humans. On the average, LH may be slightly higher during REM sleep compared with the other sleep stages, but the individual secretory episodes of LH are randomly distributed throughout both day and night. FSH levels are generally more stable than LH; FSH is also secreted episodically throughout the 24-hr period, apparently independently from LH. In some women the midcycle ovulatory surge of LH may begin in the latter hours of sleep or at the time of awakening.

Prolactin has a prominent circadian rhythm, with blood levels beginning to climb shortly after sleep onset and reaching maximum values in the last hour or two of sleep. Like GH, the prolactin rhythm is quite dependent on sleep. Early awakening fore-shortens the sleep-related prolactin increase; partial or complete reversal of the sleep–wake cycle causes an immediate shift of prolactin secretion to the new sleep schedule; and daytime naps result in prolactin release. The individual secretory episodes of prolactin appear to be entrained to REM *versus* non-REM sleep staging, with nadirs of prolactin occurring during REM and peaks during non-REM (Parker *et al.*, 1974).

TSH, the sixth anterior pituitary hormone, is not depicted in Fig. 1. Blood levels of TSH are quite stable, although episodic release has been suggested by rapid blood sampling. Several studies have defined a circadian TSH rhythm, with highest levels occurring at various times during the sleep period — either early, like GH, or late, like ACTH and prolactin.

The elucidation of the specific circadian rhythms for each of the anterior pituitary hormones now permits further investigation of their control of target organ hormones. ACTH is the main influence on cortisol secretion by the adrenal cortex, and indeed cortisol secretion patterns parallel ACTH patterns quite closely (Gallagher *et al.*, 1973). On the other hand, aldosterone, a mineralocorticoid also secreted by the adrenal cortex, is considered to be released primarily by two stimuli: increased potassium levels and increased renin and angiotensin II levels (Laragh, 1973). How-ever, aldosterone is known to be secreted episodically, it has a prominent circadian rhythm similar to ACTH and cortisol (Fig. 1), and, during sleep, bursts of aldosterone are synchronous with bursts of cortisol (Katz *et al.*, 1972). Therefore, it is reasonable to consider that ACTH may play a prominent role in aldosterone regulation, at least during sleep. Complicating this question is the observation that plasma renin activity peaks may coincide with aldosterone peaks, but renin activity at night is not higher than during the day (Katz *et al.*, 1972). However, plasma angiotensin II levels do have a circadian rhythm similar to aldosterone (Kala *et al.*, 1973). Thus, the hierarchy of importance of factors influencing aldosterone secretion — potassium, renin–angiotensin, ACTH — and the consistency of their influence throughout the 24-hr period are still unsettled.

Another area in which the pituitary regulation of a target organ hormone is emerging as a more complex relationship than formerly believed, is the gonadotropin regulation of testosterone release by the testis. Classically, LH has been considered to be the stimulant for testosterone release by the Leydig cells, with a straightforward negative feedback relationship between the two hormones. As mentioned earlier, LH has no specific circadian rhythm, whereas testosterone definitely increases during sleep. The circadian rhythm of testosterone looks quite similar to that of prolactin, as shown in Fig. 1. Recent simultaneous studies of LH, FSH, prolactin and testosterone during sleep suggest that testosterone secretion lags behind LH by 60–80 min on the average (Rubin *et al.*, 1973b; Judd *et al.*, 1974a). However, testosterone levels also correlate with prolactin levels, with testosterone again lagging behind prolactin by about 60 min (Rubin *et al.*, unpublished data). There is evidence from animal studies that both FSH and prolactin augment testosterone secretion (Hafiez *et al.*, 1972; Odell *et al.*, 1973). Thus, there may be an interplay of the 3 pituitary hormones — LH, FSH, prolactin — in the regulation of testosterone release by the testis in the adult male; the specific contribution of each hormone awaits further study.

The final hormone depicted in Fig. 1 is antidiuretic hormone (vasopressin-ADH), a posterior pituitary hormone. Like the anterior pituitary hormones, ADH is secreted episodically. In young adult males, the secretory episodes bear no relationship to sleep stages, nor is there a change in baseline levels during the night (Rubin *et al.*, 1974b). These ADH data contrast with the findings of an earlier sleep study, in which older men with indwelling urethral catheters were found to have transiently decreased urine volume and increased urine osmolality during REM sleep episodes (Mandell *et al.*, 1966). On the basis of these urine changes it had been hypothesized that ADH was released in conjunction with REM sleep; the recent direct measurements of ADH suggest either that other hormonal or autonomic nervous system mechanisms were responsible for the changes in urine volume and concentration, or that ADH release in older men may be linked to REM sleep, whereas it is not in young men. Here, too, considerable future research will be required to elucidate all the factors influencing renal function during sleep.

One aspect of sleep neuroendocrinology that is receiving considerable current interest is patterns of hormone release during puberty (Swerdloff and Rubin, 1975). Greatly elevated levels of GH, LH, and testosterone during sleep compared with waking hours have been demonstrated in pubertal children (Finkelstein *et al.*, 1972; Judd *et al.*, 1974b). These marked sleep-associated hormone patterns during puberty tend to "soften" as the adolescent enters adulthood. Slow-wave sleep-related GH release is not as striking, LH secretion becomes spread out over the entire 24-hr period, and the nocturnal rise of testosterone is percentage-wise not as great, although absolute levels of testosterone are higher at all times of the day and night in the adult male.

Hormones that are generally thought to be stable and regulated solely by metabolic factors rather than by the CNS are being investigated for possible episodic release patterns and circadian variation; one example is parathyroid hormone (PTH). PTH exhibits a circadian rhythm in adults, with fairly constant blood levels during the day and a nocturnal rise, highest levels occurring at 2–4 a.m. (Jubiz *et al.*, 1972). In this study, non-protein-bound calcium levels were constant at night, and the PTH rhythm persisted in spite of a calcium infusion which raised total calcium to high normal levels. These data were interpreted as a changing rate of PTH secretion at night; the mechanism for such a change is not understood.

An aspect of all these studies that merits greater attention in the future is the statistical analysis of the individual hormone secretion patterns. Most studies report correlations between sleep stages and hormone levels by visual inspection, whereas simple statistical tests such as Kendall's coefficient of concordance (Gibbons, 1971) can be used across subjects to ascertain whether sleep staging is at baseline values as well as whether hormone values correlate significantly with sleep stages (Rubin *et al.*,

References p. 78–80

1973c). The presence of circadian or ultradian rhythms is often mistakenly tested with a two-way analysis of variance (subjects and time as main effects), without the recognition that the time periods are correlated. Special adjustments must be made for this correlation; these include reducing the degrees of freedom for the F ratio, using a multivariate test such as Hotelling's T^2, and curve-fitting to individual subjects' data with the construction of contrasts for tests of significance (Rubin and Lubin, 1974).

Finally, it should be pointed out that very little is understood about the physiological and metabolic significance of the pulsatile episodic release patterns of the various hormones, their unique circadian and ultradian rhythms, and their relationship to the sleep–wake cycle and sleep staging. The importance of sleep for the initiation of the hormonal events of puberty has been discussed, but, as yet, only speculative hypotheses may be applied to the hormonal patterns seen in the normal adult. Their significance in normal physiological functioning remains to be explored.

SUMMARY

Sleep is an excellent paradigm for the study of the CNS control of endocrine functioning in humans, with sleep staging representing large, recurring shifts of CNS activity. During sleep the anterior and posterior pituitary hormones have unique secretion patterns, with pulsatile episodes of release contributing to an overall 24-hr pattern. Some hormones, like GH and prolactin, are closely linked to the sleep–wake cycle, whereas others, such as ACTH, have considerable inertia to their circadian rhythm and are not closely linked to sleep. Still others, such as LH, FSH, and ADH, appear to have neither a relationship to sleep staging nor a circadian rhythm in the adult. The physiological and metabolic importance of these hormone patterns remains to be explored.

ACKNOWLEDGEMENTS

This study was supported by NIMH Research Scientist Development Award K01-MH-47363 and Office of Naval Research Contract N00014-73-C-0127.

REFERENCES

DE LACERDA, L., KOWARSKI, A. AND MIGEON, C. J. (1973) Integrated concentration and diurnal variation of plasma cortisol. *J. clin. Endocr.*, **36**, 227–238.

DE WIED, D. AND DE JONG, W. (1974) Drug effects and hypothalamic–anterior pituitary function. *Ann. Rev. Pharmacol.*, **14**, 389–412.

FINKELSTEIN, J. W., ROFFWARG, H. P., BOYAR, R. M., KREAM, J. AND HELLMAN, L. (1972) Age-related change in the twenty-four-hour spontaneous secretion of growth hormone. *J. clin. Endocr.*, **35**, 665–670.

GALLAGHER, T. F., YOSHIDA, K., ROFFWARG, H. D., FUKUSHIMA, D. K., WEITZMAN, E. D. AND HELLMAN, L. (1973) ACTH and cortisol secretory patterns in man. *J. clin. Endocr.*, **36**, 1058–1068.

GIBBONS, J. D. (1971) *Nonparametric Statistical Inference*. McGraw-Hill, New York, N.Y., pp. 250–257.

HAFIEZ, A. A., LLOYD, C. W. AND BARTKE, A. (1972) The role of prolactin in the regulation of testis function: The effects of prolactin and luteinizing hormone on the plasma levels of testosterone and androstenedione in hypophysectomized rats. *J. Endocr.*, **52**, 327–332.

HALÁSZ, B. (1969) The endocrine effects of isolation of the hypothalamus from the rest of the brain. In *Frontiers in Neuroendocrinology*, W. F. GANONG AND L. MARTINI (Eds.), Oxford University Press, New York, N.Y., pp. 307–342.

JOUVET, M. (1972) The role of monoamines and acetylcholine-containing neurons in the regulation of the sleep–waking cycle. *Ergebn. Physiol.*, **64**, 166–307.

JUBIZ, W., CANTERBURY, J. M., REISS, E. AND TYLER, F. H. (1972) Circadian rhythm in serum parathyroid hormone concentration in human subjects: Correlation with serum calcium, phosphate, albumin, and growth hormone levels. *J. clin. Invest.*, **51**, 2040–2046.

JUDD, H. L., PARKER, D. C., RAKOFF, J. S., HOPPER, B. R. AND YEN, S. S. C. (1974a) Elucidation of mechanism(s) of the nocturnal rise of testosterone in men. *J. clin. Endocr.*, **38**, 134–141.

JUDD, H. L., PARKER, D. C., SILER, T. M. AND YEN, S. S. C. (1974b) The nocturnal rise of plasma testosterone in pubertal boys. *J. clin. Endocr.*, **38**, 710–713.

KALA, R., FYHRQUIST, F. AND EISALO, A. (1973) Diurnal variation of plasma angiotensin II in man. *Scand. J. clin. Lab. Invest.*, **31**, 363–365.

KATZ, F. H., ROMFH, P. AND SMITH, J. A. (1972) Episodic secretion of aldosterone in supine man: Relationship to cortisol. *J. clin. Endocr.*, **35**, 178–181.

KLEITMAN, N. (1969) Basic rest–activity cycle in relation to sleep and wakefulness. In *Sleep: Physiology and Pathology*, A. KALES (Ed.), Lippincott, Philadelphia, Pa., pp. 33–38.

LARAGH, J. H. (1973) Potassium, angiotensin, and the dual control of aldosterone secretion. *New Engl. J. Med.*, **289**, 745–747.

MANDELL, A. J., CHAFFEY, B., BRILL, P., MANDELL, M. P., RODNICK, J., RUBIN, R. T. AND SHEFF, R. (1966) Dreaming sleep in man: changes in urine volume and osmolality. *Science*, **151**, 1558–1560.

MASON, J. W. (1971) A re-evaluation of the concept of "non-specificity" in stress theory. *J. psychiat. Res.*, **8**, 323–333.

MORGANE, P. J. AND STERN, W. C. (1972) Relationship of sleep to neuroanatomical circuits, biochemistry, and behavior. *Ann. N. Y. Acad. Sci.*, **193**, 95–111.

ODELL, W. D., SWERDLOFF, R. S., JACOBS, H. S. AND HESCOX, M. A. (1973) FSH induction of sensitivity to LH: One cause of sexual maturation in the male rat. *Endocrinology*, **92**, 160–165.

PARKER, D. C., ROSSMAN, L. G. AND VANDERLAAN, E. F. (1974) Relation of sleep-entrained human prolactin release to REM–nonREM cycles. *J. clin. Endocr.*, **38**, 646–651.

REICHLIN, S. (1974) Neuroendocrinology. In *Textbook of Endocrinology*, 5th ed., R. H. WILLIAMS (Ed.), Saunders, Philadelphia, Pa., pp. 774–831.

RUBIN, R. T. AND MANDELL, A. J. (1966) Adrenal cortical activity in pathological emotional states: a review. *Amer. J. Psychiat.*, **123**, 387–400.

RUBIN, R. T., MANDELL, A. J. AND CRANDALL, P. H. (1966) Corticosteroid responses to limbic stimulation in man: Localization of stimulus sites. *Science*, **153**, 767–768.

RUBIN, R. T., GOUIN, P. R. AND POLAND, R. E. (1973a) Neuroendocrine correlates of sleep stages in man. In *Pharmacology and the Future of Man (Proc. 5th Int. Congr. Pharmacology, San Francisco 1972, Vol. 4)*, Karger, Basel, pp. 124–133.

RUBIN, R. T., GOUIN, P. R., POLAND, R. E. AND ARENANDER, A. T. (1973b) Luteinizing hormone and testosterone secretion during sleep in normal adult men. *Sleep Res.*, **2**, 198.

RUBIN, R. T., GOUIN, P. R., KALES, A. AND ODELL, W. D. (1973c) Luteinizing hormone, follicle stimulating hormone, and growth hormone secretion in normal adult men during sleep and dreaming. *Psychosom. Med.*, **35**, 309–321.

RUBIN, R. T. AND LUBIN, A. (1974) Review: Integrated concentration and circadian variation of plasma testosterone in normal men (DE LACERDA, L. *et al.* (1973), *J. clin. Endocr.*, **37**, 366–371). *Sleep Res.*, **3**, in press.

RUBIN, R. T., POLAND, R. E., RUBIN, L. E. AND GOUIN, P. R. (1974a) The neuroendocrinology of human sleep. *Life Sci.*, **14**, 1041–1052.

RUBIN, R. T., POLAND, R. E., RAVESSOUD, F., GOUIN, P. R. AND TOWER, B. B. (1974b) Antidiuretic hormone secretion during sleep in adult men. Paper presented at the *Fifth Int. Congr., Int. Soc. Psychoneuroendocrinol., Utrecht, 24–27 July, 1974.*

SASSIN, J. F. (1974) Hormones and human sleep. *J. nat. med. Ass. (N.Y.)*, **66**, 45–48.

SCHALLY, A. V., ARIMURA, A. AND KASTIN, A. J. (1973) Hypothalamic regulatory hormones. *Science*, **179**, 341–350.

SWERDLOFF, R. S. AND RUBIN, R. T. (1975) The psychoneuroendocrinology of puberty. In *Handbook of Psychoneuroendocrinology*, F. BRAMBILLA AND E. ENDRÖCZI (Eds.), Plenum, New York, N.Y., in press.

TAKAHASHI, Y. (1974) Growth hormone secretion during sleep: A review. In *Biological Rhythms in Neuroendocrine Activity*, M. KAWAKAMI (Ed.), Igaku-Shoin, Tokyo, pp. 316–325.

WEITZMAN, E. D., NOGEIRE, C., PERLOW, M., FUKUSHIMA, D., SASSIN, J., MCGREGOR, P., GALLAGHER, T. F. AND HELLMAN, L. (1974) Effects of a prolonged 3-hour sleep–wake cycle on sleep stages, plasma cortisol, growth hormone and body temperature in man. *J. clin. Endocr.*, **38**, 1018–1030.

WYATT, R. J. (1972) The serotonin-catecholamine-dream bicycle: A clinical study. *Biol. Psychiat.*, **5**, 33–64.

Twenty-four-Hour Cortisol Secretory Patterns
in Depressed and Manic Patients

EDWARD J. SACHAR

Department of Psychiatry, Albert Einstein College of Medicine, 1300 Morris Park Avenue, Bronx,
N.Y. 10461 (U.S.A.)

There are several reasons for suspecting that 24-hr hormonal secretory patterns might be affected in the depressive and manic depressive illnesses. Many clinical features of depressive illness suggest hypothalamic involvement — particularly disturbances in mood, appetite, sexual and aggressive drives, and autonomic function. Hypothalamic neuroendocrine regulation might well be involved as well. Furthermore, there is considerable suggestive evidence that the affective disorders are associated with abnormalities in the metabolism of brain indoleamines and catecholamines (Davis, 1970; Sachar and Coppen, 1975), neurotransmitters which also play a major role in neuroendocrine regulation (Anton-Tay and Wurtman, 1971). In addition, depressive illness is usually associated with significant sleep disturbance, and often with a diurnal variation in the intensity of symptomatology, clinical features which might well find their correlates in altered 24-hr secretory patterns of those hormones closely associated with circadian and sleep–wake cycles. Study of hormonal secretory patterns in depression and mania might help illuminate hypothalamic function in those conditions, and provide clues as to possible neurotransmitter abnormalities. In this paper, I shall focus primarily on patterns of cortisol secretion in depressed and manic patients.

That many depressed patients hypersecrete cortisol has been apparent for some years. Undoubtedly, such "non-specific" stress factors as the anxiety associated with hospitalization (Sachar, 1967), defensive decompensation (Sachar, 1970), suicidal impulses (Bunney *et al.*, 1969) and the illness itself (Sachar *et al.*, 1970a) contribute significantly to the adrenocortical activation in many patients; however, even taking these factors into account, there remains evidence that the cortisol hypersecretion may reflect a more primary neuroendocrine disturbance, particularly in patients judged to be severely depressed (Carroll, 1972a).

Roffwarg and I, with colleagues from Albert Einstein College of Medicine, have been studying the 24-hr secretory pattern of cortisol in depressed patients, sampling blood every 20 min through an intravenous cannula and, during the night, simultaneously monitoring sleep patterns by EEG (electroencephalogram) and EOG (electrooculogram). We have been exploring the precise way the "extra" cortisol is secreted in hypersecreting depressed patients.

The normal 24-hr secretory pattern for cortisol has been well described by Weitzman, who pioneered in this research (Weitzman *et al.*, 1971). Normally, subjects who sleep from 11:00 p.m. to 7:00 a.m. manifest a period of minimal secretion during the evening and early morning, lasting about 6 hr, and plasma cortisol concentration approaches zero. About 2:00 a.m., a series of discrete major secretory episodes begin, the largest occurring from about 5:00 to 9:00 a.m., and usually totaling about 7–9 for the day. These episodes, apparent in sharp peaks of plasma cortisol concentration with "decay curves" following, are believed to be stimulated by bursts of ACTH (corticotropin) secretion (Berson and Yalow, 1968), which in turn are probably secondary to pulses of corticotropin-releasing factor (CRF) secretion. The plasma cortisol curve is thus inferred to reflect, indirectly, pulses of hypothalamic neuro-endocrine activity.

I shall report here on our findings in a group of 7 depressed patients with no previous history of mania. All had been hospitalized for at least a week, were unmedicated, and had previously been adapted to the sleep laboratory and the apparatus for 2 nights. Data from 5 of these patients had been reported previously (Sachar *et al.*, 1973). Figs. 1 and 2 illustrate typical plasma cortisol patterns before and after clinical recovery in two patients. The pervasive disturbances in cortisol patterns during illness are apparent. Detailed analysis of the 7 curves permit us to characterize some of the abnormalities.

(1) During illness, mean 24-hr plasma cortisol concentration was substantially

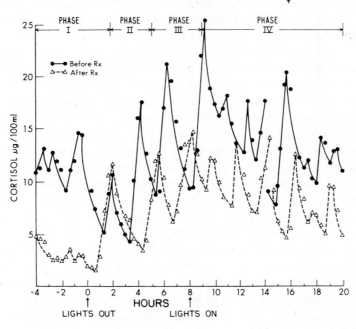

Fig. 1. Twenty-four-hour plasma cortisol patterns in a unipolar depressed 52-year-old woman before and after clinical recovery. Zero time represents the time of lights out for sleep.

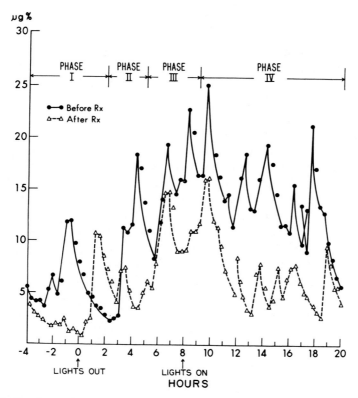

Fig. 2. Twenty-four-hour plasma cortisol patterns in a unipolar depressed 42-year-old woman. Zero time represents time of lights out for sleep.

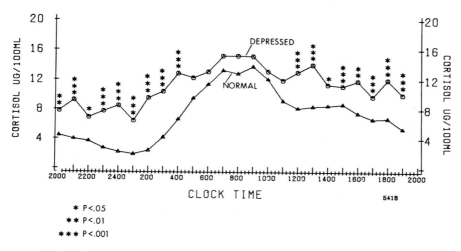

Fig. 3. Mean hourly plasma cortisol concentration over a 24-hr period for 7 unipolar depressed patients compared with the mean for 54 normal subjects. Each dot represents the mean cortisol concentration during the preceding hour. Asterisks indicate the significance of differences between depressed and normal values for each hour.

References p. 90–91

increased above normal: for the 7 depressed patients, 11.25 μg%, S.D. 1.83; for 54 normal subjects, studied by Weitzman and his colleagues, it was 7.28 μg%, S.D. 1.87 ($P < 0.001$).

Cortisol concentration in the depressives was pervasively elevated, both at the beginning and end of secretory episodes, and through both day and night. Fig. 3 compares a composite of the 24-hr plasma cortisol curves in the depressives with a composite of 54 curves from Weitzman's normal subjects. Although the composite irons out individual secretory episodes, it is apparent that mean values for the depressives were higher at every hour, especially in the evening and early morning.

(2) There was active cortisol secretion even during the evening and early morning hours when normally secretion virtually ceases. In contrast to the normals during this period, plasma cortisol concentration *never* approached zero; of over 500 samples from the 7 depressed patients, only *one* had a cortisol concentration of less than 2 μg% (1.9 μg%). This failure to turn off cortisol secretion in the evening is evident in a relative flattening of the curve for depressives in Fig. 3. This alteration is made more apparent in Fig. 4, in which cortisol concentrations for each subject are converted into percent deviation from his 24-hr mean concentration, and then averaged with similar measures for others of his group. While for the depressives relative cortisol concentration continued to be lowest in late evening, and highest in the morning, the spread was diminished compared to the normals.

(3) After clinical recovery, cortisol secretory patterns normalized (Figs. 1 and 2).

The altered secretory patterns seem to suggest an excessive driving or disinhibition of the neuroendocrine pathways regulating ACTH secretion. One might ask whether

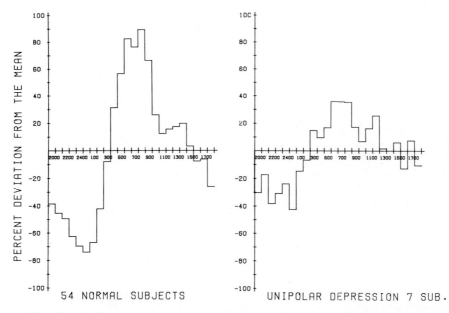

Fig. 4. Mean hourly plasma cortisol concentration expressed as percent deviation from the mean 24-hr cortisol concentration. Means for depressed (right) and normal (left) subjects are compared.

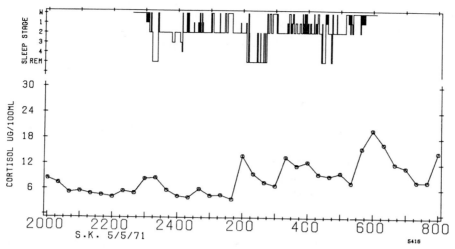

Fig. 5. Plasma cortisol concentrations and sleep pattern from 20:00 to 8:00 hr in a unipolar depressed 62-year-old woman. Note the frequent awakenings and virtual absence of stage 3 and 4 sleep. Note also that plasma cortisol concentration ranges from 4 to 20 μg%.

this neuroendocrine disturbance is a reflection of a non-specific stress response, or a more fundamental neuroendocrine abnormality. A definitive answer cannot be given, but it seems unlikely that all the data could fit a simple stress model.

(1) The disturbances also occur, albeit less commonly, in patients with apathetic depressions and little manifest anxiety — as in the case illustrated in Fig. 2.

(2) A stress response associated with manifest anxiety would be expected to be limited to waking hours, while the increased secretion in the depressed patients persists during hours of sleep as well. However, a complicating factor is that depressed patients sleep poorly, with a decrease in slow-wave sleep (stages 3 and 4) and frequent awakenings (Fig. 5; Mendels and Hawkins, 1972). An analysis of the relation between sleep patterns and changes in plasma cortisol in 8 previously studied depressed patients suggested a tendency for cortisol concentration to increase in association

TABLE I

PLASMA CORTISOL CONCENTRATION (μg%) IN DEPRESSED AND NORMAL SUBJECTS WHILE ASLEEP

Time	Normals			Depressed			P
	N	Cortisol	S.D.	N	Cortisol	S.D.	
23:00–24:00	54	2.7	2.9	4	5.5	1.2	NS
24:00–01:00	54	2.2	2.6	5	6.2	2.4	< 0.001
01:00–02:00	54	1.9	2.1	6	4.4	1.7	< 0.001
02:00–03:00	54	2.4	2.5	6	9.1	4.2	< 0.001
03:00–04:00	54	4.2	2.9	7	11.8	3.5	< 0.001
04:00–05:00	54	6.7	3.9	4	9.9	0.6	NS
05:00–06:00	54	9.5	3.7	5	10.8	4.4	NS

References p. 90–91

with spontaneous awakenings (Roffwarg *et al.*, 1970). This might be consistent with an effect of waking anxiety.

To approach this question another way in the present group of patients, we sorted out, hour-by-hour, those nocturnal cortisol values that were determined from samples drawn while the patients were actually asleep. Table I indicates that depressed patients *while asleep* have substantially higher plasma cortisol levels than do sleeping normals for comparable hours of the night, especially from 24:00 to 04:00.

Such gross correlations of plasma cortisol with sleep pattern are fraught with pitfalls, of course. Because the half-life of cortisol in plasma is roughly 60–70 min, cortisol concentration may remain relatively elevated after an earlier secretory episode, which may have occurred during a previous waking period. More to the point, there is a lag of several minutes between a pulse of ACTH secretion and the plasma cortisol response. Indeed, a definitive answer will probably have to await a plasma CRF assay.

Could the sleep deprivation and frequent awakenings, which depressed patients characteristically experience, itself be a stress, stimulating cortisol production, even during sleep periods? To study this question, we systematically deprived two normal subjects of NREM (non-rapid eye movement), and of REM sleep, each for a period of 8 successive days. There was remarkably little change from the baseline cortisol secretory pattern (Fig. 6), suggesting that awakenings and sleep deprivation alone do not produce hypersecretion (Ellman *et al.*, 1970). A similar lack of effect of 205 hr of total sleep deprivation on urinary corticosteroid excretion has been reported by Rubin *et al.* (1969).

(3) Further data suggesting that the cortisol hypersecretion is not a simple stress response are provided by reports that depressed patients were relatively resistant to dexamethasone suppression tests (Carroll 1972b; Stokes 1972). Although these findings have been disputed by certain laboratories (Carpenter and Bunney, 1971; Shopsin and Gershon, 1971), it is impressive that in a number of patients, even after

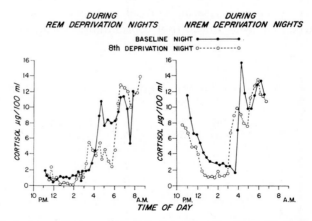

Fig. 6. Nocturnal plasma cortisol concentrations in a normal subject. The left graph compares a baseline night with the eighth successive night of REM sleep deprivation. The right graph compares a baseline night with the eighth successive night of non-REM sleep deprivation.

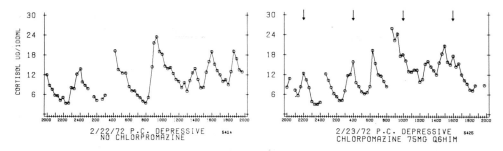

Fig. 7. Twenty-four-hour plasma cortisol patterns in a unipolar depressed 65-year-old woman before (left) and during (right) chlorpromazine therapy (75 mg every 6 hr, i.m.). Arrows indicate times of injections.

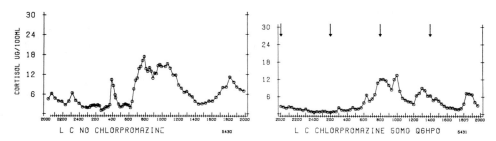

Fig. 8. Twenty-four-hour plasma cortisol patterns in a normal young man before (left) and during (right) chlorpromazine administration (50 mg every 6 hr orally). Arrows indicate times of injections.

doses of 8 mg of dexamethasone, morning plasma cortisol concentration remained relatively elevated (Stokes, 1972).

(4) Were the hypersecretion purely a manifestation of anxiety-associated stress response, one would expect reduced cortisol production in these patients after sedative or anti-anxiety medication. However, Stokes has shown that doses up to 350 mg of barbiturates failed to reduce daytime plasma cortisol levels in his cases (Stokes, 1972). We have found the same to be true after chlorpromazine. Thus (Fig. 7), the hypersecretion of a depressed woman was unaffected by 75 mg of chlorpromazine given i.m. every 6 hr. Her average 24-hr plasma cortisol concentration was 10.8 $\mu g\%$ before, and 11.4 $\mu g\%$ during chlorpromazine treatment. In contrast only 50 mg of chlorpromazine given orally every 6 hr reduced the average cortisol concentration of a normal unanxious subject by 26%, from 6.8 $\mu g\%$ to 4.2 $\mu g\%$ (Fig. 8).

While the question of the contribution of non-specific stress factors to the cortisol hypersecretion certainly remains open, it does appear, in our view, that a substantial part of the hypersecretion in severely depressed patients represents a more fundamental, intrinsic neuroendocrine disturbance: a pervasive hyperactivity or disinhibition of the neuroendocrine pathways stimulating CRF and ACTH release, which may be part of a central hypothalamic dysfunction associated with depressive illness.

It is relevant to point out that one of the major psychobiological hypotheses of the chemical pathology of depressive illness posits a functional depletion in brain noradrenaline (Davis, 1970; Sachar and Coppen, 1975), and that there is considerable evidence that a noradrenergic system normally tonically inhibits the secretion of ACTH (Van Loon, 1973). It is tempting to speculate that the hypersecretory cortisol pattern of the severely depressed patients is an endocrine reflection of depleted hypothalamic noradrenergic activity.

This formulation is certainly simplistic. The central nervous system (CNS) regulation of ACTH is quite complex, and probably involves several neurotransmitter systems. Similarly, indoleaminergic and cholinergic systems, as well as catecholaminergic systems, have been implicated in affective disorders. Nevertheless, it should be noted that several laboratories have reported diminished human growth hormone (HGH) responses to hypoglycemia in depressed patients (Sachar *et al.*, 1971; Mueller *et al.*, 1972; Carroll, 1972c; Sachar *et al.*, 1975). Since this response appears to be catecholaminergically mediated (Martin, 1973), its reduction in depressed patients might be interpreted as a neuroendocrine reflection of central catecholamine depletion.

I would like to conclude by describing briefly studies of 24-hr cortisol secretory patterns in manic patients. Here our work becomes quite anecdotal and empiric.

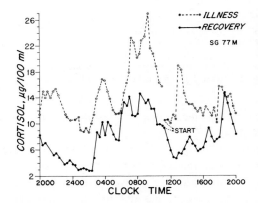

Fig. 9. Twenty-four-hour plasma cortisol patterns in a severely manic 77-year-old man, before and after lithium-induced recovery.

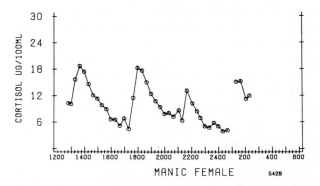

Fig. 10. Plasma cortisol concentrations in a severely manic 66-year-old woman, from 12:00 to 02:00 hr.

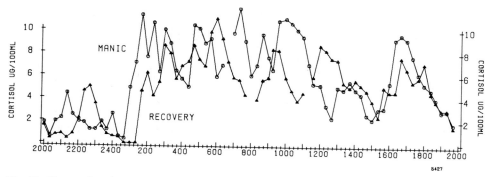

Fig. 11. Twenty-four-hour plasma cortisol patterns in a moderately manic 50-year-old man, before and after lithium-induced recovery.

It is anecdotal because the technical problems of maintaining an intravenous cannula in acutely manic patients are exceedingly difficult, and we have only 3 patients to report; it is empiric, because the neurochemical basis of mania is even more obscure than that of depression, and because it is virtually impossible to separate the endocrine effects of mania *per se* from the generalized arousal which is an integral part of the clinical syndrome of mania. In a previous investigation, we had shown that total 72-hr urinary cortisol production was not significantly increased in mildly manic (hypomanic) patients during illness as compared with recovery values (Sachar *et al.*, 1972). However, the 24-hr plasma cortisol pattern in a severely manic man (Fig. 9) was markedly disturbed, showing the same type of hypersecretion seen in severely depressed patients; the pattern normalized after lithium-induced clinical recovery. Lithium therapy of itself does not affect cortisol production (Sachar *et al.*, 1970b). A similar hypersecretory pattern was apparent in an acutely manic woman who could be studied for only 14 hr (Fig. 10). On the other hand, there was only a slight disturbance in the plasma cortisol pattern of a hypomanic man studied before and after lithium-induced recovery (Fig. 11).

One might speculate that cortisol hypersecretion is associated with severe mania, but not with hypomania. (A similar relation to severity of illness has been noted in depression (Carroll, 1972a).) This is a problem which will require the investigative cooperation of several clinical research groups, because of the difficulty of any individual center assembling a large enough series of these fascinating, but extraordinarily taxing cases.

SUMMARY

The 24-hr secretory pattern of cortisol is significantly disturbed in both severely depressed and severely manic patients. With regard to the depressed patients, it appears likely that the hypersecretion cannot be accounted for entirely by generalized stress or arousal factors alone, and may well reflect a central neuroendocrine abnormality associated with the illness. If this is so, the study of hormonal secretory patterns

References p. 90–91

and responses in the affective disorders may help illuminate the nature of hypothalamic dysfunction and central neurotransmitter disturbance in these conditions.

ACKNOWLEDGEMENTS

This work was supported by U.S. PHS Grants Nos. MH 25133 and 5 K2 MH-22613.
In addition to the collaborators cited in the text and bibliography, Peter H. Gruen and Norman Altman participated in this research.

REFERENCES

ANTON-TAY, F. AND WURTMAN, R. J. (1971) Brain monoamines and endocrine function. In *Frontiers of Neuroendocrinology*, L. MARTINI AND W. F. GANONG (Eds.), Oxford University Press, New York, N.Y., pp. 45–66.
BERSON, S. A. AND YALOW, R. S. (1968) Radioimmunoassay of ACTH in plasma. *J. clin. Invest.*, **47**, 2725–2751.
BUNNEY, W. E., FAWCETT, J. A., DAVIS, J. M. AND GIFFORD, S. (1969) Further evaluation of urinary 17-hydroxycorticosteroids in suicidal patients. *Arch. gen. Psychiat. (Chic.)*, **21**, 138–150.
CARPENTER, W. T. AND BUNNEY, W. E. (1971) Adrenal cortical activity in depressive illness. *Amer. J. Psychiat.*, **128**, 31–40.
CARROLL, B. J. (1972a) Plasma cortisol levels in depression. In *Depressive Illness: Some Research Studies*, B. DAVIES, B. J. CARROLL AND R. M. MOWBRAY (Eds.), Thomas, Springfield, Ill., pp. 69–86.
CARROLL, B. J. (1972b) Control of plasma cortisol levels in depression: studies with the dexamethasone suppression test. In *Depressive Illness: Some Research Studies*, B. DAVIES, B. J. CARROLL AND R. M. MOWBRAY (Eds.), Thomas, Springfield, Ill., pp. 87–148.
CARROLL, B. J. (1972c) Studies with hypothalamic–pituitary–adrenal stimulation tests in depression. In *Depressive Illness: Some Research Studies*, B. DAVIES, B. J. CARROLL AND R. M. MOWBRAY (Eds.), Thomas, Springfield, Ill., pp. 149–201.
DAVIS, J. M. (1970) Theories of biological etiology of affective disorders. *Int. Rev. Neurobiol.*, **12**, 145–175.
ELLMAN, S. J., ROFFWARG, H. P., SACHAR, E. J., FINKELSTEIN, J., CURTI, J. AND HELLMAN, L. (March, 1970) Effects of REM deprivation on cortisol and growth hormone levels. Presented to *Association for the Psychophysiological Study of Sleep, Santa Fé, New Mexico*.
MARTIN, J. (1973) Neural regulation of growth hormone secretion. *New Engl. J. Med.*, **288**, 1384–1393.
MENDELS, J. AND HAWKINS, D. R. (1972) Sleep studies in depression. In *Recent Advances in the Psychobiology of the Depressive Illnesses*, T. A. WILLIAMS, M. M. KATZ AND J. A. SHIELD (Eds.), DHEW Publ. 70-9053, Washington, D.C., pp. 147–170.
MUELLER, P. S., HENINGER, G. R., McDONALD, P. K. (1972) Studies on glucose utilization and insulin sensitivity in affective disorders. In *Recent Advances in the Psychobiology of the Depressive Illnesses*, T. A. WILLIAMS, M. M. KATZ AND J. A. SHIELD (Eds.), DHEW Publ. 70-9053, Washington, D.C., pp. 235–245.
ROFFWARG, H. P., SACHAR, E. J., FINKELSTEIN, J., CURTI, J., ELLMAN, S., KREAM, J., FISHMAN, R., GALLAGHER, T. F. AND HELLMAN, L. (1970) Sleep stage pattern in depression in relation to nocturnal plasma cortisol and human growth hormone. *Psychophysiology*, **7**, 323–324.
RUBIN, R. T., KOLLAR, E. J., SLATER, G. S. AND CLARK, B. R. (1969) Excretion of 17-hydroxycorticosteroid and vanillylmandelic acid during 205 hours of sleep deprivation in man. *Psychosom. Med.*, **31**, 68–79.
SACHAR, E. J. (1967) Corticosteroids in depressive illness. I. A reevaluation of control issues and the literature. *Arch. gen. Psychiat. (Chic.)*, **17**, 544–553.
SACHAR, E. J. (1970) Psychological factors relating to activation and inhibition of the adrenal cortical stress response in man. A review. In *Pituitary, Adrenal and the Brain, Progress in Brain Research*, *Vol. 32*, D. DE WIED AND J. A. W. WEIJNEN (Eds.), Elsevier, Amsterdam, pp. 316–324.

SACHAR, E. J., ALTMAN, N., GRUEN, P. H. AND SASSIN, J. (1975) Growth hormone responses to hypo-glycemia in postmenopausal depressed women. *Arch. gen. Psychiat. (Chic.)*, **32**, 31–33.

SACHAR, E. J. AND COPPEN, A. (1975) Biological aspects of affective psychoses. In *Biology of Brain Dysfunction*, G. GAULL (Ed.), Plenum Press, New York, N.Y., in press.

SACHAR, E. J., FINKELSTEIN, J. AND HELLMAN, L. (1971) Growth hormone responses in depressive illness: response to insulin tolerance test. *Arch. gen. Psychiat. (Chic.)*, **24**, 263–269.

SACHAR, E. J., HELLMAN, L., FUKUSHIMA, D. K. AND GALLAGHER, T. F. (1970a) Cortisol production in depressive illness. *Arch. gen. Psychiat. (Chic.)*, **23**, 289–298.

SACHAR, E. J., HELLMAN, L., FUKUSHIMA, D. K. AND GALLAGHER, T. F. (1972) Cortisol production in mania. *Arch. gen. Psychiat. (Chic.)*, **26**, 137–139.

SACHAR, E. J., HELLMAN, L., KREAM, J., FUKUSHIMA, D. K. AND GALLAGHER, T. F. (1970b) Effect of lithium carbonate therapy on adrenocortical activity. *Arch. gen. Psychiat. (Chic.)*, **22**, 304–307.

SACHAR, E. J., HELLMAN, L., ROFFWARG, H. P., HALPERN, F. S., FUKUSHIMA, D. K. AND GALLAGHER, T. F. (1973) Disrupted 24-hour patterns of cortisol secretion in psychotic depression. *Arch. gen. Psychiat. (Chic.)*, **28**, 19–24.

SHOPSIN, B. AND GERSHON, S. (1971) Plasma cortisol response to dexamethasone suppression in depressed and control patients. *Arch. gen. Psychiat. (Chic.)*, **24**, 320–326.

STOKES, P. E. (1972) Studies on the control of adrenocortical function in depression. In *Recent Advances in the Psychobiology of Depressive Illnesses*, T. A. WILLIAMS, M. M. KATZ AND J. A. SHIELD (Eds.), DHEW Pub. 70-9053, Washington, D.C., pp. 199–220.

VAN LOON, G. R. (1973) Brain catecholamines and ACTH secretion. In *Frontiers in Neuroendocrinology*, W. F. GANONG AND L. MARTINI (Eds.), Oxford University Press, New York, N.Y., pp. 209–247.

WEITZMAN, E. D., FUKUSHIMA, D., NOGEIRE, C., ROFFWARG, H. P., GALLAGHER, T. F. AND HELLMAN, L. (1971) Twenty-four hour pattern of the episodic secretion of cortisol in normal subjects. *J. clin. Endocr.*, **33**, 14–22.

Neuro-endocrine Pattern of Secretion during the Sleep–Wake Cycle of Man

ELLIOT D. WEITZMAN

Department of Neurology, Montefiore Hospital and Medical Center, and The Albert Einstein College of Medicine, Bronx, N.Y. 10467 (U.S.A.)

In this report I will describe two separate studies dealing with the problem of stability and environmental influence on the 24-hr pattern of the episodic secretion of cortisol in normal subjects.

The first study is a comparison of the 24-hr cortisol and growth hormone (GH) secretory patterns during ambulatory functional activity and minimal activity at bed rest. This work was done in collaboration with Stephanie Erlich and Peter McGregor.

Recent studies have demonstrated that the 24-hr pattern of ACTH (corticotropin)–cortisol secretion consists of a sequence of temporally ordered episodic secretory patterns throughout the entire 24-hr period and that the "circadian" cycle results from the temporal clustering of episodic secretion (Weitzman *et al.*, 1966; Hellman *et al.*, 1970; Weitzman *et al.*, 1971). A "basal level" or "steady state" of cortisol concentration was not found for any extended time period of the day. Only when the concentration falls to near zero, generally during the 4 hr in proximity to sleep onset, is there any prolonged period of constancy. There is considerable variability in lag time between secretory episodes and the plasma concentration at which the episodes are initiated. These findings have led us to suggest that the temporal sequence of episode initiation appears to be under CNS control as a "programmed" sequence of events, and that with a stable repetitive daily life pattern, the association of the ACTH-adrenal secretory events with the sleep–waking cycle is part of a general program of biological rhythms. In these studies specific environmental factors such as conversations, reading, carrying out usual daily activities, etc. were not carefully controlled.

In order to evaluate some of these factors, we recently performed a study to determine differences in the 24-hr cortisol secretory pattern between a condition of normal ambulatory "*activity*" and one of minimal activity, "*basal*". Each of 6 normal young adult male subjects (medical students, ages 20–25) spent the waking 16 hr on two separate occasions either on a normal *activity* schedule of classes, meals, etc. or on strict bed rest (lights on) without reading, conversing or other external stimulation. During this latter *basal* condition they were fed a liquid diet given in 150 ml amounts at approximately hourly intervals. They were allowed to sleep undisturbed for as long as they pleased during this period and were polygraphically monitored during the entire "basal" day to define all daytime sleep periods. On both experimental nights

References p. 101–102

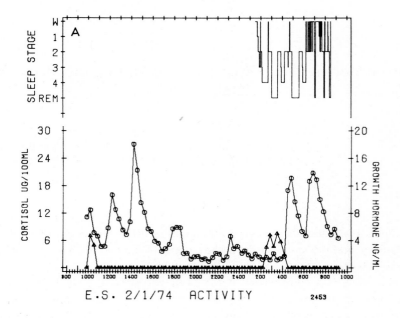

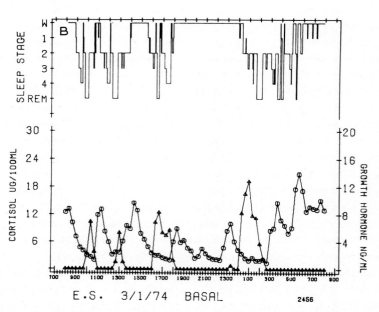

Fig. 1. Twenty-four-hour plasma concentration pattern of cortisol and growth hormone in one subject during the "*activity*" (A) and "*basal*" (B) experimental condition. Samples were obtained every 20 min from an intravenous catheter. The polygraphically defined sleep stage pattern is depicted for each sleep period. Cortisol, open circles; growth hormone, triangles.

TABLE I

COMPARISON OF THE MEAN CONCENTRATION OF PLASMA CORTISOL $\pm$ S.D. (μg/100 ml) OF 8-hr CLOCK TIMES FOR THE "ACTIVITY" AND "BASAL" EXPERIMENTAL CONDITIONS FOR 6 SUBJECTS

Clock time	Activity	Basal
Noon–8 p.m.	10.7 ± 1.1	7.2 ± 1.1*
8 p.m.–4 a.m.	4.6 ± 1.1	4.6 ± 2.2**
4 a.m.–noon	11.2 ± 3.6	10.9 ± 2.1**

* $P < 0.001$ (t-test).
** N.S.

they slept in the laboratory (12 p.m.–8 a.m.) with polygraphic recording. Twenty-four-hour plasma sampling, every 20 min, was carried out with an indwelling i.v. catheter during both the "activity" and "basal" experimental 24-hr period. All subjects took naps in the "basal" condition with total sleep time during the 16 hr lights on period ranging from 131 to 408 min.

In 5 of the 6 subjects, higher peak concentrations of cortisol were found during the 16-hr waking portion of the 24-hr curve on the activity than on the basal days. This difference was not present during the 8-hr sleep portion of the curve. An episodic secretory pattern was clearly present for all subjects on both the "activity" and "basal" 24-hr periods, and all subjects demonstrated the typical circadian rhythmicity for the cortisol concentrations during both periods. Statistical analysis of the mean concentrations of cortisol of the 8-hr time periods comparing "activity" with "basal" days, demonstrated that a highly significant difference was present for the clock time segment from noon to 8 p.m. (activity day, 10.7 ± 1.1 μg/100 ml; basal day 7.2 ± 1.1 μg/100 ml; $P < 0.001$) (Table I). The other 8-hr segments (8 p.m.–4 a.m. and 4 a.m.–noon) were not significantly different for the two behavioral conditions. These results indicate that a significant difference in the concentration of secreted cortisol occurs when subjects are either in a quiet, relaxed state or actively involved in usual daytime activities. In spite of this difference, the episodic ultradian and circadian patterns of hormone secretion were clearly preserved.

We also measured the 24-hr pattern of GH in each of the subjects under the two different experimental conditions. All subjects secreted GH shortly after sleep onset at night as expected (Takahashi et al., 1968; Sassin et al., 1969; Pawel et al., 1972). There were 8 secretory episodes at night (midnight–8 a.m.) for the "activity" condition and 6 episodes at night for the "basal" condition. A major difference in amount and pattern of GH secretion was present during the 16-hr day. There were a total of 11 secretory episodes summed across subjects on the "activity" day, as compared with 18 on the "basal" day. Since the subjects took daytime naps which were polygraphically defined on the "basal" day, we determined the relation between the GH episodes and a sleep period. It was found that 15 of the 18 episodes were clearly associated with a daytime sleep period. An estimate of the integrated area under the GH curve for the two conditions showed an activity/basal ratio of 2–3. Therefore, more GH was secreted under basal "rest" conditions than when the subjects were actively engaged in normal daytime waking activities. This difference could clearly be accounted for by the presence of naps taken in the basal experimental conditions.

The second study is one that concerns the seasonal pattern of sleep stages and the secretion of cortisol and growth hormone during 24-hr periods in Northern Norway. This study was done in collaboration with Drs. Andries S. deGraaf, Jon F. Sassin, Tormar Hansen, Ole B. Godtlibsen and Leon Hellman.

Life within the Arctic Circle carries with it exposure to marked seasonal changes. Extreme shifts in the ratio of light to darkness during the course of the year is a prominent feature in these areas, ranging between the polar night and the midnight sun. There is abundant evidence that these fluctuations affect plants and animals but very little precise information about the degree to which humans are affected. Numerous complaints are heard among the general population of all age groups about disturbances in their sleep pattern, especially during the dark period of the Arctic winter (Kleitman and Kleitman, 1953).

The present experiment was designed to investigate not only seasonal variation in sleep but also alterations in the secretion of cortisol and growth hormone of 7 young men in relation to the different seasons in a subarctic region. Tromsö (Norway), at about 70° N. latitude, was selected because it is the world's northernmost neurological center with facilities for polygraphic recording.

The investigations were performed during the following 4 seasonal intervals: (1) April–May, 1971; (2) July–August, 1971; (3) October–November, 1971; (4) January–February, 1972. During each period, polygraphic recordings were made on 3 consecutive nights. Over the last 24 hr, blood samples were collected every 20 min with an indwelling catheter.

The subjects, 7 healthy men, members of the technical staff of the Norwegian Air Force and stationed at Bardufoss Air Force Base, about 70 miles from Tromsö, participated in the study. Their ages were between 22 and 40 years. Most of them were born in northern Norway and all of them had been living there during the preceding years. Each had a private room where he could relax, listen to the radio, watch T.V. A regular hospital diet was served at 8 a.m., noon and 5 p.m. Coffee and food were not served after 8 p.m. Naps were not allowed and drugs were not used.

Each subject slept in his own sound-attenuated room which was well ventilated and darkened by black curtains. Collection of blood samples was begun at 9 a.m. on the third day of each period and then sequentially sampled at 20-min intervals for the next 24 hr. The plasma was obtained and immediately frozen. Within 2 weeks after each interval, the frozen samples were packed in a container provided with freezing elements and flown to New York for the hormone determination.

Although there is some variation of total sleep time among the subjects, the sleep stage percents were quite consistent across subjects for each night for stages 1, 2, and REM sleep. Stages 3 and 4 were more variable. The subjects demonstrated a decrease from approximately 20 to 15% in REM sleep on the night of the plasma sampling as well as a small increase in waking time from approximately 5 to 12%.

There was *no* significant difference found when sleep stage patterns of the 7 subjects

TABLE II

SLEEP STAGE PERCENT OF TOTAL SLEEP TIME, AVERAGED FOR EACH SEASON

N = night; REM = rapid eye movement.

	Spring			Summer			Autumn			Winter		
	N1	N2	N3	N1	N2	N3	N1	N2	N3	N1	N2	N3
Sleep time (total) (% of total time of 8 hr)	96	97	83	95	95	88	98	98	88	95	93	88
Stage 1	5	6	10	5	7	11	7	6	11	7	6	8
Stage 2	58	55	60	62	57	61	54	59	61	58	57	59
Stage 3	10	10	11	8	10	9	11	9	12	9	9	9
Stage 4	7	6	5	5	5	4	6	5	3	6	6	7
REM	20	23	13	20	21	15	21	20	14	20	20	16

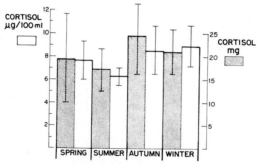

Fig. 2. Bar graph of the mean and standard deviation of both the total amount of cortisol secreted (mg) and the average concentration (μg/100 ml) for 24-hr periods for all subjects as a function of yearly season.

TABLE III

MEAN PLASMA CORTISOL CONCENTRATIONS (μg/100 ml) DURING 6-hr DAY SEGMENTS FOR THE SEASON

Clock time	Spring	Summer	Autumn	Winter
02:00–08:00	5.2	5.0	6.7	6.5
08:00–14:00	5.8	4.1	4.8	5.5
14:00–20:00	1.8	2.8	3.4	3.1
20:00–02:00	2.3	0.6	1.9	1.6

were compared as a function of yearly season. The seasonal variation in sleep stage amounts was less than that found among the individual subjects (Table II).

All subjects demonstrated the characteristic pattern of episodic secretion of cortisol for all the 24-hr periods of measurement (Hellman *et al.*, 1970; Weitzman *et al.*, 1971). Calculation of the 24-hr mean concentration of cortisol revealed that there was a significant difference between the winter and summer and the autumn and summer values ($P < 0.01$, < 0.02, respectively) (Fig. 2). Calculation of the mean concentration as a function of 6-hr clock segments indicated that the hours from 8 p.m. to 2 a.m. had the greatest difference between summer and the 3 other seasons (Table III). A difference was also present during spring for the 2 p.m. to 8 p.m. clock time period. The mean 24-hr concentration and secretory amount among the individual subjects revealed no significant differences, although one subject had an unusually high mean value for both. Calculation of the mean total time spent in secretion of cortisol during the 24-hr measured periods revealed that the winter period had the highest value. However, because of the large variability across seasons and among the subjects, no statistical difference was recognized. No significant difference in the number of secretory episodes per 24 hr was found for season or subjects.

The percent deviation of each hour's mean cortisol concentration from the 24-hr mean value was calculated and plotted as a graphic display (Fig. 3). The curves for each of the 4 seasons are remarkably similar and almost superimposable and, therefore,

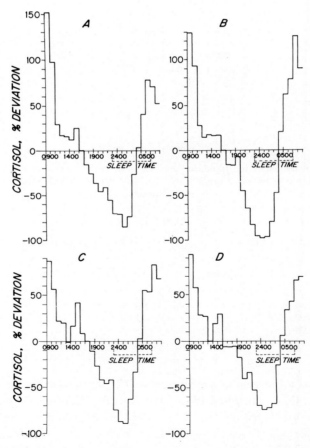

Fig. 3. The 24-hr pattern of plasma cortisol concentration expressed as percent deviation of the mean daily concentration. A, spring; B, summer; C, autumn; D, winter.

TABLE IV

MEAN DURATION (min) OF CORTISOL INTER-EPISODE INTERVALS FOR CLOCK TIME AND SEASONS

Clock time	Spring	Summer	Autumn	Winter	Mean
20:00–02:00	175	184	272	151	196
02:00–08:00	107	110	107	108	108
08:00–14:00	113	106	108	108	108
14:00–20:00	167	176	202	93	105
				173	180
Mean	141	144	172	131	

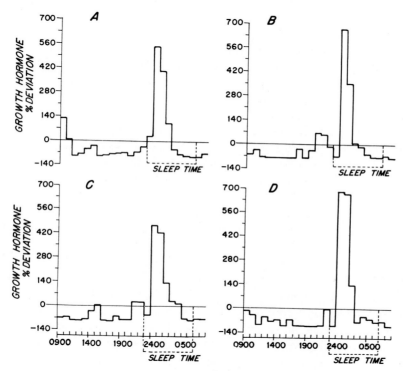

Fig. 4. The 24-hr pattern of plasma growth hormone concentration expressed as percent deviation of the mean daily concentration. A, spring; B, summer; C, autumn, D, winter.

do not demonstrate any major difference in pattern. An estimate of the length of the inter-secretory episode interval as a function of the time of the day demonstrated that the hours from 2 a.m. to 8 a.m. had a remarkably similar value across seasons whereas it was much greater and more variable between 8 p.m. and 2 a.m. (Table IV).

All subjects secreted GH shortly after onset of sleep with a peak occurring approximately 2 hr after sleep onset (about 1 a.m.) (Takahashi *et al.*, 1968; Sassin *et al.*, 1969; Pawel *et al.*, 1972). No difference in timing of release was found with regard to season of the year (Fig. 4). In addition, no difference was found regarding the sporadic

References p. 101–102

waking daytime releases of GH as a function of season. The sleep onset related GH release was the major release of the 24 hr for all 7 subjects studied. On only 2 out of 28 occasions did a daytime GH peak concentration exceed the peak at sleep onset at night.

In a study carried out in Tromsö during the summer of 1951, Kleitman reported that previous anecdotal information, indicating that the residents slept very little during the all light summer months, was highly inaccurate (Kleitman and Kleitman, 1953). He found in interviews that time spent in bed during the summer months averaged 7 hr and 26 min, and 8 hr and 25 min, during winter months. Although there was considerably greater variability of the time of going to bed in the winter as compared to the summer, the time of getting up in the morning was the same for the two seasons.

The data from the present study clearly support Dr. Kleitman's survey in that essentially no difference was found for polygraphically monitored sleep between the seasons. The choice of a relatively stable group of air force personnel in our study decreased the possibility of variable life styles producing deviations of the diurnal routine of the sleep–wakefulness pattern. Therefore, it does not appear that any seasonal sleep pattern difference in man in the arctic is an obligatory direct requirement of that environment, but rather suggests that if a change does occur, the effect is an indirect one mediated through seasonally altered social and work schedules.

The reproducibility and lack of difference of the 24-hr temporal pattern of cortisol and GH secretion within and across subjects is also in agreement with previous studies. All subjects had stage 3 during the first 2 hr on each of the nights of plasma sampling and had a concomitant release of GH at that time. Previous studies indicate that the stage 2–3 electroencephalographic pattern of sleep is correlated with the triggering of a GH release (Pawel et al., 1972).

The clear consistent synchronization of the 24-hr cortisol and GH patterns with the stability of the sleep stage patterns and sleep–waking 24-hr rhythm is in full agreement with the concept that social and sleep cues are the dominant determinants in man of circadian phase relationships (Aschoff et al., 1971).

The finding of a small but significant increase in the 24-hr mean plasma concentration and 24-hr output of cortisol during the autumn and winter months in the arctic has not been reported previously to the best of our knowledge and suggests the possibility of a circannual rhythm. The major difference in mean concentration during the afternoon and evening hours (2 p.m.–2 a.m.) suggests that waking behavioral activity in relation to increased environmental demands during the winter and autumn seasons may have contributed to this seasonal difference.

SUMMARY

In order to study the stability of the 24-hr pattern of the episodic secretion of cortisol and growth hormone (GH) in relation to the sleep–waking cycle of man, two studies were performed. The first is a comparison of the 24-hr cortisol and GH secretory pattern during ambulatory functional activity and minimal activity at bed rest. Each of 6 normal young adult male subjects (medical students, ages 20–25) spent the waking 16 hr on two separate occasions either on a normal *activity* schedule of classes, meals, etc. or on strict bed rest (lights on) without reading, conversing or other external stimulation. They were allowed to sleep undisturbed for as long as they pleased during this period and were polygraphically monitored during the entire "basal" day to define all daytime sleep periods. On both experimental nights they slept in the laboratory (12 p.m.–8 a.m.) with polygraphic recording. Twenty-four-hour plasma sampling, every 20 min, was carried out with an indwelling i.v. catheter during both the "activity" and "basal" experimental 24-hr period. All subjects took naps in the "basal" condition with total sleep time during the 16-hr lights on period ranging from 131 to 408 min. In 5 of the 6 subjects, higher peak concentrations of cortisol were found during the 16-hr waking portion of the 24-hr curve on the activity than on the basal days. An episodic secretory pattern was clearly present for all subjects on both the "activity" and "basal" 24-hr periods, and all subjects demonstrated the typical circadian rhythmicity for the cortisol concentrations during both periods. All subjects secreted GH shortly after sleep onset at night as expected. A major difference in amount and pattern of GH secretion was present during the 16-hr day. More GH was secreted under basal "rest" conditions than when the subjects were actively engaged in normal daytime waking activities. This difference could clearly be accounted for by the presence of naps taken in the basal experimental conditions.

In a second study, a group of 7 healthy male subjects were studied in regard to sleep stages and, 24-hr plasma cortisol and GH patterns during the 4 seasons of the year in an arctic environment (Tromsö, Norway). No difference in total sleep or sleep stage percents was found for any of the yearly seasons. A small but statistically significant increase in mean plasma cortisol concentration and amount secreted for 24 hr was found for the autumn–winter seasons, as compared with the spring and summer. However, no difference in the circadian curve of cortisol hormonal pattern was found. All subjects secreted GH shortly after sleep onset at night and no difference was found as a function of season of the year.

REFERENCES

ASCHOFF, J., FATRANSKA, M., GIEDKE, H., DOERR, P., STAM, D. AND WISSER, H. (1971) Human circadian rhythms in continuous darkness entrainment by social cues. *Science*, **171**, 213–215.
HELLMAN, L., NAKADA, F., CURTI, J., WEITZMAN, E. D., KREAM, J., ROFFWARG, H., ELLMAN, S., FUKUSHIMA, D. K. AND GALLAGHER, T. F. (1970) Cortisol is secreted episodically by normal man. *J. clin. Endocr.*, **30**, 411–422.
KLEITMAN, N. AND KLEITMAN, H. (1953) Sleep–wakefulness pattern in arctic. *Scient. Monthly*, **76**, 349–356.
PAWEL, M. A., SASSIN, J. F. AND WEITZMAN, E. D. (1972) The temporal relation between HGH release and sleep stage changes at nocturnal sleep onset in man. *Life Sci.*, **11**, 587–593.
SASSIN, J., PARKER, D. C., MACE, J. W., GOTLIN, R. W., JOHNSON, L. C. AND ROSSMAN, L. G. (1969) Human growth hormone release: relation to slow wave sleep at sleep–waking cycles. *Science*, **165**, 513–515.

TAKAHASHI, Y., KIPNIS, D. M. AND DAUGHADAY, W. H. (1968) Growth hormone secretion during sleep. *J. clin. Invest.*, **47**, 2079–2090.

WEITZMAN, E. D., SCHAUMBURG, H. AND FISHBEIN, W. (1966) Plasma 17-hydroxycorticosteroid levels during sleep in man. *J. clin. Endocr.*, **26**, 121–127.

WEITZMAN, E. D., FUKUSHIMA, D., NOGEIRE, C., ROFFWARG, H., GALLAGHER, T. F. AND HELLMAN, L. (1971) Twenty-four hour pattern of the episodic secretion of cortisol in normal subjects. *J. clin. Endocr.*, **33**, 14–22.

Twenty-four-Hour Patterns of Luteinizing Hormone Secretion in Humans: Ontogenetic and Sexual Considerations

SHELDON KAPEN, ROBERT M. BOYAR,
LEON HELLMAN and ELLIOT D. WEITZMAN

Departments of Neurology, Oncology and the Institute of Steroid Research, Montefiore Hospital and Medical Center and The Albert Einstein College of Medicine, Bronx, N. Y. 10467 (U.S.A.)

Much progress has been made in recent years in understanding factors controlling gonadotropin secretion in humans. This progress has been made possible primarily by 3 technical advances: (1) the development of sensitive and specific assays for LH (luteinizing hormone) and FSH (follicle-stimulating hormone), especially radio-immunoassay (Midgley, 1966); (2) frequent blood sampling by techniques which interfere as little as possible with the subject's waking and sleeping activity (VanKirk and Sassin, 1969); and (3) polygraphic recording of the EEG (electroencephalogram), EOG (electrooculogram), and EMG (electromyogram) during sleep so that sleep onset and offset can be precisely determined and correlations can be made with sleep stages (Rechtschaffen and Kales, 1968). Previous work had determined that plasma LH concentrations during the follicular phase of the menstrual cycle are characterized by rising values on a day-to-day basis (Ross *et al.*, 1970). Several days prior to ovulation, LH secretion greatly increases, the LH surge, and this rise lasts approximately 24 hr. Concentrations during the luteal phase are lower than those during the follicular phase. FSH is also characterized by a mid-cycle surge, lower than that of LH and, in addition, there is a peak at the beginning of the follicular phase, which is probably responsible for the initiation of growth of a new crop of follicles.

Using the methods enumerated in the foregoing paragraph, we will describe findings from this laboratory which deal with 24-hr LH secretory patterns in men and women from childhood to adulthood. We will examine the question of the presence or absence of circadian or ultradian rhythms and the influence of sleep and waking states on these LH secretory patterns.

(1) Adult men

The LH secretory pattern in adult men is characterized by the occurrence of 10–15 secretory episodes per 24-hr period (Boyar *et al.*, 1972b). The episodes have a sharp rise and a slower fall, suggesting a massive release of LH over a short time period followed by minimal secretion until the next episode (Fig. 1). Analysis of the data from our laboratory reveals no statistical difference between diurnal and nocturnal secretion. However, Nankin and Troen (1972) felt that there was an enhanced secre-

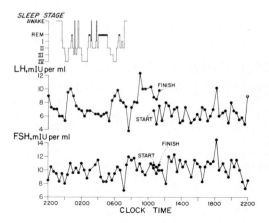

Fig. 1. Twenty-four-hour secretory patterns of LH and FSH in a 22-year-old male derived from 20-min interval plasma sampling and measurement by double-antibody radioimmunoassay. Both hormones are expressed in terms of mIU (milli-International Units) of the second IRP–HMG (International Reference Preparation–Human Menopausal Gonadotropin) standard. Sleep and waking stages are plotted in the upper left-hand corner of the plot. REM = rapid eye movement; I through IV = slow-wave sleep stages. The gonadotropins are secreted episodically both during sleep and wakefulness.

tion of LH towards the end of the nocturnal sleep period. Furthermore, our data reveal no apparent correlation with individual sleep stages although Rubin *et al.* (1972), using Kendall's coefficient of concordance, reported a 14% higher concentration of plasma LH during REM (rapid eye movement) periods than during non-REM periods. Our finding of the lack of a circadian rhythm or sleep-related changes in man was confirmed by Krieger *et al.* (1972).

(II) Adult women

As in men, LH is secreted in women in discrete episodes. These episodes are irregular in timing and unequal in amplitude; however, there is an average frequency of about 100 min, which suggests a possible relationship with the REM–non-REM sleep cycle of 90–100 min.

During the early follicular phase, LH secretion transiently falls after sleep onset (Kapen *et al.*, 1973b). The magnitude of this fall varies from subject to subject but can be as great as 65% when compared to the 24-hr mean LH concentration (Fig. 2). Hour-by-hour analysis was made of the combined data from a group of 5 subjects and the results were expressed as average percentage change from the 24-hr mean. This analysis showed that a significant negative deviation from the 24-hr mean occurred during the third hour after stage 2 sleep onset (Fig. 3). A similar analysis of a comparable group of 5 male subjects did not reveal a significant variation during either the sleep or waking periods.

In order to determine whether the above decrease in LH secretion is sleep-related or is driven by the light–dark cycle, a group of 6 women were studied during the early

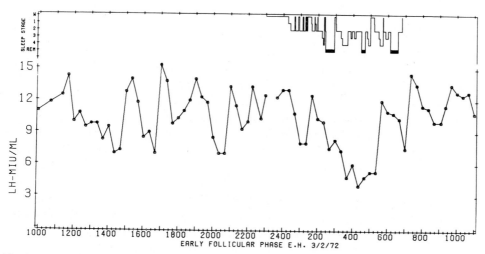

Fig. 2. Twenty-two-year-old woman. Early follicular phase. LH is plotted in 20-min intervals. There is a marked decrease in plasma LH concentrations shortly following sleep onset.

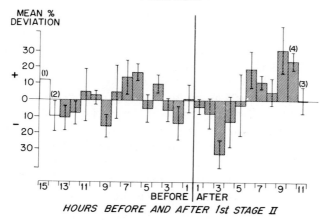

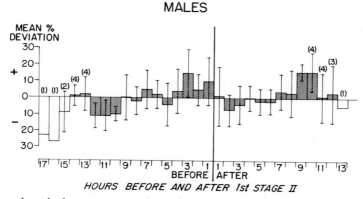

Fig. 3. Average hour-by-hour percentage change from the 24-hr mean LH concentration for a group of 5 normal women (above) and 5 normal men (below). The female plot is marked by a large fall in LH concentrations in the third hour following sleep onset.

References p. 111–113

follicular phase (Kapen and Weitzman, 1974b). The subjects underwent a baseline 24-hr study following which, one to several months later, an acute 180° reversal of the sleep–wake cycle was carried out. After remaining awake for 1 night, the subjects slept from 11:00 to 19:00 with simultaneous polygraphic recording. Hour-by-hour analysis was done using, as the definition of sleep onset, the first 10 min of uninterrupted stage 2 which was followed by stage 3. In the baseline studies, the greatest percentage decrease from the 24-hr mean for each subject for the first 4 hr after sleep onset ranged from 27.2 to 52.4%. The range for the reversal studies was from 15.4 to 51.0%. The average hourly percentage decrease for the first 4 hr of sleep was 14% for the baseline group and 13% for the reversal group. There was no correlation for individual subjects between the magnitude of the fall in the baseline study and that in the reversal. However, there was a rough direct correlation between minutes of slow-wave sleep (stages 3 and 4 combined) and the percentage of decrease in LH secretion during the same time period. One of the subjects, during her reversal study, awoke for 2.5 hr before falling asleep again. Each sleep onset was associated with a major decrease in plasma LH concentrations.

Further insight into the mechanisms relating sleep and LH secretion was gained by analyzing plasma LH values in another woman who was part of a larger study of cortisol and growth hormone secretion in individuals on a 3-hr sleep–wake cycle (Weitzman *et al.*, 1974). This subject had a baseline study during the early follicular phase. She then began the 3-hr sleep–wake protocol which lasted 10 days, during which she remained awake for 2 hr and was allowed to sleep for 1 hr with continual monitoring. On the eighth day of this regimen, an intravenous catheter was inserted in the morning and blood samples were collected every 20 min for the next 24 hr.

The baseline study was characterized by a marked decrease in LH secretion during the early part of her sleep period. The data from the ultradian study are strongly suggestive of a decrease in LH concentrations during each sleep episode, with the major falls occurring when slow-wave sleep was predominant and a lesser or no fall occurring when REM sleep made up the major part of her sleep time.

These data indicate that LH secretion decreases during the early part of a nocturnal or diurnal sleep period. They also suggest that slow-wave sleep, which is predominant during the first half of sleep, plays a critical role. The mechanism for this phenomenon is unclear. One could postulate some kind of change in estrogen feedback or the possible role of prolactin as a gonadotropin inhibitor (Friesen *et al.*, 1973), since prolactin secretion increases during sleep (Sassin *et al.*, 1972, 1973). The possibility that two related indoleamines, serotonin and/or melatonin, could be involved, is also a strong consideration. Serotonin has been implicated by Jouvet (1969) and others in the initiation and maintenance of slow-wave sleep and is a possible inhibitor of gonadotropin secretion in rats (Fraschini, 1971). Melatonin, in turn, inhibits LH secretion in rats (Fraschini, 1971), causes synchronization of the EEG and behavioral sleep in chickens (Barchas *et al.*, 1967; Hishikawa *et al.*, 1969), cats (Marczynski *et al.*, 1964) and humans (Anton-Tay *et al.*, 1971), and undergoes an enhanced synthesis by the pineal gland in rats during the dark period (Wurtman *et al.*, 1963).

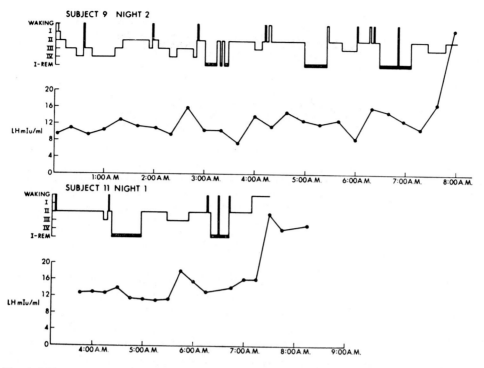

Fig. 4. LH concentration is plotted for two women in the late follicular phase. The LH surge for each woman begins just as the sleep period ends.

(III) Periovulatory secretory patterns

The episodic mode of LH secretion, seen in women and men, continues during the LH surge which precedes ovulation (Midgley and Jaffe, 1971; Yen *et al.*, 1972; Kapen *et al.*, 1973b). Data from the beginning of the LH surge in 3 women suggest that the augmentation of LH secretion, which characterizes the surge, begins towards the end of the nocturnal sleep period (Kapen *et al.*, 1973b) (Fig. 4). This suggests that the triggering of the LH surge in humans is entrained to a factor associated with the latter part of nocturnal sleep or to the interface between dark and light. This would not be too surprising a finding because the light–dark cycle plays a role in the secretion of ovulation inducing hormone in chickens (Fraps, 1965). Furthermore, there is a periodicity for the preovulatory rise of LH secretion on the day of proestrous in the rat (Everett and Sawyer, 1950; Everett, 1956).

(IV) Prepubertal patterns

The absolute concentrations of plasma LH are low prior to puberty. There is little fluctuation and no difference in secretion between sleep and waking (Fig. 5).

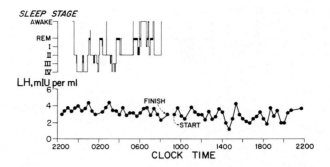

Fig. 5. Prepubertal 9-year-old girl. The LH secretory pattern, as compared with the adult, is marked by small fluctuations and low concentrations. No difference exists in mean concentration between sleep and wakefulness.

(V) Puberty

Several groups of investigators have followed the rising pattern of LH and FSH during the pubertal process in cross-sectional studies based on single blood samples from individual children (Root *et al.*, 1970; Wieland *et al.*, 1970; August *et al.*, 1972). Little information was available until recently about the processes initiating puberty in humans but animal work has led to the hypothesis that around the time of puberty, the hypothalamic threshold for negative feedback by gonadal steroids rises which leads to an increased synthesis and release of gonadotropin-releasing factor (Hohlweg, 1936; Byrnes and Meyer, 1951; Ramirez and McCann, 1963). There is also evidence in the literature that the pineal gland, as well as certain regions of the telencephalon, may play important roles in the initiation of puberty (Kitay and Altschule, 1954; Wurtman *et al.*, 1963; Bar-Sela and Critchlow, 1966; Wurtman, 1967).

The importance of environmental factors, especially the light–dark cycle, has been emphasized in many studies (Tanner, 1962) but the possible influence of sleep on pubertal mechanisms was given little scientific attention until the report of Boyar *et al.* (1972a) who showed an augmentation of LH and FSH secretion during sleep which was evident as early as the P2 stage of Tanner (1962) (Fig. 6). All normal children during puberty have shown this feature, which can be employed as an index of delayed puberty in order to differentiate this condition from hypogonadotropic hypogonadism (Boyar *et al.*, 1973b). This association of augmented LH secretion and sleep in normal individuals is confined to puberty while progression of puberty to adulthood is characterized by an increase of daytime secretion until the adult 24-hr pattern is attained (Boyar *et al.*, 1972b). Inspection of the pattern of LH secretion during sleep suggests that the augmented LH secretion is related to slow-wave sleep (stages 2 through 4) because there appears to be a strong correlation between REM periods and a fall in LH concentration (Boyar *et al.*, 1972a).

An experiment involving acute 180° sleep reversal was carried out by our laboratory in order to study the effects of this procedure on LH secretion (Kapen *et al.*, 1974a). The results were consistent with the hypothesis that augmented secretion of LH

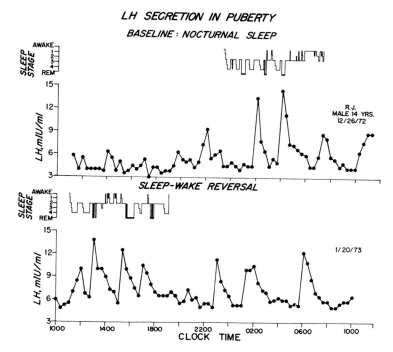

Fig. 6. Fourteen-year-old pubertal boy. The baseline study above shows plasma LH values when the subject sleeps at night. Note the enhanced secretion during sleep. Below is the pattern following an acute 180° sleep–wake inversion. The nocturnal waking period is characterized by larger secretory episodes than during diurnal waking in the baseline study.

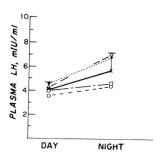

Fig. 7. Mean waking LH concentrations for each of 4 pubertal boys in the baseline study ("day") and in the reversal study ("night"). The heavy line represents the mean for all subjects. The short vertical lines denote 1 S.D. The difference between diurnal waking and nocturnal waking is significant.

during puberty is correlated with sleep. The 4 boys whom we studied, aged 14–15, all had LH concentrations during diurnal sleep higher than those during nocturnal waking (Fig. 6). This finding after acute sleep–wake reversal is comparable to the findings reported for growth hormone and prolactin secretion after reversal (Sassin *et al.*, 1969, 1973). However, there is a major difference between the characteristics of pubertal LH secretion during sleep reversal and those of growth hormone and

References p. 111–113

prolactin and this is the significantly higher secretion of LH during the nocturnal waking period than during daytime waking (Figs. 6, 7). Such a phenomenon suggests that, in addition to sleep, LH secretion during puberty may be influenced by the light–dark cycle.

In order to show whether the pubertal LH secretory pattern would be present in cases of precocious puberty, 3 patients were studied in our laboratory. All had precocious puberty from the following causes: idiopathic, hypothalamic tumor, and adrenal hyperplasia. Each of these patients had enhanced LH secretion during sleep (Boyar *et al.*, 1973a). The findings from the patient with adrenal hyperplasia, in particular, suggest that adrenarche may normally have an important role in the initiation of puberty. In this regard, another set of patients with gonadal dysgenesis is important in demonstrating the lack of dependence of the pubertal LH secretory program on ovarian function. Three patients with this condition were studied, two being of pubertal age. These two patients had the sleep-related augmentation of LH secretion while a third patient, who was 22 years old, did not (Boyar *et al.*, 1973c). It can be concluded that sleep-related augmentation of LH secretion at puberty is a result of an autonomous CNS program, unrelated to steroid feedback by ovarian hormones (although the adrenal gland may play a role).

(VI) Abnormal LH secretory patterns: preliminary results

(A) Chiari–Frommel syndrome
We have studied one patient with Chiari–Frommel syndrome (post-parturitional amenorrhea and galactorrhea) (Kapen *et al.*, 1973a). Two 24-hr studies were carried out on this patient, the first prior to and the second following clomiphene citrate therapy. LH and FSH secretion were markedly depressed during the evening and night-time hours of both studies while prolactin secretion was characterized by a sleep-related rise similar to that found in normal subjects (Sassin *et al.*, 1972). The reciprocal nature nocturnally of the secretion of LH and FSH on the one hand, and of prolactin on the other, suggests an impairment of the hypothalamic dopaminergic secretory system (Ganong, 1972). The findings in this patient further bring to mind the decrease in LH secretion after sleep onset in normal women (Kapen *et al.*, 1973c) and raise the possibility that they were due to an exaggeration of this phenomenon.

(B) Galactorrhea and pituitary tumors
In a diverse group of patients with galactorrhea, we have found that the sleep–waking difference in prolactin secretion is obliterated in cases with pituitary tumors (Boyar *et al.*, 1974a). This may be one of the earliest pathological signs of this condition.

(C) Anorexia nervosa
A group of patients with anorexia nervosa had patterns similar to those of pubertal subjects in whom sleep is marked by a significant increase in LH secretion (Boyar *et al.*, 1974b). The striking difference in the relationship of LH secretion to sleep from

that of normal adult women is obvious. One patient with anorexia nervosa showed a return to the expected normal pattern when she was studied a second time after she improved clinically. It may be surmised that the pubertal pattern in these patients with amenorrhea represents evidence in favor of a reversion to the pubertal state from the standpoint of the hypothalamo–hypophyseal–gonadal axis.

SUMMARY

The twenty-four-hour patterns of LH (luteinizing hormone) secretion are characterized by major changes with ontogenetic development and by marked gender differences. Thus, sleeping activity is distinguished during puberty by an augmentation of LH secretion while, conversely, LH secretion decreases during the sleep of adult women. Adult men do not show such sleep-related changes in LH secretion. Underlying these, group differences must be major differences in the way the central nervous system controls the synthesis and release of this hormone. The importance of understanding the 24-hr secretory patterns of LH is underscored by abnormalities in these patterns which have been found in some diseases of the hypothalamo–hypophyseal–gonadal axis. The latter include Chiari–Frommel syndrome, pituitary tumors and anorexia nervosa.

REFERENCES

ANTON-TAY, F., DIAZ, J. L. AND FERNANDEZ-GUARDIOLA, A. (1971) On the effect of melatonin upon human brain. Its possible therapeutic implications. *Life Sci.*, **10**, 841–850.

AUGUST, G. P., GRUMBACH, M. M. AND KAPLAN, S. L. (1972) Hormonal changes in puberty. III. Correlation of plasma testosterone, LH, FSH, testicular size, and bone age with male pubertal development. *J. clin. Endocr.*, **34**, 319–326.

BARCHAS, J., DeCOSTA, F. AND SPECTER, S. (1967) Acute pharmacology of melatonin. *Nature (Lond.)*, **214**, 919–920.

BAR-SELA, M. AND CRITCHLOW, V. (1966) Delayed puberty following electrical stimulation of amygdala in female rats. *Amer. J. Physiol.*, **211**, 1103–1107.

BOYAR, R., FINKELSTEIN, J., ROFFWARG, H., KAPEN, S., WEITZMAN, E. D. AND HELLMAN, L. (1972a) Synchronization of augmented luteinizing hormone secretion with sleep during puberty. *New Engl. J. Med.*, **287**, 582–586.

BOYAR, R., PERLOW, M., HELLMAN, L., KAPEN, S. AND WEITZMAN, E. D. (1972b) Twenty-four hour pattern of luteinizing hormone secretion in normal men with sleep stage recording. *J. clin. Endocr.*, **35**, 73–81.

BOYAR, R. M., FINKELSTEIN, J., DAVID, R., ROFFWARG, H., KAPEN, S., WEITZMAN, E. D. AND HELLMAN, L. (1973a) Twenty-four hour patterns of plasma luteinizing hormone and follicle-stimulating hormone in sexual precocity. *New Engl. J. Med.*, **289**, 282–286.

BOYAR, R., KAPEN, S., ROFFWARG, H. AND WEITZMAN, E. D. (1973b) Positive identification of "delayed" puberty. *Endocrine Society, Annual Meeting, June, 1973, Chicago, Ill.*, p. A-199 (abstract).

BOYAR, R., FINKELSTEIN, J., ROFFWARG, H., KAPEN, S., WEITZMAN, E. D. AND HELLMAN, L. (1973c) Twenty-four luteinizing hormone and follicle-stimulating hormone secretory patterns in gonadal dysgenesis. *J. clin. Endocr.*, **37**, 521–525.

BOYAR, R., KAPEN, S., FINKELSTEIN, J., PERLOW, M., SASSIN, J., FUKUSHIMA, D., WEITZMAN, E. D. AND HELLMAN, L. (1974a) Hypothalamic–pituitary function in diverse hyperprolactinemic states. *J. clin. Invest.*, **53**, 1588–1598.

BOYAR, R., KAPEN, S., FINKELSTEIN, J., FUKUSHIMA, D., WEITZMAN, E. D. AND HELLMAN, L. (1974b) Delineation of the luteinizing hormone and cortisol abnormalities in anorexia nervosa. *J. clin. Invest.*, **53**, 9A.

BYRNES, W. W. AND MEYER, R. K. (1951) Effect of physiological amounts of estrogen on secretion of follicle stimulating and luteinizing hormone. *Endocrinology*, **49**, 449–460.

EVERETT, J. W. AND SAWYER, C. H. (1950) A 24-hour periodicity in the "LH release apparatus" of female rats, disclosed by barbiturate sedation. *Endocrinology*, **47**, 198–218.

EVERETT, J. W. (1956) The time of release of ovulating hormone from the rat hypophysis. *Endocrinology*, **59**, 580–585.

FRAPS, R. M. (1965) Twenty-four hour periodicity in the mechanism of pituitary gonadotrophin release for follicular maturation and ovulation in the chicken. *Endocrinology*, **77**, 5–18.

FRASCHINI, J. (1971) Role of indoleamines in the control of the secretion of pituitary gonadotropins. In *Neurochemical Aspects of Hypothalamic Function*, L. MARTINI AND J. MEITES (Eds.), Academic Press, New York, N.Y., pp. 141–159.

FRIESEN, H., TOLIS, G., SHIU, R., HWANG, P. AND HARDY, J. (1973) Studies on human prolactin: chemistry, radioreceptor assay and clinical significance. In *International Symposium on Human Prolactin*, J. C. PASTEELS AND C. ROBYN (Eds.), Excerpta Medica, Amsterdam, p. 19.

GANONG, W. F. (1972) Pharmacological aspects of neuroendocrine integration. In *Topics in Neuroendocrinology, Progress in Brain Research, Vol. 38*, J. A. KAPPERS AND J. P. SCHADÉ (Eds.), Elsevier, Amsterdam, pp. 46–47.

HISHIKAWA, Y., CRAMER, H. AND KUHLO, W. (1969) Natural and melatonin-induced sleep in young chickens — a behavioral and electrographic study. *Exp. Brain Res.*, **7**, 84–94.

HOHLWEG, W. (1936) Der Mechanismus der Wirkung von gonadotropen Substanzen auf das Ovar der infantilen Ratte. *Klin. Wschr.*, **15**, 1832–1835.

JOUVET, M. (1969) Biogenic amines and the states of sleep. *Science*, **163**, 32–41.

KAPEN, S., BOYAR, R., FREEMAN, R., HELLMAN, L. AND WEITZMAN, E. D. (1973a) Amenorrhea-galactorrhea: Nocturnal inhibition of gonadotropin secretion in a patient with Chiari–Frommel syndrome. *Sleep Res.*, **2**, 196 (abstract).

KAPEN, S., BOYAR, R., HELLMAN, L. AND WEITZMAN, E. D. (1973b) Episodic release of luteinizing hormone at mid-menstrual cycle in normal adult women. *J. clin. Endocr.*, **36**, 724–729.

KAPEN, S., BOYAR, R., PERLOW, M., HELLMAN, L. AND WEITZMAN, E. D. (1973c) Luteinizing hormone: Changes in secretory pattern during sleep in adult women. *Life Sci.*, **13**, 693–701.

KAPEN, S., BOYAR, R., FINKELSTEIN, J., HELLMAN, L. AND WEITZMAN, E. D. (1974a) Effect of sleep–wake cycle reversal on luteinizing hormone secretory pattern in puberty. *J. clin. Endocr.*, **39**, 259–265.

KAPEN, S. AND WEITZMAN, E. D. (1974b) The relationship of LH secretion to sleep in women during the early follicular phase. *Endocrine Society, Annual Meeting, Atlanta, Ga., June, 1974*, p. A-194 (abstract).

KITAY, J. J. AND ALTSCHULE, M. D. (1954) *The Pineal Gland — A Review of the Physiologic Literature*, Harvard Univ. Press, Cambridge, Mass.

KRIEGER, D. T., OSSOWSKI, R., FOGEL, M. AND ALLEN, W. (1972) Lack of circadian periodicity of human serum FSH and LH levels. *J. clin. Endocr.*, **35**, 619–623.

MARCZYNSKI, T. J., YAMAGUCHI, N., LING, G. M. AND GRODZENSKA, L. (1964) Sleep induced by the administration of melatonin (5-methoxy-N-acetyl-tryptamine) to the hypothalamus in unrestrained cats. *Experientia (Basel)*, **20**, 435–437.

MIDGLEY, JR., A. R. (1966) Radioimmunoassay: a method for human chorionic gonadotropin and human luteinizing hormone. *Endocrinology*, **79**, 10–18.

MIDGLEY, JR., A. R. AND JAFFE, R. B. (1971) Regulation of human gonadotropins. X. Episodic fluctuation of LH during the menstrual cycle. *J. clin. Endocr.*, **33**, 962–969.

NANKIN, H. R. AND TROEN, P. (1972) Overnight patterns of serum luteinizing hormone in normal men. *J. clin. Endocr.*, **35**, 705–710.

RAMIREZ, V. D. AND MCCANN, S. M. (1963) Comparison of the regulation of luteinizing hormone (LH) secretion in immature and adult rats. *Endocrinology*, **72**, 452–464.

RECHTSCHAFFEN, A. AND KALES, A. (1968) *A Manual of Standardized Terminology, Techniques, and Scoring System for Sleep Stages of Human Subjects*, U.S. Dept. of Health, Education and Welfare, Public Health Service, National Institutes of Health, National Institutes of Neurological Disease and Blindness, Neurological Information Network, Bethesda, Md.

ROOT, A. W., MOSHANG, JR., T., BONGIOVANNI, A. M. AND EBERLEIN, W. R. (1970) Concentrations of plasma luteinizing hormone in infants, children, and adolescents with normal and abnormal gonadal function. *Pediat. Res.*, **4**, 175–186.

ROSS, G. T., CARGILLE, C. M., LIPSETT, M. B., RAYFORD, P. C., MARSHALL, J. R., STROTT, C. A. AND RODBARD, D. (1970) Pituitary and gonadal hormones in women during spontaneous and induced ovulatory cycles. *Recent Progr. Hormone Res.*, **26**, 1–62.

RUBIN, R. T., KALES, A., ADLER, R., FAGAN, T. AND ODELL, W. (1972) Gonadotropin secretion during sleep in normal adult men. *Science*, **175**, 196–198.

SASSIN, J. F., PARKER, D. C., MACE, J. W., GOTLIN, R. W., JOHNSON, L. C. AND ROSSMAN, L. G. (1969) Human growth hormone release: relation to slow-wave sleep and sleep–waking cycles. *Science*, **165**, 513–515.

SASSIN, J. F., FRANTZ, A. G., WEITZMAN, E. D. AND KAPEN, S. (1972) Human prolactin: 24-hour pattern with increased release during sleep. *Science*, **177**, 1205–1207.

SASSIN, J. F., FRANTZ, A. G., KAPEN, S. AND WEITZMAN, E. D. (1973) The nocturnal rise of human prolactin is dependent on sleep. *J. clin. Endocr.*, **37**, 436–440.

TANNER, J. M. (1962) *Growth at Adolescence*, Blackwell Scientific Publications, Oxford.

VANKIRK, K. AND SASSIN, J. F. (1969) Technique for serial blood sampling during sleep recording. *Amer. J. EEG Technol.*, **9**, 143–146.

WEITZMAN, E. D., NOGEIRE, C., PERLOW, M., FUKUSHIMA, D., SASSIN, J., MCGREGOR, P., GALLAGHER, T. F. AND HELLMAN, L. (1974) Effects of a prolonged 3-hour sleep–wake cycle on sleep stages, plasma cortisol, growth hormone and body temperature in man. *J. clin. Endocr.*, **38**, 1018–1030.

WIELAND, R. G., YEN, S. S. C. AND POHLMAN, C. (1970) Serum testosterone levels and testosterone binding affinity in prepubertal and adolescent males; correlation with gonadotropins. *Amer. J. med. Sci.*, **259**, 358–360.

WURTMAN, R. J., AXELROD, J. AND PHILLIPS, L. S. (1963) Melatonin synthesis in the pineal gland: control by light. *Science*, **142**, 1071–1073.

WURTMAN, R. J. (1967) Effects of light and visual stimuli on neuroendocrine function. In *Neuroendocrinology, Vol. 2*, L. MARTINI AND W. F. GANONG (Eds.), Academic Press, New York, N.Y., pp. 19–59.

YEN, S. S. C., TSAI, C. C., NAFTOLIN, F., VANDENBERG, G. AND AJABOR, L. (1972) Pulsatile patterns of gonadotropin release in subjects with and without ovarian function. *J. clin. Endocr.*, **34**, 671–675.

Sleep–Waking Cycle of the Hypophysectomized Rat

JEAN-LOUIS VALATX, GUY CHOUVET AND MICHEL JOUVET

Département de Médecine Expérimentale, Université Claude Bernard, 8 Avenue Rockefeller, 69373 Lyon (France)

INTRODUCTION

The role of pituitary hormones in the sleep–waking cycle is not yet clearly defined. The hypophysis is not essential to trigger sleep: in the chronic pontile cat without hypothalamus or hypophysis, paradoxical sleep occurs during the first 5 days of survival (Jouvet, 1965). However, prolonged survival up to 2 months requires chronic administration of corticotropin (ACTH) or vasopressin (ADH).

On the other hand, pituitary hormones seem to be effective in the behavior of hypophysectomized rats (de Wied, 1969; Lissák and Bohus, 1972). Acquisition and retention of passive or active avoidance reaction is facilitated by ACTH or ADH administration.

Since the first work of Lucero (1970), Leconte *et al.* (1973), Smith *et al.* (1972) and Pagel *et al.* (1973) have demonstrated a close relation between sleep (paradoxical sleep) and learning. Impairment of learning in the hypophysectomized rat might be due to an alteration of the sleep cycle.

Thus, this work has been undertaken to study the sleep–waking cycle of the hypophysectomized rat and the effects of ACTH upon sleep. The problem is to separate specific from non-specific effects of hypophysectomy on sleep mechanisms and learning.

METHODS

We have studied 30 OFA male rats, 10 weeks old at the time of transaural hypophysectomy, performed by the "Centre d'Elevage des Oncins" (IFFA-CREDO).

Under Nembutal anesthesia (30 mg/kg, i.p.), cortical and muscular electrodes were implanted 2 weeks after hypophysectomy. Cerebellar temperature was recorded by means of a thermistor, chronically implanted (Valatx *et al.*, 1973). After surgery animals were placed in a plexiglass cylinder with food and water *ad lib*. The ambient temperature was constant (24 $\pm$ 1 °C) and the lighting schedule consisted of 12 hr light (7.00–19.00) and 12 hr darkness (19.00–7.00). The electrode cable was attached 10 days before the beginning of the electroencephalogram (EEG) recording.

References p. 120

After a period of 5 consecutive days to study the baseline of the sleep–waking cycle, a heat test (30 °C) was performed during 24 hr. The effect of a long-acting preparation of ACTH (corticotropin Z, Organon) was also tested, and the results were compared to those obtained after treatment with placebo (zn-phosphate).

At the end of experimentation, animals were sacrificed. Ablation of the hypophysis was checked and the adrenals were dissected and weighed. Sleep states were scored by visual analysis of 30-sec epochs. Quantitative analysis has been completed by studying the circadian sleep–wakefulness rhythm. By means of spectral analysis methods, the analysis of periodicity within the temporal characteristics of sleep records has been done. For each state of sleep, a time series was computed from the sleep duration within each consecutive hour during 4 or 5 consecutive days (X_i, $i = 1, \ldots N$, i representing the rank of the corresponding hour from the beginning of the experiment). Considering this time series as representing a periodic sampling of the probability of occurrence of a given sleep state *versus* time, it is then possible to compute the spectral density by means of a Fast Fourier Transform (FFT). The spectrum is divided by the experimental variance of observations (s^2) to normalize the results and to allow further comparisons. For each frequency, the following are computed:

$$\frac{A_N^2(\omega_p) + B_N^2(\omega_p)}{2s^2} \tag{1}$$

with

$$A_N(\omega_p) = \sqrt{\frac{2}{N}} \sum_{i=1}^{N} X_i \cos i\omega_p$$

$$B_N(\omega_p) = \sqrt{\frac{2}{N}} \sum_{i=1}^{N} X_i \sin i\omega_p$$

$$\omega_p = \frac{2\pi p}{N} \quad (p = 1, 2 \ldots N/2) \text{ angular frequency}$$

If the X_i's are independent and normally distributed, the numerator in equation (1) has a distribution proportional to χ^2 with 2 *df* ($s^2\chi^2(2)$). The value (1) is then similar to a $\chi^2(2)/2$. Each value of (1) greater than $\chi^2_{0.05}(2)/2 = 3$ indicates a correlation between the observations at the corresponding frequency with an error risk of 5%.

RESULTS

Qualitative data

In the isolated hypophysectomized rat, motor activity during wakefulness was reduced; sleep behavior (posture) was unchanged; EEG patterns of sleep were normal. One

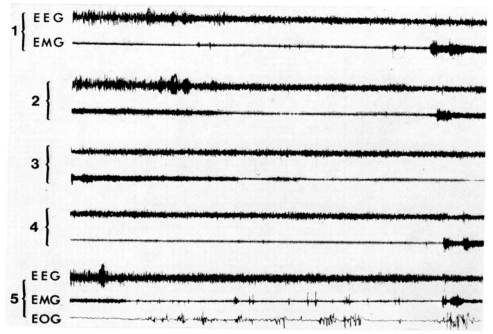

Fig. 1. Polygraphic samples of slow-wave sleep (SWS) and paradoxical sleep (PS) from normal rat (1) and hypophysectomized rat (2–5). Note important muscular activity during SWS (2) and numerous eye movements during PS (5) in hypophysectomized rat. Note narcoleptic episode (3–4) characterized by direct transition from wakefulness to paradoxical sleep. EEG = electroencephalogram; EMG = electromyogram; EOG = electro-oculogram.

month after hypophysectomy, episodes of narcolepsy were observed: paradoxical sleep occurred directly after wakefulness or a few seconds of slow-wave sleep (SWS) (Fig. 1).

Cerebellar temperature presented approximately the same fluctuations during sleep–waking cycle as in control rats but the mean level was over 2 °C lower than normal (34–35 °C *versus* 36.5–37.5 °C).

Quantitative data

(1) Sleep–waking cycle at 25 °C

We have observed some variations among series of hypophysectomized rats, but overall sleep duration was always reduced. The total sleep time per day was 604 ± 15 min *versus* 715 ± 18 min in control rats. SWS duration was reduced (−10%) less than paradoxical sleep (PS) (−50%). Thus the PS/SWS ratio was smaller (PS/SWS = 8) than in control animals (PS/SWS = 14.4) (Fig. 2). The mean duration of the PS phase tends to increase while the number of phases is drastically reduced. The diminution of sleep time was preferentially observed during daytime.

The day–night difference of PS duration was not as important (15 min) as in the control rat (50 min). The circadian sleep rhythm is completely altered (Fig. 3).

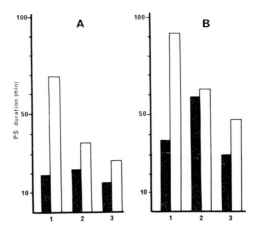

Fig. 2. Paradoxical sleep (PS) duration during night (black bars) and during day (white bars) at 25°C (A) and 30°C (B) ambient temperature in normal rat (1) and in hypophysectomized rat, 30 days (2) and 60 days (3) after ablation of the hypophysis.

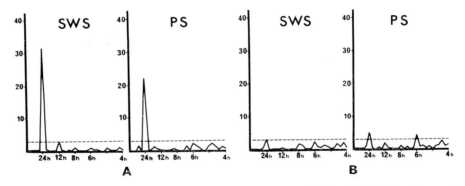

Fig. 3. Spectral analysis of slow-wave sleep (SWS) and paradoxical sleep (PS) rhythm of normal rat (A) and hypophysectomized rat (B). The computed values ($A^2_N + B^2_N/2s^2$) in arbitrary units (ordinates) are plotted against the frequency (abscissae). Dotted lines represent $\chi^2_{0.05} (2)/2 = 3$, *i.e.*, the limit of confidence of the spectrum amplitude. Note the lack of circadian rhythm (24 hr) in hypophysectomized rat.

Some subjects presented progressive alterations in sleep with a maximal diminution 2 months after ablation of the hypophysis (Fig. 2). This maximal diminution was often observed at the beginning of EEG recording (2–3 weeks after hypophysectomy).

(2) Effects of ambient temperature (30 °C)

Twenty four hours of exposure at 30 °C increased sleep duration (SWS and PS) as in normal rats. The augmentation started within the first several hours of heat exposure. Return to 25°C immediately stopped this alteration. The PS variation (+66%) was more important than that of SWS (+5%) and was due to the increase in the number of episodes. The mean duration of each episode remained unchanged.

TABLE I

ADRENAL WEIGHT (mg)

Number of rats	Intact	Hypox*-placebo	Hypox-ACTH
5	31.4	9.1	18.3

* Hypophysectomized.

(3) Effect of ACTH

Corticotropin Z was always administered at 18:00 hr (5 injections of 3 I.U./2 days) by the subcutaneous route. Some rats received placebo. The augmentation of adrenal weight after the fifth injection was a criterion for effectiveness of the injections (see Table I).

PS duration increased progressively after the second or third injection of ACTH. The maximum was observed after the fourth injection (80 min *versus* 45 min before injection).

The narcolepsy syndrome seemed to be unaffected by ACTH. Cerebellar temperature increased progressively with ACTH administration (up to 36 °C) and then returned gradually to 34 °C when ACTH injections were stopped.

DISCUSSION

The sleep–waking cycle of the hypophysectomized rat is markedly disturbed in our experimental conditions from 3 weeks to 2 months after ablation of the hypophysis. In order to obtain a stable baseline of sleep, it was not possible to start recordings earlier than 3 weeks after ablation, the time taken for recovery from surgery and implantation and habituation to the recording cable.

Alteration of the circadian rhythm of PS has been observed by Kawakami *et al.* (1972). However our results showed an important reduction of PS duration at 25 °C. This variation might be due to hypothermia observed in hypophysectomized rats. Therefore heat exposure (30 °C) increases central temperature and provokes an augmentation of PS duration as in normal rats. Neurochemical mechanisms of the action of heat exposure on the sleep cycle are not yet clearly understood (see refs. in Valatx *et al.*, 1973).

On the other hand, the action of ACTH upon sleep might be explained by non-specific effects. The progressive action of ACTH on sleep and cerebral temperature could be the consequence of improvement of health due to the increased adrenal activity. The physiological doses used in our experiments (3 I.U./2 days) alter sleep and temperature in hypophysectomized rats but not in normal animals.

However, heat exposure and ACTH have a common specific effect: the preferential increase of paradoxical sleep. The utilization of ACTH analogs without hormonal

References p. 120

activity could solve this problem. Narcolepsy occurs 1 month after hypophysectomy. This delay might be due to the degeneration of nerve fibers of the hypophysis or hypothalamus coming from the brain stem. In fact, surgical technique for ablation of the hypophysis might destroy a small part of the hypothalamus.

SUMMARY

Hypophysectomy provokes a diminution of total sleep time in the albino rat. The reduction of paradoxical sleep is more important than that of slow-wave sleep.

Heat exposure (30 °C) immediately reverses this diminution. ACTH administration progressively increases the duration of paradoxical sleep. In both cases cerebral temperature increases. These findings seem to be partly due to non-specific effects on sleep mechanisms.

These results indicate that the basic mechanisms of sleep are not altered in the hypophysectomized rat, but only the regulation or triggering of sleep.

ACKNOWLEDGEMENTS

This work was supported by INSERM (U.52), CNRS LA162 and DRME No. 73198.

The generous supply of ACTH by Organon Comp., Oss, The Netherlands, is gratefully acknowledged.

The authors are very indebted to Mrs. Luce Paut for technical assistance.

REFERENCES

JOUVET, M. (1965) Étude de la dualité des états de sommeil et des mécanismes de la phase paradoxale. In *Aspects Anatomo-fonctionnels de la Physiologie du Sommeil*, CNRS, Paris, pp. 397–449.

KAWAKAMI, M., YAMAOGA, S. AND YAMAGUCHI, T. (1972) Influence of light and hormones upon circadian rhythm of EEG slow wave and paradoxical sleep. In *Advances in Climatic Physiology*, S. ITOH, K. OGATA AND H. YOSHIMURA (Eds.), Igaku Shoin, Tokyo, pp. 349–366.

LECONTE, P., HENNEVIN, E. ET BLOCH, V. (1973) Analyse des effets d'un apprentissage et de son niveau d'acquisition sur le sommeil paradoxal consécutif, *Brain Res.*, **49**, 367–379.

LISSAK, K. AND BOHUS, B. (1972) Pituitary hormones and avoidance behavior of the rat. *Int. J. Psychobiol.*, **2**, 103–115.

LUCERO, M. (1970) Lengthening of REM sleep duration consecutive to learning in the rat. *Brain Res.*, **20**, 319–322.

PAGEL, J., PEGRAM, V., VAUGHAN, S., DONALDSON, P. AND BRIDGERS, W. (1973) The relationship of REM sleep with learning and memory in mice. *Behav. Biol.*, **9**, 383–388.

SMITH, C. T., KITAHAMA, K., VALATX, J.-L. ET JOUVET, M. (1972) Sommeil paradoxal et apprentissage chez deux souches consanguines de souris. *C.R. Acad. Sci. (Paris)*, **275**, 1283–1286.

VALATX, J.-L., ROUSSEL, B. ET CURE, M. (1973) Sommeil et température cérébrale du rat au cours de l'exposition chronique en ambiance chaude. *Brain Res.*, **55**, 107–122.

WIED, D. DE (1969) Effects of peptides hormones on behavior. In *Frontiers in Neuroendocrinology*, W. F. GANONG AND L. MARTINI (Eds.), Oxford Univ. Press, New York, N.Y., pp. 97–140.

Free Communications

Sleep EEG stages and growth hormone levels in endogenous and exogenous hyper-cortisolemia or ACTH elevation

D. T. KRIEGER — *Division of Endocrinology, Department of Medicine, Mount Sinai School of Medicine, City University of New York, New York City, N.Y. (U.S.A.)*

Studies of nocturnal sleep EEG stages and plasma growth hormone (GH) and cortisol levels (used as indices of central nervous system (CNS) function) were performed in subjects with endogenous or exogenous elevation of plasma corticosteroid or ACTH levels, and in patients with hypothalamic tumors. These studies were designed to determine if there was any evidence of altered CNS function that was unique to Cushing's disease, independent of any effects of hypercortisolemia *per se*.

The findings of the same marked reduction of sleep EEG stages III–IV and of the nocturnal GH rise in 4 treated (remission 5 months to 2 years) and 6 untreated patients with Cushing's disease (clinically active 2 months to 10 years duration); in 4 "eu-corticoid" patients with hypothalamic tumors; and the presence of normal sleep EEG stages and nocturnal GH rise in a patient with Cushing's syndrome 16 months following removal of an adrenal adenoma, as well as normal sleep EEG stages and lessened decrements in nocturnal GH rise in 7 patients receiving chronic prednisone therapy (15–60 mg daily for 4 months to 10 years) support the concept that altered CNS function may be involved in the pathophysiology of Cushing's disease. The finding of suppression of stage III–IV sleep in the patient with the adrenal adenoma and lack of such suppression in patients receiving chronic prednisone therapy suggests differential effects of exogenous and endogenous steroids. The presence of normal percentages of stage III–IV sleep following the removal of the adrenal adenoma suggests, however, that cortisol excess also plays some role in the observed sleep EEG and GH changes. The presence of normal sleep EEG stages in 4 patients with Cushing's disease who have subsequently developed Nelson's syndrome of 1–9 years duration additionally suggests a role of this peptide in the genesis of sleep EEG stages.

Antidiuretic hormone secretion during sleep in adult men

ROBERT T. RUBIN, RUSSELL E. POLAND, FERNANDO RAVESSOUD, PAUL R. GOUIN AND BARBARA B. TOWER — *Department of Psychiatry and Pharmacology, U.C.L.A. School of Medicine, Harbor General Hospital Campus, Torrance, Calif. 90509 (U.S.A.)*

Decreased urine volume and increased osmolality have been noted in older men (with indwelling urethral catheters) in close relationship to REM sleep episodes[1]. The postulated mechanism was ADH release from the posterior pituitary during REM sleep. However, the specific study of sleep-related ADH release has awaited the recent development of a sensitive ADH radioimmunoassay[2].

We studied 8 normal young adult men on two consecutive nights with blood sampling every 20 min from 23:00 to 07:00 according to an established protocol[3]. Water restriction began at 19:00. ADH was released episodically in all subjects. However, in contrast to the postulated mechanism of REM-activated ADH release, there was no increase of ADH during REM sleep. For the 8 subjects, Kendall's coefficient of concordance for wake + stage I, stage II, stage III + IV, and stage REM was only 0.08. Thus, the REM-related decreases in urine volume noted in the earlier study[1] do not appear to be related to ADH release, although that study was done in older men, and this one in young men.

1 MANDELL, A. J., CHAFFEY, B., BRILL, P., MANDELL, M. P., RODNICK, J., RUBIN, R. T., AND SCHEFF, R., Science, 151 (1966) 1558–1560.
2 SKOWSKY, W. R., ROSENBLOOM, A. A., AND FISHER, D. A., J. clin. Endocr. Metab., 38 (1974) 278–287.
3 RUBIN, R. T., GOUIN, P. R., KALES, A., AND ODELL, W. D., Psychosom. Med., 35 (1973) 309–321.

Session III

HORMONES ON LEARNING AND MEMORY FUNCTIONS

Chairmen: D. DE WIED (Utrecht)
J. L. McGAUGH (Irvine, Calif.)

Mechanism of Steroid Hormone Actions on Motivated Behavioral Reactions

E. ENDRÖCZI

Research Division, Postgraduate Medical School, Budapest (Hungary)

Individual variability of behavioral reactions may be determined by genetic factors, both humoral and neuronal influences occurring in perinatal life and also by social environment in randomly bred animals. It is known that strain differences are important in behavioral responses to psychotropic drugs, antiadrenergic and cholinergic agents (Bovet *et al.*, 1969; Fontenay *et al.*, 1970; Evans, 1971; Oliverio *et al.*, 1973). Individual variations of pituitary–adrenal response to different stress situations have been observed in earlier studies (Lissák and Endröczi, 1965; Endröczi, 1972a). An asymmetric U-shape correlation of plasma corticosterone response levels to the exploratory activity in a novel situation could be observed in randomly bred rats. Moreover, it was found that the daily rhythms of the plasma corticosterone concentration and the exploratory activity show opposite phases.

Both ACTH (corticotropin) and corticosteroids exert an influence on the brain functions and there are observations which indicated opposite influences on the conditioned reflex behavior (Lissák and Endröczi, 1965; de Wied, 1967; Bohus, 1970; Endröczi, 1972a). Concerning the neuroanatomical substrate sensitive for pituitary–adrenocortical hormones much attention was paid to the role of hippocampal–hypothalamic–brain stem connections in these events. Numerous observations have been accumulated in the literature which support the hypothesis that the hippocampus exerts a modifying influence on the exploratory activity, the acquisition and extinction of conditioned responses and the memory consolidation (Scoville, 1954; Milner, 1959; Douglas, 1967; Jarrard and Isaacson, 1965; Endröczi, 1972a and b). Ablation studies revealed that hippocampectomy is followed by an impairment of the acquisition and extinction of conditioned responses when the withdrawal of responding was the task for the animal (see the review of Endröczi, 1972a). In stimulation studies it was found that the electrical stimulation of dorsal hippocampus 30 sec after the end of a partial acquisition of the approaching response (at a current intensity which did not induce after-discharges) led to a marked facilitation of the performance 24 hr later (Stein and Chorover, 1968; Erickson and Patel, 1969; McGaugh, 1972; Destrade *et al.*, 1973). These observations led to the assumption that the activation of hippocampus in the form of driven theta rhythm is followed by a long-lasting change in the excitability state of the central nervous system which is involved in memory consolidation and retrieval. From a biochemical point of view it is worth mentioning that the RNA synthesis in the hippocampal cells of rats with "poor performance level" is less than that of the "high performers" (Izquierdo *et al.*, 1972). Moreover, it was found that topically applied RNA precursors in the hippocampus produced an increase in the acquisition of conditioned response (Ott and Matthies, 1973). In the light of ablation and stimulation studies as well as on the basis of the biochemical and pharmacological findings we may assume that the hippocampus is involved in decoding environmental signals, on the one hand, and in memory consolidation and retrieval, on the other.

McEwen *et al.* (1970) have reported that hippocampal cells have the property of accumulating corticosterone to a greater extent than other parts of the brain. This specific uptake of corticosteroids by the hippocampus and its role in controlling the hippocampus-adjusted behavioral reactions were already the subjects of speculations (see the review of Endröczi, 1972a and b). Moreover, the hippocampus exerts an inhibitory role on the pituitary–adrenal axis and the hippocampectomy is followed by the abolition of daily rhythm of pituitary ACTH release.

In the present investigations we have studied the correlations between the corticosterone binding capacity of hippocampus and elementary behavioral reactions, on the one hand, and the influence of ACTH on the binding property of the limbic structures for corticosterone, on the other hand.

METHODS

The uptake of $[4\text{-}^{14}C]$corticosterone was studied under *in vitro* conditions: the tissue slices were incubated in Tyrode solution in a shaking-thermostat at $37\,^\circ C$ for 60 min. In some experiments the tissue was homogenized before the addition of labeled steroid in ice-cooled Tyrode solution, then the homogenate was incubated at the $37\,^\circ C$ for 15 min; afterwards the tubes were cooled and the separation of the nuclear and cytosol fractions as well as that of the free and bound steroids was performed according to the technique of Baulieu *et al.* (1970). The radioactivity was measured with a Packard 314 EX liquid scintillation spectrometer.

The uptake of the $[\text{methylene-}^{14}C]$noradrenaline was measured after incubation of tissue slices with 2 nmoles labeled noradrenaline in Tyrode solution which contained 0.1% ascorbic acid. The tissue was homogenized and the pellet was washed 3 times with buffer to remove free ligand, and after the addition of Soluene (Packard solubilizer) the radioactivity was measured in a Packard liquid scintillation spectrometer. More details of the procedure have been described elsewhere (Préda *et al.*, 1975).

The exploratory activity was tested in a 12-cell maze and scored according to the number of gates in the wall crossed by the animal during time units. In most experiments the exploratory activity was tested for 10 min and the scores were recorded in 1-min intervals. For studying the habituation of exploratory activity the testing was repeated 5 times in morning and late afternoon sessions. The animals were sacrificed 24 hr after the end of the behavioral observation in order to study the biochemical parameters.

Adrenalectomy was performed under ether anesthesia 2 or 14 days prior to the behavioral experiments. The 2-day adrenalectomy was aimed to avoid a possible effect of the endogenous ACTH secretion, and to eliminate the influence of endogenous corticosterone production on the uptake of labeled corticosterone. The findings on 2-day adrenalectomized rats were compared to those of sham-operated animals.

RESULTS AND DISCUSSION

Two weeks after adrenalectomy the exploratory activity was significantly greater than that of the intact male rats. For comparison of drive intensity one group of rats was deprived of water for 23.5 hr during 2 consecutive days and then tested on the morning of the third day for exploration. The basal exploratory activity of the thirsty rats was about the same as had been observed for normal animals.

When intact, adrenalectomized and water-deprived rats were tested for exploratory activity during the course of 5 successive sessions (morning and late afternoon sessions were alternated), a significant habituation could be observed in intact groups and only a moderate habituation in the adrenalectomized or water-deprived rats.

Two to 3 hr after the end of the first exploratory test the intact rats showed a significant loss of the exploratory activity which could not be observed 16–24 hr

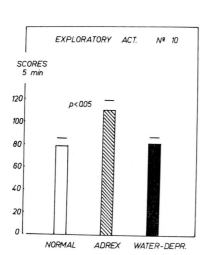

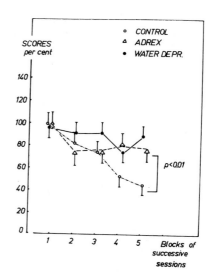

Fig. 1. Exploratory activity of intact (normal), adrenalectomized (adrex) and water-deprived rats in a 12-cell maze. Mean and standard errors are shown.

Fig. 2. Decrease of exploratory activity during the course of repeated tests: each session corresponds to a 5-min test, the testing was performed morning and late afternoon (for abbreviations, see Fig. 1).

References p. 133–134

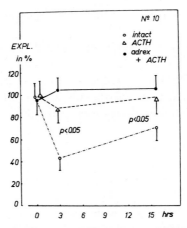

Fig. 3. Changes of exploratory activity 3 hr after the end of the first testing in intact and ACTH treated, and adrenalectomized (adrex) + ACTH treated rats.

later. After the administration of 10 I.U. ACTH to intact or adrenalectomized rats before the first testing, the transient decrease of exploration was absent. With regard to the time course of the observation these findings resemble the discovery of Kamin (1957) who found that rats were unable to reproduce a previously acquired two-way active avoidance response on an intermediate retention test while the performance was excellent both immediately and 24 hr after the initial aversive conditioning experience. In relation to these findings the importance of ACTH in memory retrieval was already

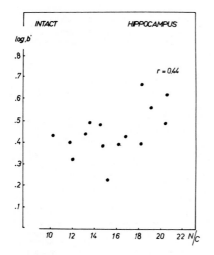

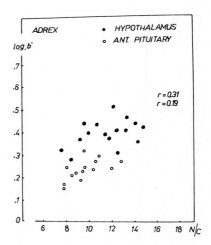

Fig. 4. Insignificant correlation between the ratio of the corticosterone uptake by the nuclear and cytosol fractions (N/C) and the slopes of the habituation to a new environment in intact rats.

Fig. 5. Insignificant correlations between the corticosterone uptake by the nuclear and cytosol fractions of the hypothalamus and the anterior (ant.) pituitary and the slope of habituation to a new environment in adrenalectomized (adrex) rats.

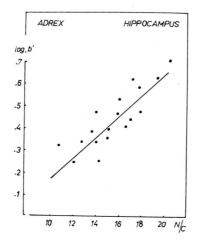

Fig. 6. Significant correlation ($P = 0.05$) between the slope of the habituation of exploratory activity in a new environment and the N/C ratios in the hippocampal uptake of corticosterone in adrenalectomized rats. $r = 0.89$.

suggested by several investigators (Brush and Levine, 1966; Bintz, 1970; Klein and Spear, 1970). Present observations about the suppression of the exploratory drive in the intermediate test 2–3 hr after the initial testing led to the assumption that a retention deficit in avoidance conditioning occurring in the intermediate test is not necessarily related to the suppression of memory retrieval. With regard to ACTH administration producing a beneficial effect on the exploratory activity in both intact and adrenalectomized rats, a direct influence of ACTH on brain function seems to be very likely.

When the habituation of exploratory activity was tested in 5 consecutive sessions the corticosterone-binding capacity of the hypothalamus, the anterior pituitary gland and the hippocampus showed no significant correlation with the slope of the habituation. The binding capacity was expressed by the ratio of the nuclear (N) to the cytosol (C) uptake.

In contrast to these observations, the habituation of exploratory activity of adrenalectomized rats was significantly correlated to the N/C ratios.

The present study revealed that the corticosterone uptake of the hippocampus is greater in rats with a faster habituation to a novel environment than in rats with slower habituation. Moreover, the rats were adrenalectomized prior to the study and the individual differences in the uptake of corticosterone as well as its correlation to the behavioral processes seem to be intrinsic properties of the limbic structures. Nevertheless, further studies are required to understand whether biochemical and behavioral parameters are causally related or independent phenomena.

In studying the direct effect of ACTH on the limbic system, we found that the intravenous injection of 10 I.U. of ACTH produced a significant change in the corticosterone uptake in intact and adrenalectomized rats. The influence of ACTH on corticosterone binding was opposite in adrenalectomized animals. While, as a

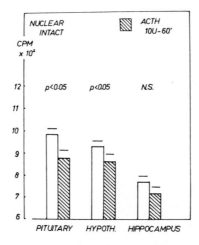

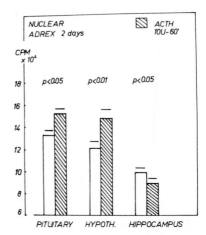

Fig. 7. Effect of ACTH administration on the corticosterone uptake of the nuclear fractions by the limbic structure and the pituitary gland in intact rats.

Fig. 8. Effect of ACTH administration on the corticosterone uptake of the nuclear fraction by the anterior pituitary and the limbic structures (hypothalamus and hippocampus) in adrenalectomized rats.

result of the endogenous corticosterone production the ACTH induced a decrease of the corticosterone uptake by the nuclear fraction in intact rats, an inverse effect has been observed in 2-day adrenalectomized groups. The hippocampal uptake was suppressed by ACTH treatment in both intact and adrenalectomized rats. An increase of the corticosterone-binding capacity of the cytosol fraction may be observed in the hippocampus of both intact and adrenalectomized rats while the other structures did not show similar alterations.

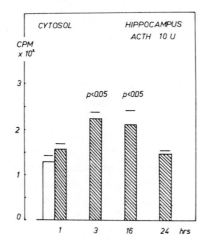

Fig. 9. Changes of cytosol-binding capacity of the hippocampus after ACTH treatment at different intervals in adrenalectomized rats.

A very characteristic time course of the changes of corticosterone uptake by the hippocampal cytosol fraction could be observed following ACTH injection in adrenalectomized rats. An increase of the binding capacity was already present 1 hr after ACTH administration, and this was followed by a peak lasting for 6–12 hr.

It is worth mentioning that the effect of ACTH under *in vitro* conditions could not be replicated, which might be due to inactivation of hormone or to involvement of other factors present under *in vivo* conditions.

In further experiments we have studied the effects of pituitary–adrenocortical hormones on the noradrenaline uptake of limbic structures. It was found that the administration of 5 mg corticosterone acetate did not induce alterations in the noradrenaline-binding capacity of the hypothalamus, brain stem hippocampus and neocortex when the rats were sacrificed 2 hr after the injection. The observations were performed in 2-day adrenalectomized male rats.

In contrast to these findings the administration of ACTH to 2-day adrenalectomized rats resulted in a significant decrease of the noradrenaline uptake in all structures studied in the present investigations.

The specificity of the uptake was controlled by *in vitro* saturation with 10^{-7} M noradrenaline and dopamine: both monoamines produced a marked suppression of the uptake of labeled noradrenaline. In other studies the saturation with serotonin, histamine and different adrenocortical and sex steroids proved unsuccessful.

The effect of ACTH on the noradrenaline uptake of the hippocampus showed a characteristic time course. Thus, the suppressive action may be observed as long as 12 hr after ACTH administration in the hippocampus and the neocortex.

The present study supports the hypothesis that ACTH exerts an influence on brain

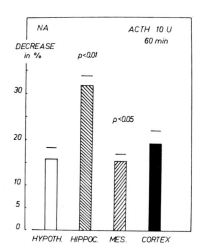 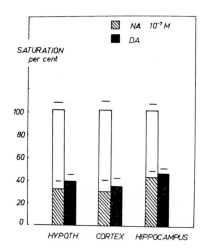

Fig. 10. Percentual decrease of the labeled noradrenaline pool of the hypothalamus, hippocampus, brain stem (MES.) and neocortex after ACTH treatment.

Fig. 11. Replacement of labeled noradrenaline by noradrenaline (NA) and dopamine (DA) in different brain tissues.

References p. 133–134

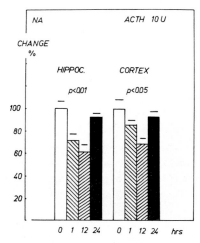

Fig. 12. Changes in the labeled noradrenaline (NA) pool of the hippocampus and the neocortex after ACTH administration at different intervals.

and behavior relations, and it modifies the hormone-sensitive receptor field of the limbic structures for both corticosteroids and catecholamines. A long-lasting effect of ACTH and its fragments on brain function was already recognized in both animal experiments and human studies (Endröczi et al., 1970; Endröczi, 1972a). The present data have suggested that the involvement of ACTH in controlling the corticosterone uptake by the limbic structures may be important in the homeostatic balance of neuroendocrine adaptation. Moreover, the influence of ACTH on catecholamine storage of limbic structures raised the possibility that such biochemical changes play a role in ACTH-adjusted behavioral reactions such as mood changes, exploratory activity, learning behavior and memory consolidation.

SUMMARY

Numerous observations indicate that both ACTH and corticosteroids can induce changes in habituation, learning and memory functions. The effect of corticosteroids seems to be mediated through the limbic system and specific binding receptors for corticosterone are involved in this mechanism. Recent observations revealed that ACTH administration produced changes in the binding capacity of the cytosol and nuclear compartment at the brain and pituitary level. It is assumed that ACTH plays a role in controlling the transfer of the steroid–receptor complex from cytosol to nuclear receptors. Similarly, the pituitary gonadotropins exert an influence on the estradiol uptake by the brain, pituitary and uterine receptors. After a transient increase of the binding sites as a result of the adrenalectomy and gonadectomy respectively, the binding capacity of target organs shows a decline which can be attributed to an increase of the pituitary tropic hormones.

Individual differences could be observed in the intensity of habituation to a new environment in rats. Accumulation of labeled corticosterone by hippocampal cells did not show significant differences in rats showing variable intensity of habituation. In contrast to this finding, the ratio of cytosol to nuclear binding sites was inversely correlated to the speed of habituation.

It is assumed that the accumulation of sex or adrenocortical hormones depends not only on the saturation of binding sites but the pituitary tropic hormones play a role in controlling the mechanism of binding at the target cell level.

REFERENCES

BAULIEU, E. E., RAYNAUD, J. P. AND MILGROM, E. (1970) Measurement of steroid binding proteins. In *Karolinska Symposia on Research Methods in Reproductive Endocrinology, Geneva*, WHO and Ford Found., Stockholm, pp. 104–121.

BINTZ, J. (1970) Time-dependent memory deficits of aversively motivated behavior. *Learning and Motivation*, **1**, 405–406.

BOHUS, B. (1970) The medial thalamus and the opposite effect of corticosteroids and adrenocorticotrophic hormone on avoidance extinction in the rat. *Acta physiol. Acad. Sci. hung.*, **38**, 217–223.

BOVET, D., BOVET-NITTI, F. AND OLIVERIO, A. (1969) Genetic aspects of learning and memory in mice. *Science*, **163**, 139–148.

BRUSH, F. R. AND LEVINE, S. (1966) Adrenocortical activity and avoidance learning as a function of time after fear conditioning. *Physiol. Behav.*, **1**, 309–311.

DESTRADE, C., SOUMIREU-MOURAT, B. AND CARDO, B. (1973) Effects of posttrial hippocampal stimulation on acquisition of operant behavior in the mouse. *Behav. Biol.*, **8**, 713–724.

DOUGLAS, R. J. (1967) The hippocampus and behavior. *Psychol. Bull.*, **67**, 416–442.

ENDRÖCZI, E. (1972a) *Limbic System, Learning and Pituitary–Adrenal Function*, Akadémiai Kiadó, Budapest.

ENDRÖCZI, E. (1972b) Pavlovian conditioning and adaptive hormones. In *Hormones and Behavior*, S. LEVINE (Ed.), Academic Press, New York, N.Y., pp. 173–207.

ENDRÖCZI, E., LISSÁK, K., FEKETE, T. AND DE WIED, D. (1970) Effects of ACTH on EEG habituation in human subjects. In *Pituitary, Adrenal and the Brain, Progress in Brain Research, Vol 32*, D. DE WIED AND W. M. H. WEIJNEN (Eds.), Elsevier, Amsterdam, pp. 254–263.

ERICKSON, C. K. AND PATEL, J. B. (1969) Facilitation of avoidance learning by posttrial hippocampal electrical stimulation. *J. comp. physiol. Psychol.*, **68**, 400–406.

EVANS, H. L. (1971) Behavioral effects of metamphetamine and methyltyrosine in the rat. *J. Pharmacol. exp. Ther.*, **176**, 244–254.

FONTENAY, M. J., LeCORNEC, M., ZACZINSKA, M. C., DEBARLE, P. ET BOISSIER, S. et J. R. (1970) Problèmes posés par l'utilization de trois tests de comportement du rat pour l'étude des médicaments psychotropes. *J. Pharm. Chim. Paris*, **1**, 243–254.

IZQUIERDO, I., ORSINGHER, O. A. AND OGURA, A. (1972) Hippocampal facilitation and RNA build-up in response to stimulation in rats with a low inborn learning ability. *Behav. Biol.*, **3**, 699–707.

JARRARD, L. E. AND ISAACSON, R. L. (1965) Hippocampal ablation in rats: effects of intertrial interval. *Nature (Lond.)*, **207**, 109–110.

KAMIN, L. J. (1957) Retention of an incompletely learned avoidance response. *J. comp. physiol. Psychol.*, **50**, 457–460.

KLEIN, S. B. AND SPEAR, N. E. (1970) Forgetting by the rat after intermediate intervals ("Kamin effect") as retrieval failure. *J. comp. physiol. Psychol.*, **71**, 165–170.

LISSÁK, K. AND ENDRÖCZI, E. (1965) *The Neuroendocrine Control of Adaptation*, Pergamon Press, London, p. 196.

McEWEN, B. S., WEISS, J. M. AND SCHWARTZ, L. S. (1970) Retention of corticosterone by cell nuclei from brain regions of adrenalectomized rats. *Brain Research*, **17**, 471–482.

McGAUGH, J. L. (1972) Impairment and facilitation of memory consolidation. *Activ. nerv. sup. (Praha)*, **14**, 64–74.

MILNER, B. (1959) The memory defect in bilateral hippocampal lesions. *Psychiat. Res. Rep.*, **11**, 43–52.

OLIVERIO, A., ELEFTHERIOU, B. E. AND BAILEY, D. W. (1973) Exploratory activity: genetic analysis of its modification by scopolamine and amphetamine. *Physiol. Behav.*, **10**, 893–899.

OTT, T. AND MATTHIES, H. (1973) Some effects of RNA precursors on development and maintenance of long-term memory: hippocampal and cortical pre- and post-training application of RNA precursors. *Psychopharmacologia (Berl.)*, **28**, 195–204.

PRÉDA, I., KÁRPÁTI, P. AND ENDRÖCZI, E. (1975) Studies on noradrenaline uptake after coronary occlusion in rats. *Acta physiol. Acad. Sci. hung.*, in press.

SCOVILLE, W. B. (1954) The limbic loci in man. *J. Neurosurg.*, **11**, 64–66.

STEIN, D. G. AND CHOROVER, S. (1968) Effects of posttrial electrical stimulation of hippocampus and caudate nucleus on maze learning in the rat. *Physiol. Behav.*, **3**, 787–791.

WIED, D. DE (1967) Opposite effects of ACTH and glucocorticoids on extinction of conditioned avoidance behavior. In *Hormonal Steroids*, L. MARTINI, F. FASCHINI AND M. MOTTO (Eds.), Mouton, The Hague, pp. 945–951.

The Role of Vasopressin in Memory Processes

Tj. B. van WIMERSMA GREIDANUS, B. BOHUS and D. de WIED

Rudolf Magnus Institute for Pharmacology, University of Utrecht, Medical Faculty, Utrecht (The Netherlands)

During the last 10 years evidence has accumulated that peptides from pituitary origin play an important role in acquisition and/or extinction of conditioned avoidance behavior. Administration of pitressin, a crude vasopressin preparation extracted from posterior pituitary tissue, induces resistance to extinction of a shuttlebox avoidance response. A subcutaneous injection of pitressin tannate in oil every other day either during acquisition or during extinction increases resistance to extinction of the conditioned avoidance response (CAR) (de Wied and Bohus, 1966). No or only minor extinction was found in pitressin-treated animals, in contrast to placebo-treated rats, in which the response extinguished during the period of observation. These results suggest that pitressin has a "long-term" effect on the preservation of a CAR irrespective of the time of treatment.

The principle present in pitressin responsible for this "long-term" effect seemed to be vasopressin and proof of this assumption was obtained in experiments in which a pole jump avoidance response was studied. A single subcutaneous injection of graded doses (0.6 and 1.8 μg) of synthetic lysine-8-vasopressin (LVP), immediately after the first extinction session, appeared to exhibit a dose-dependent long-term inhibitory effect on extinction of the pole jumping avoidance response (van Wimersma Greidanus *et al.*, 1973). Other structurally and physiologically related peptides like oxytocin, angiotensin, insulin or growth hormone failed to affect the rate of extinction of the CAR following administration of comparable amounts (de Wied, 1971).

Closely related peptides, such as arginine-8-vasopressin (AVP), the rat's naturally occurring antidiuretic principle, and desglycinamide–lysine-8-vasopressin (DG–LVP), a peptide isolated from hog pituitaries (Lande *et al.*, 1971) which has only minor antidiuretic, pressor and ACTH releasing activities, have a similar effect on avoidance behavior as LVP (de Wied *et al.*, 1974). Thus, the behavioral effect of vasopressin is not related to its effects on water and salt metabolism nor on the circulation.

LVP not only affects active avoidance behavior, but also passive avoidance behavior, as studied in a simple "step through" passive avoidance situation. This situation uses the innate response of rats in preferring darkness to light. The apparatus consists of a dark box connected to an illuminated elevated platform (Ader *et al.*, 1972). Rats are placed on the platform and latency to enter the dark box is recorded. This latency generally amounts to a few seconds. One trial is given on day 1; three such trials on day 2. At the end of the third trial on day 2, animals receive an electric footshock (EFS). Latency to enter is subsequently determined 24 and 48 hr after the learning trial during extinction sessions with an observation time of maximally 300 sec.

Avoidance latency is a function of intensity and duration of the EFS (Ader *et al.*, 1972). Following low shock intensities (0.25 mA, 1 sec), latencies to enter the black box were approximately 25 sec. Subcutaneous injection of LVP 1 hr prior to the first extinction session or immediately after the learning (shock) trial markedly increases avoidance latency, *i.e.* preserves passive avoidance behavior (Ader and de Wied, 1972). Indeed, avoidance latency is still augmented during the second extinction (retention) trial, 48 hr after the learning trial. Thus, long-term preservation of avoidance behavior is also observed in a passive avoidance situation.

The significance of vasopressin for the consolidation of learned behavior is also demonstrated by experiments in rats with hereditary hypothalamic diabetes insipidus (DI) (Brattleboro strain), which lack the ability to synthesize vasopressin (Valtin and Schroeder, 1964). It appeared that homozygous DI rats in contrast to heterozygous littermates were unable to retain the passive avoidance response. Whereas avoidance latency in heterozygous animals increased with the intensity of the EFS 24 and 48 hr after the learning trial, homozygous rats failed to exhibit significant passive avoidance behavior. Even a high shock intensity of 1 mA presented for up to 10 sec during the learning trial was unable to induce passive avoidance behavior compared to hetero-zygous DI rats. A single subcutaneous injection of 1 μg AVP or DG–LVP to homo-zygous DI rats immediately after the learning trial restored avoidance latency towards the same values as those found in heterozygous animals. The responsiveness to EFS of homozygous and heterozygous DI rats appeared to be similar. No difference was found between the shock thresholds for the response categories flinch or jerk,

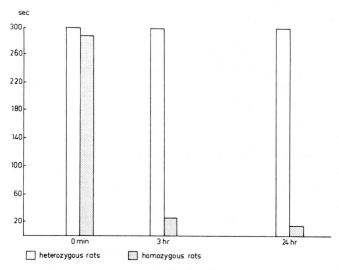

Fig. 1. Retention of passive avoidance behavior in rats homozygous or heterozygous for hereditary diabetes insipidus.

jump and run in homozygous and heterozygous Brattleboro rats. Moreover a single injection of DG–LVP did not affect the responsiveness to EFS. In addition, gross behavior as measured in an open field was the same in homozygous and heterozygous DI animals.

In order to determine whether vasopressin affects learning or memory processes, homozygous DI rats were trained in the passive avoidance test and retention was measured immediately after the learning trial (1 mA for 3 sec) and at 3 and 24 hr after the EFS. The animals showed complete passive avoidance behavior when retested immediately after the learning trial. Avoidance latency of all animals was maximal and lasted during the total observation period of 300 sec. Passive avoidance behavior was markedly reduced at 3 hr after the learning trial and not present at 24 hr after the shock trial (Fig. 1). Thus, the absence of vasopressin does not affect learning *per se*, but memory consolidation.

Acquisition of a shuttle-box and pole jump avoidance response was not so much disturbed as passive avoidance behavior in homozygous DI rats. Although these rats were inferior in acquiring a shuttle-box avoidance response as compared to heterozygous controls the learning criterion of 80% CARs was eventually achieved by the homozygous DI rats. Extinction was, however, facilitated in homozygous DI animals. Acquisition of a pole jumping avoidance response did not differ between the two categories of animals, but extinction was more rapid in homozygous than in heterozygous DI rats. The results of these studies are in agreement with those obtained from previous experiments in posterior lobectomized rats.

Removal of the posterior pituitary from Wistar rats facilitates extinction of a shuttle-box avoidance response in these animals (de Wied, 1965) although acquisition of the response is normal. This again indicates that posterior pituitary principles are involved in the consolidation of behavioral experiences. Pitressin and LVP normalize extinction of shuttle-box avoidance behavior in posterior lobectomized rats (de Wied, 1965). Posterior lobectomy does not completely remove vasopressin since part of the structure in the anterior hypothalamus responsible for its synthesis remains intact.

Central blockade of available vasopressin might be obtained by using serum containing specific antibodies against vasopressin, administered directly into the lateral ventricle of the brain.

Antibodies against AVP were raised by coupling AVP to thyroglobulin by ethylcarbodiimide according to Skowsky and Fisher (1972) and the product was emulsified in Freund's complete adjuvant and injected i.m. into young adult New Zealand rabbits. An initial dose of antigen corresponding to 0.4 mg AVP (300 I.U./mg) was given, followed by a booster of half this amount every 3 weeks. The first collection of antiserum was performed 18 weeks after the initial injection.

Undiluted antiserum was administered in an amount of 1 μl into the lateral ventricle either 0.5 hr before or immediately after the learning trial of 0.75 mA for 3 sec in passive avoidance conditioning. Retention sessions were performed at 24 and 48 hr after the learning trial. No passive avoidance response was found in animals treated with antibodies against AVP, while a control group, treated with normal rabbit

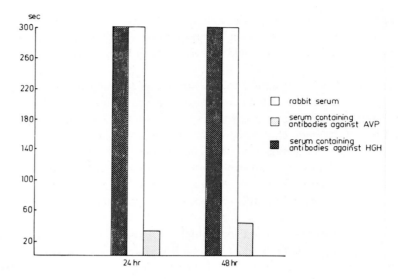

Fig. 2. Retention of passive avoidance behavior in rats following intraventricular injection of anti-AVP serum, anti-HGH (human growth hormone) serum or rabbit serum immediately after the learning trial.

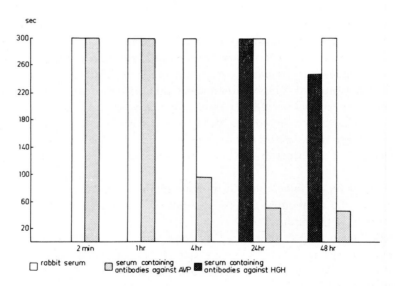

Fig. 3. Retention of passive avoidance behavior in rats following intraventricular injection of anti-AVP serum, anti-HGH (human growth hormone) serum or rabbit serum 30 min prior to the learning trial.

serum, showed the maximal latency score of 300 sec. Treatment with antibodies against growth hormone resulted in a passive avoidance behavior no different from that of controls (Fig. 2). Also in this situation the absence of vasopressin induced a disturbance in memory consolidation rather than in learning, because passive avoidance behavior was present when the rats treated with antibodies against AVP were tested for avoidance latency scores at 2 min or 1 hr after the learning trial. All animals showed the maximal latency score, when tested at these time intervals between learning and retention trial. Passive avoidance behavior was markedly reduced at 4 hr and absent at 24 and 48 hr after the learning trial (Fig. 3).

The median latency score of the animals which received 1 μl of rabbit serum containing anti-AVP antibodies into the lateral ventricle was 93 sec for the retention trial at 4 hr after the learning trial, and 49 and 44 sec during the retention trials at 24 or 48 hr, respectively. The latency scores of rats treated with normal rabbit serum reached the maximum time of 300 sec, independent of the time interval between the learning trial and the retention trial. When this anti-serum against AVP was intraventricularly administered 0.5 hr before the acquisition sessions of a pole jumping avoidance response, it appeared that the acquisition of this active response did not differ from that of rats injected with normal rabbit serum. However, extinction of the pole jumping avoidance response was markedly facilitated in the animals treated with anti-AVP serum, although the treatment was not continued during extinction (Fig. 4).

These findings clearly demonstrate that vasopressin and/or vasopressin analogues are involved in memory consolidation. Rats which lack vasopressin show a severe deficit in one-trial passive avoidance behavior which can be restored by the administration of vasopressin and a moderate deficit in active avoidance behavior in which multiple learning trials are used. On the other hand, exogenous vasopressin and vasopressin analogues can induce resistance to extinction of a once acquired response

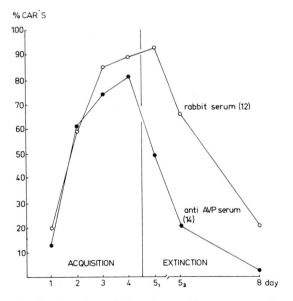

Fig. 4. Acquisition and extinction of a pole jumping avoidance response in rats following intraventricular injection of anti-AVP serum or rabbit serum during acquisition.

References p. 141

regardless of whether preservation of the response has any physiological advantage or not. The mechanisms by which vasopressin affects memory processes are not well understood and remain to be elucidated. Recent observations on the protective effect of DG–LVP on puromycin-induced memory loss in mice (Lande *et al.*, 1972) point to interference with protein synthesis. It may be that vasopressin or closely related peptides affect protein synthesis in neurons belonging to the midbrain limbic circuit, which is probably the site of behavioral action of this neuropeptide (van Wimersma Greidanus *et al.*, 1975) and in this way enhance the storage and/or retrieval of recently acquired information or experience.

SUMMARY

It has been established that vasopressin stimulates the consolidation of conditioned avoidance behavior. Administration of vasopressin and vasopressin analogues induces resistance to the extinction of active and passive avoidance behavior. In fact, removal of the posterior and intermediate lobe of the pituitary facilitates extinction of a shuttle-box avoidance response and this abnormal behavior can be normalized by administration of vasopressin. Similar observations were made in rats with hereditary diabetes insipidus (D.I.) (Brattleboro strain) which lack the ability to synthesize vasopressin. Homozygous D.I. rats, in contrast to heterozygous controls, failed to display retention of a one-trial passive avoidance response even at high shock intensity punishment, indicating a severe memory deficit, which can be restored by administration of vasopressin or vasopressin analogues. No difference was found between these two groups of animals in responsiveness to inescapable footshock and in behavior in an open field. Acquisition of multitrial active avoidance behavior was not severely disturbed in homozygous D.I. rats, although extinction was facilitated.

Administration of antibodies against vasopressin directly into the lateral ventricle of the brain of Wistar rats, or immediately after the learning trial of a passive avoidance response, induces the same memory deficit as in homozygous D.I. rats, whereas this treatment during acquisition of a pole jumping avoidance response again facilitates extinction. These results support the hypothesis implicating an important role for vasopressin in memory processes.

ACKNOWLEDGEMENTS

The authors thank Dr. Lesley H. Rees (Department of Chemical Pathology, Bartholomews Hospital, London) for supplying anti-HGH serum; Angèle Balvers and Ruud Buys for their excellent technical help, and Linda Philbert-Hutzezon for her secretarial work.

REFERENCES

ADER, R. AND WIED, D. DE (1972) Effects of lysine vasopressin on passive avoidance learning. *Psychon. Sci.*, **29**, 46–48.

ADER, R., WEIJNEN, J. A. W. M. AND MOLEMAN, P. (1972) Retention of a function of the intensity and duration of electric shock. *Psychon. Sci.*, **26**, 125–128.

LANDE, S., WITTER, A. AND WIED, D. DE (1971) Pituitary peptides: an octapeptide that stimulates conditioned avoidance acquisition in hypophysectomized rats. *J. biol. Chem.*, **246**, 2058–2062.

SKOWSKY, W. R. AND FISHER, D. A. (1972) The use of thyroglobulin to induce antigenicity to small molecules. *J. Lab. clin. Med.*, **80**, 134–144.

VALTIN, H. AND SCHROEDER, H. A. (1964) Familial hypothalamic diabetes insipidus in rats (Brattleboro strain). *Amer. J. Physiol.*, **206**, 425–430.

WIED, D. DE (1965) The influence of the posterior and intermediate lobe of the pituitary and pituitary peptides on the maintenance of a conditioned avoidance response in rats. *Int. J. Neuropharmacol.*, **4**, 157–167.

WIED, D. DE AND BOHUS, B. (1966) Long term and short term effect on retention of a conditioned avoidance response in rats by treatment respectively with long acting pitressin or α-MSH. *Nature (Lond.)*, **212**, 1484–1488.

WIED, D. DE (1971) Long term effect of vasopressin on the maintenance of a conditioned avoidance response in rats. *Nature (Lond.)*, **232**, 58–60.

WIED, D. DE, BOHUS, B. AND WIMERSMA GREIDANUS, TJ. B. VAN (1974) The hypothalamic neuro-hypophyseal system and the preservation of conditioned avoidance behavior in rats. In *Integrative Hypothalamic Activity*, *Progr. Brain Res.*, Vol. *41*, D. F. SWAAB AND J. P. SCHADÉ (Eds.), Elsevier, Amsterdam, pp. 417–428.

WIMERSMA GREIDANUS, TJ. B. VAN, BOHUS, B. AND WIED, D. DE (1973) Effects on peptide hormones on behavior. In *Progress in Endocrinology, Proc. 4th Int. Congr. Endocrinol., Washington, D.C., 1972*, Excerpta Medica International Congress Series No. 273, Excerpta Medica, Amsterdam, pp. 197–201.

WIMERSMA GREIDANUS, TJ. B. VAN, BOHUS, B. AND WIED, D. DE (1975) CNS sites of action of ACTH, MSH and vasopressin, in relation to avoidance behavior. In *Anatomical Neuroendocrinology, Proc. Conference on Neurobiology of CNS–Hormone Interactions, Chapel Hill, N. C., 14–16 May, 1974*, W. E. STUMPF AND L. D. GRANT (Eds.), Karger, Basel, in press.

Behavioral and Electrographic Changes in Rat and Man after MSH

ABBA J. KASTIN, CURT A. SANDMAN, LOIS O. STRATTON,
ANDREW V. SCHALLY AND LYLE H. MILLER

Veterans Administration Hospital and Tulane University School of Medicine, and University of New Orleans, New Orleans, La., Ohio State University, Columbus, Ohio, and Temple University, Philadelphia, Pa. (U.S.A.)

Our approach to the actions of melanocyte-stimulating hormone (MSH) on the central nervous system (CNS) has been two-fold: first, to determine whether MSH has any effect on the CNS of man; second, to attempt to identify the behavioral systems which are involved by also studying animals. A remarkable part of this second aspect involves special attention to the role of MSH during development of the organism. Each part of this general approach is different from that taken by others. The early clinical studies (Lerner and McGuire, 1961, 1964) with MSH were concerned mainly with its pigmentary effects. Among the early animal studies of the effects of MSH on the nervous system, one group of investigators looked only at the spinal cord and electric discharge (Krivoy and Guillemin, 1961; Krivoy et al., 1962). Another group, using a neurophysiological approach, tested only stretching activity and yawning for several years (Ferrari et al., 1961; Gessa et al., 1967). A more extensive behavioral effort was made by de Wied and his collaborators (1967, 1969) but, for the most part, until recently (Garrud et al., 1974) they almost exclusively restricted themselves to the conditioned avoidance response, and, like the earlier investigations of Murphy and Miller (1955) and Miller and Ogawa (1962), initially approached the problem from a focus on ACTH (corticotropin) rather than MSH itself. All of these excellent pioneering approaches contributed greatly to our knowledge in this area of study.

Initially, in our animal studies, we examined the effects of MSH in appetitive tasks. In the first such study, hungry rats were placed in a T-maze and trained to run to the arm of the maze which contained food. During extinction, the animals did so more often and faster if they received MSH than if they were injected with diluent (Sandman et al., 1969). Similarly, hungry rats trained to press a lever in order to obtain food on a fixed ratio of reinforcement and injected with synthetic α-MSH were found to have delayed extinction of the task as compared with control rats (Kastin et al., 1974). Our findings with an appetitive task have been confirmed recently by de Wied and his collaborators (Garrud et al., 1974).

Each of the appetitive tasks mentioned above was performed in a relatively simple apparatus. Although the major effect of MSH was observed during extinction, there was a tendency in one of these appetitive experiments toward facilitated acquisition of the task (Sandman *et al.*, 1969), and this was seen in an experiment involving avoidance (Sandman *et al.*, 1973a). It seemed possible (Kastin *et al.*, 1973b) that the difficulty of the task might interact with the effects of MSH, as we had found previously in a different type of study (Stratton and Kastin, 1973a). We reasoned that perhaps a complex maze which could provide more choices to the rat would make a slight effect of MSH on initial learning more readily apparent. This possibility was tested with hungry rats placed in a 12-choice Warden maze. MSH was found to increase running speed as well as reduce the variability and number of errors during acquisition of the maze (Stratton and Kastin, submitted).

Although speed of running may indicate increased motivation, it can also reflect a general increased motor activity. Under basal laboratory conditions, we have previously shown that MSH does not affect activity as measured by an instrument designed to detect movements of a rat across tuned electromagnetic resonant circuits (Kastin *et al.*, 1973c) or by time spent in light or dark alleys of a T-maze (Stratton *et al.*, 1973b). This tended to rule out increased motor activity as a complete explanation for the behavioral effects of MSH. However, the activity detected by these methods may be more "aimless" than that shown by the more exploratory tests of open field behavior. A tendency toward increased activity was found in one study of open field behavior involving animals previously receiving 0.8 mA electric shock and α-MSH (Nockton *et al.*, 1972), but not β-MSH or $ACTH_{1-10}$ (Weijnen and Slangen, 1970). In another study in which rats were tested in a large drum, a statistically significant effect of MSH on the number of quadrants entered by the rat was observed (Brown *et al.*, 1974). In a third study, rats treated with MSH showed significantly greater open field activity and hind-leg rearing behavior than control animals. An injection of D-amphetamine together with MSH had a greater effect on this activity than injection with either MSH or D-amphetamine alone (Sandman *et al.*, in preparation-a).

If it is possible that rats injected with MSH might be more active, then this might account at least in part for delayed extinction of the conditioned avoidance response, but it probably could not account for the inhibition of a passive avoidance response which we observed in a two-chambered shuttle box (Sandman *et al.*, 1971b). However, one might object that even in such a passive avoidance task, a rat receiving MSH could be more active in the "safe" chamber and yet still be considered "passive" because it did not enter the second chamber where it previously had received electric shock. This possibility was rendered unlikely by one of the activity studies (Kastin *et al.*, 1973c) and was ruled out by the use of a small platform in place of one of the chambers. In this type of restricted passive avoidance task, administration of MSH still resulted in increased resistance to extinction as evidenced by a longer time on the platform, regardless of whether the MSH was injected during acquisition, extinction, or both (Dempsey *et al.*, 1972). Moreover, pigmented rats were tested in this "restricted" passive avoidance task whereas albinos were tested in the two-chamber task.

When albino rats were tested in a simple reversal procedure involving escape from shock in a Y maze, MSH was found to hasten performance of the reversal task (Sandman *et al.*, 1972). In a somewhat similar procedure involving a slightly different apparatus and avoidance rather than escape from shock, MSH was again associated with a faster reversal of the brightness discrimination task in albino rats (Sandman *et al.*, 1973a). However, the tendency for hooded rats to reverse faster after MSH was not statistically significant, a finding which may have been influenced by the faster acquisition and reversal by the hooded than the albino rats. Differences between strains of rats were also found for dark preference (Stratton *et al.*, 1973b). It is likely that the genetic differences and the lighting conditions under which the rats were reared are more important predisposing factors for maximal MSH effects than the color of their skin. The illumination used when the animals are tested must also be considered (Sandman *et al.*, 1971b, 1972; Stratton *et al.*, 1973b), since light probably inhibits the release of MSH (Kastin *et al.*, 1967).

The level of electric shock used in avoidance tasks is also an important variable. If rats were trained in a two-way shuttle box to avoid shock presented at two levels of intensity, MSH was found to facilitate learning at low but not at high levels of shock (Stratton and Kastin, 1974). This finding emphasizes that we have found facilitation of acquisition of avoidance tasks (Sandman *et al.*, 1973a; Stratton and Kastin, 1974) as well as appetitive tasks (Stratton and Kastin, submitted) after administration of MSH.

The stage of development of the rat may also influence the response to MSH. Infant albino rats were injected with MSH once a day from the age of 2–7 days in two studies conducted at Ohio State University. In one of these studies (Beckwith *et al.*, in preparation), the rats were tested at the age of 33 days in a difficult operant task. After being trained to press a lever for food, these hungry animals could only be reinforced again with food if they waited for 20 sec between responses. An efficiency ratio of responses to reinforcements was calculated for each day on this "DRL 20" task. In the beginning, the rats which had previously been injected with MSH made significantly more responses than either the rats injected with diluent or the uninjected controls. This probably contributed to the poor initial efficiency ratio of the rats receiving MSH. However, by the time that half of the training on the DRL 20 schedule had been received, the animals injected with MSH showed superior efficiency.

In the second study involving rats injected with MSH from the age of 2–7 days, a different type of task was used (Sandman *et al.*, in preparation-b). These animals were tested for the first time when they were 90 days old with a brightness discrimination problem in a modified Y-maze (Thompson–Bryant box). The original visual problem involved discrimination between black and white cues. After this task was acquired, the problem was reversed but still involved black and white. Subsequently the rats were required to learn an extradimensional shift in which brightness was not relevant, but rather position (*e.g.* right or left). Although injections of MSH facilitated performance of the discrimination problem, the results appeared to be complicated by differences between male and female rats. What is striking, however, is that administration of MSH to rats in the first few days of life seems to exert effects which persist into adulthood. This implies the possibility of a permanent organizational effect of MSH on the brain. Whether any inferences can be drawn from this finding which can be applied to the human being is not known, but MSH has been found in the pituitary of every human fetus in which it was measured (Kastin *et al.*, 1968b).

Another variable which modulates the effects of MSH on behavior is the degree of training. This was demonstrated in a similar task with albino rats treated with MSH or a control solution of diluent and tested with a visual discrimination problem in the Thompson–Bryant box. After acquisition of the original visual discrimination problem, half the rats were overtrained and all the animals were tested with a spatial discrimination rather than the visual type of problem. Not only did overtraining significantly disrupt performance during this spatial or extradimensional shift, but overtraining together with MSH treatment resulted in even poorer performance on the changed extradimensional dimension (Sandman *et al.*, 1974). The effect of MSH on an intradimensional shift to cues of the same type of visual problem had previously been tested in the Thompson–Bryant box. It was found that administration of MSH resulted in facilitation of the shift (Sandman *et al.*, 1973a). This pattern of improved performance on the intradimensional shift but deteriorated performance on the extra-dimensional shift after administration of MSH to rats is similar to the pattern we found in normal human beings tested with an active fragment of MSH (α-MSH$_{4-10}$ = ACTH$_{4-10}$) in intradimensional and extradimensional shifts (Sandman *et al.*, in preparation-b).

α-MSH$_{4-10}$ was given to 10 healthy young men 21–30 years old and the results compared with those obtained from a similar group of 10 men given diluent in a "double-blind" procedure in which neither the investigators nor the subjects knew the contents of the solutions which were infused i.v. at a constant rate for 4 hr. Behavioral tests were conducted three times: during the first 2 hr of the infusion; during the second 2 hr of the infusion; and during a 1-hr period after the infusion was completed. Blood samples were obtained before and after the infusion for determination of plasma cortisol. Since no significant difference in cortisol levels was noted between the two groups of subjects, it seemed reasonable to conclude that any changes found after infusion of α-MSH$_{4-10}$ were not due to an action of this peptide on the adrenal cortex. Earlier studies of the CNS actions of ACTH in animals and man were usually extremely difficult to interpret because they did not adequately take into consideration the secondary effects of ACTH on the adrenal gland.

In our study (Sandman *et al.*, submitted), all the men were trained on a two-choice discrimination problem in which color (*e.g.* red) was the relevant dimension of discrimination. Two objects of different color and different shape were placed before the subject. Each time this was done, he was instructed to choose one of the two objects and was immediately informed whether his choice was correct. After learning the first correct dimension, he was given three additional series of tests. In the first, a simple reversal problem, color remained the relevant dimension but the reinforced cue shifted to the second color (*e.g.* from red to green). In the next test, the intra-dimensional shift, neither red nor green was correct but rather another color such as blue. For the third test, the extradimensional shift, color was no longer reinforced, but instead the shape of the test object (*e.g.* square, regardless of color). At no time was the subject told when the "rules" had changed so that he was receiving another of the three types of test. He was required to realize without instruction that previously rewarded cues were no longer being reinforced and to attempt to determine a newly defined correct response.

In the initial testing, both groups of normal men performed the intradimensional shift relatively rapidly and the extradimensional shift more slowly, as expected. After the infusion, the normal subjects not receiving the MSH peptide improved on the extradimensional shift. In contrast, the subjects receiving α-MSH$_{4-10}$ did better on the intradimensional shift and worse on the extradimensional shift, similar to the performance of rats tested with equivalent problems.

These concept formation procedures involving visual discrimination are considered to be very sensitive indicators of the state of attention of the subject (MacIntosh 1965, 1969). That MSH or its active component affects attention in normal men was further supported by the results from the Benton Visual Retention Test in which a subject is instructed to reproduce geometric forms shown briefly a few seconds previously. After receiving α-MSH$_{4-10}$, the subjects improved significantly in this test. α-MSH$_{4-10}$ also resulted in better performance in the Rod and Frame test, in which the subject is asked to align a vertical pole within a square frame which is placed in several different spatial configurations.

The improvement in the Benton Visual Retention Test in man after α-MSH$_{4-10}$ confirmed our earlier finding of a similar improvement in normal as well as hypo-pituitary subjects after infusion of α-MSH (Kastin *et al.*, 1971). No improvement in verbal retention as measured by the Wechsler Memory Scale was found in that study. In this investigation also, infusion for 4 hr of 10 mg α-MSH, essentially equivalent to ACTH$_{1-13}$, did not stimulate the release of cortisol. By placing disc EEG electrodes over the right somatosensory cortical area and elsewhere on the scalp and administering threshold electrical stimulation of the median nerve, we were able to measure averaged somatosensory cortical evoked responses in a computer of average transients. The increases in the averaged somatosensory evoked responses were so great that they could be seen directly on single trials of the EEG. They were greatest when the subjects were attentive to the electric stimulation. The changes in EEG frequency were not as dramatic as those seen in the first clinical study of the effects of MSH on the CNS. In that study performed in 1966 (Kastin *et al.*, 1968a), half of the subjects showed EEG changes. EEG changes have also been observed in the rabbit (Dyster-Aas and Krakau, 1965), rat (Sandman *et al.*, 1971a), and frog (Denman *et al.*, 1972) after administration of MSH.

The effects of MSH on the EEG of normal men were examined more carefully in a study in which 10 mg α-MSH$_{4-10}$ was injected rapidly i.v. as a bolus (Miller *et al.*, 1974). The occipital EEG was analyzed in terms of the power output from 4 band-pass filters. The 10 subjects who received the α-MSH$_{4-10}$ exhibited a statistically significant increase in the power output of the 12+ Hz and the 7–12 Hz frequency bands as well as a slight decrease in the output of the 3–7 Hz band. They also showed significantly more 7–12 Hz activity than did controls. Whereas the

References p. 148–150

subjects receiving diluent as a control showed habituation of the EEG response arousal pattern, the subjects receiving the MSH peptide did not habituate but persisted in the arousal pattern. Endröczi *et al.* (1970) observed a similar effect with $ACTH_{1-10}$ and $ACTH_{1-24}$. We also found that injection of the MSH peptide resulted in improvement in the Benton Visual Retention Test, as was observed previously (Kastin *et al.*, 1971) and subsequently (Sandman *et al.*, submitted). In this study (Miller *et al.*, 1974) in which $\alpha\text{-MSH}_{4-10}$ was injected stat as well as in the study in which it was infused for 4 hr (Sandman *et al.*, submitted), decreased anxiety as measured by the State–Trait Anxiety Inventory was found.

It is not known whether the changes associated with the administration of exogenous MSH to rat and man represent exaggerations of physiologically occurring responses, and, at the moment, it does not seem crucial to determine this. Stress releases endogenous MSH (Kastin *et al.*, 1969), and this release can be "conditioned" (Sandman *et al.*, 1973b) and frequently separated from the release of ACTH (Gosbee *et al.*, 1970; Dunn *et al.*, 1972; Kastin *et al.*, 1969; Kastin *et al.*, 1973a; Sandman *et al.*, 1973b). Consideration of the physiologically adaptive role of MSH in the camouflage of lower vertebrates and its phylogenetic persistence makes it entirely reasonable for MSH to have an adaptive role in mammals. The fact that radioactive MSH is localized in certain areas of the brain (Dupont *et al.*, 1974; Pelletier *et al.*, submitted), that MSH affects blood flow differentially in the brain (Goldman *et al.*, submitted), or that MSH changes the turnover of certain biogenic amines in certain areas of the brain (Kostrzewa *et al.*, in preparation; Spirtes *et al.*, submitted), still does not identify the exact CNS function of MSH. Nevertheless, we believe that a logical investigative approach from several different directions is most likely to enhance our understanding of the role(s) of MSH.

SUMMARY

MSH or its active component was administered to rats and human beings in a series of studies. The behavioral and electrographic changes which were observed reinforce the concept that MSH has extra-pigmentary actions in mammals.

ACKNOWLEDGEMENTS

The $\alpha\text{-MSH}_{4-10} = ACTH_{4-10}$ was supplied by Organon International BV, The Netherlands, under the code name OI 63.

This study was supported in part by grants from the Veterans Administration and NIH (NS 07664) and the Graduate School of Ohio State University.

REFERENCES

BECKWITH, W. E., SANDMAN, C. A., HOTHERSALL, D. AND KASTIN, A. J. (1975) Effects of early injection of MSH on infant operant behavior, in preparation.

BROWN, G. M., UHLIR, I. V., SEGGIE, J., SCHALLY, A. V. AND KASTIN, A. J. (1974) Effect of septal lesions on plasma levels of MSH, corticosterone, GH and prolactin before and after exposure to novel environment: Role of MSH in the septal syndrome. *Endocrinology*, **94**, 583–587.

DEMPSEY, G. L., KASTIN, A. J. AND SCHALLY, A. V. (1972) The effects of MSH on a restricted passive avoidance response. *Horm. Behav.*, **3**, 333–337.

DENMAN, P. M., MILLER, L. H., SANDMAN, C. A., SCHALLY, A. V. AND KASTIN, A. J. (1972) Electro-physiological correlates of melanocyte-stimulating hormone activity in the frog. *J. comp. physiol. Psychol.*, **80**, 59–65.

DUNN, J. D., KASTIN, A. J., CARRILLO, A. J. AND SCHALLY, A. V. (1972) Additional evidence for dissociation of MSH and ACTH release. *J. Endocr.*, **55**, 463–464.

DUPONT, A., KASTIN, A. J., LABRIE, F., PELLETIER, G., PUVIANI, R. AND SCHALLY, A. V. (1974) Organ distribution of radioactivity after injection of $[^{125}I]$-α-melanocyte stimulating hormone in rat and mouse. *J. Endocr.*, in press.

DYSTER-AAS, K. AND KRAKAU, C. E. T. (1965) General effects of α-melanocyte stimulating hormone in the rabbit. *Acta endocr. (Kbh.)*, **48**, 609–618.

ENDRÖCZI, E., LISSÁK, K., FEKETE, T. AND DE WIED, D. (1970) Effects of ACTH on EEG habituation in human subjects. In *Pituitary, Adrenal and the Brain, Progr. Brain Res., Vol. 32*, D. DE WIED AND J. A. W. M. WEIJNEN (Eds.), Elsevier, Amsterdam, pp. 254–262.

FERRARI, W., GESSA, G. L. AND VARGIU, L. (1961) Stretching activity in dogs intracisternally injected with a synthetic melanocyte-stimulating hexapeptide. *Experientia (Basel)*, **17**, 90.

GARRUD, P., GRAY, J. A. AND DE WIED, D. (1974) Pituitary–adrenal hormones and extinction of rewarded behaviour in the rat. *Physiol. Behav.*, **12**, 109–119.

GESSA, G. L., PISANO, M., VARGIU, L., CRABAI, F. AND FERRARI, W. (1967) Stretching and yawning movements after intracerebral injection of ACTH. *Rev. canad. Biol.*, **26**, 229–236.

GOLDMAN, H., SANDMAN, C. A., KASTIN, A. J. AND MURPHY, S., MSH affects regional perfusion of the brain. *Pharm. Biochem. Behav.*, Submitted for publication.

GOSBEE, J. L., KRAICER, J., KASTIN, A. J. AND SCHALLY, A. V. (1970) A functional relationship between the pars intermedia and ACTH secretion in the rat. *Endocrinology*, **86**, 560–567.

KASTIN, A. J., SCHALLY, A. V., VIOSCA, S., BARRETT, L. AND REDDING, T. W. (1967) MSH activity in the pituitaries of rats exposed to constant illumination. *Neuroendocrinology*, **2**, 257–262.

KASTIN, A. J., KULLANDER, S., BORGLIN, N. E., DYSTER-AAS, K., DAHLBERG, B., INGVAR, D., KRAKAU, C. E. T., MILLER, M. C., BOWERS, C. Y. AND SCHALLY, A. V. (1968a) Extrapigmentary effects of MSH in amenorrheic women. *Lancet*, **i**, 1007–1010.

KASTIN, A. J., GENNSER, G., ARIMURA, A., MILLER, M. C. AND SCHALLY, A. V. (1968b) Melanocyte-stimulating and corticotrophic activities in human foetal pituitary glands. *Acta endocr. (Kbh.)*, **58**, 6–10.

KASTIN, A. J., SCHALLY, A. V., VIOSCA, S. AND MILLER, M. C. (1969) MSH activity in plasma and pituitaries of rats after various treatments. *Endocrinology*, **84**, 20–27.

KASTIN, A. J., MILLER, L. H., GONZALEZ-BARCENA, D., HAWLEY, W. D., DYSTER-AAS, K., SCHALLY, A. V., VELASCO-PARRA, M. L. AND VELASCO, M. (1971) Psycho-physiologic correlates of MSH activity in man. *Physiol. Behav.*, **7**, 893–896.

KASTIN, A. J., BEACH, G. D., HAWLEY, W. D., KENDALL, J. W., EDWARDS, M. S. AND SCHALLY, A. V. (1973a) Dissociation of MSH and ACTH release in man. *J. clin. Endocr.*, **36**, 770–772.

KASTIN, A. J., MILLER, L. H., NOCKTON, R., SANDMAN, C. A., SCHALLY, A. V. AND STRATTON, L. O. (1973b) Behavioral aspects of melanocyte-stimulating hormone (MSH). In *Drug Effects on Neuroendocrine Regulation, Progress in Brain Research, Vol. 39*, E. ZIMMERMANN, W. H. GISPEN, B. H. MARKS AND D. DE WIED (Eds.), Elsevier, Amsterdam, pp. 461–470.

KASTIN, A. J., MILLER, M. C., FERRELL, L. AND SCHALLY, A. V. (1973c) General activity in intact and hypophysectomized rats after administration of melanocyte-stimulating hormone (MSH), melatonin, and Pro-Leu-Gly-NH$_2$. *Physiol. Behav.*, **10**, 399–401.

KASTIN, A. J., DEMPSEY, G. L., LEBLANC, B., DYSTER-AAS, K. AND SCHALLY, A. V. (1974) Extinction of an appetitive operant response after administration of MSH. *Horm. Behav.*, **5**, 135–139.

KOSTRZEWA, R., KASTIN, A. J. AND SPIRTES, M. A., Effect of MSH and MIF-I on activity of catecholamine-containing neurons in rat brain. In preparation.

KRIVOY, W. A. AND GUILLEMIN, R. (1961) On a possible role of β-melanocyte stimulating hormone (β-MSH) in the central nervous system of mammalia: An effect of β-MSH in the spinal cord of the cat. *Endocrinology*, **69**, 170–175.

KRIVOY, W. A., LANE, M., CHILDERS, H. A. AND GUILLEMIN, R. (1962) On the action of β-melanocyte stimulating hormone (β-MSH) on spontaneous electric discharge of the transparent knife fish, *G. eigenmannia. Experientia (Basel)*, **18**, 521.

LERNER, A. B. AND McGUIRE, J. S. (1961) Effect of alpha- and beta-melanocyte-stimulating hormone on the skin colour of man. *Nature (Lond.)*, **189**, 176–179.

LERNER, A. B. AND McGUIRE, J. S. (1964) Melanocyte-stimulating hormone and adrenocorticotrophic hormone: Their relation to pigmentation. *New Engl. J. Med.*, **270**, 539–546.

MACKINTOSH, N. J. (1965) Selective attention in animal discrimination learning. *Psychol. Bull.*, **64**, 124–150.

MACKINTOSH, N. J. (1969) Further analysis of the overtraining reversal effect. *J. comp. physiol. Psychol. Monogr.*, **67**, 1–18.

MILLER, R. E. AND OGAWA, N. (1962) The effect of adrenocorticotrophic hormone (ACTH) on avoidance conditioning in the adrenalectomized rat. *J. comp. physiol. Psychol.*, **55**, 211–213.

MILLER, L., KASTIN, A. J., SANDMAN, C. A., FINK, M. AND VAN VEEN, W. J. (1974) Polypeptide influence on attention, memory and anxiety in man. *Pharm. Biochem. Behav.*, **2**, 663–668.

MURPHY, A. V. AND MILLER, R. E. (1955) The effect of adrenocorticotrophic hormone (ACTH) on avoidance conditioning in the rat. *J. comp. physiol. Psychol.*, **48**, 47–49.

NOCKTON, R., KASTIN, A. J., ELDER, S. T. AND SCHALLY, A. V. (1972) Passive and active avoidance responses at two levels of shock administration of melanocyte-stimulating hormone. *Horm. Behav.*, **3**, 339–344.

PELLETIER, G., LABRIE, F., KASTIN, A. J. AND SCHALLY, A. V. (1974) Autoradiographic localization of MSH in the brain after intracarotid and intraventricular injection. *Pharm. Biochem. Behav.*, Submitted.

SANDMAN, C. A., KASTIN, A. J. AND SCHALLY, A. V. (1969) Melanocyte-stimulating hormone and learned appetitive behavior. *Experientia (Basel)*, **25**, 1001–1002.

SANDMAN, C. A., DENMAN, P. M., MILLER, L. H., KNOTT, J. R., SCHALLY, A. V. AND KASTIN, A. J. (1971a) Electroencephalographic measures of melanocyte-stimulating hormone activity. *J. comp. physiol. Psychol.*, **76**, 103–109.

SANDMAN, C. A., KASTIN, A. J. AND SCHALLY, A. V. (1971b) Behavioral inhibition as modified by melanocyte-stimulating hormone (MSH) and light–dark conditions. *Physiol. Behav.*, **6**, 45–48.

SANDMAN, C. A., MILLER, L. H., KASTIN, A. J. AND SCHALLY, A. V. (1972) A neuroendocrine influence on attention and memory. *J. comp. physiol. Psychol.*, **80**, 54–58.

SANDMAN, C. A., ALEXANDER, W. D. AND KASTIN, A. J. (1973a) Neuroendocrine influences on visual discrimination and reversal learning in the albino and hooded rat. *Physiol. Behav.*, **11**, 613–617.

SANDMAN, C. A., KASTIN, A. J., SCHALLY, A. V., KENDALL, J. W. AND MILLER, L. H. (1973b) Neuroendocrine responses to physical and psychological stress. *J. comp. physiol. Psychol.*, **84**, 386–390.

SANDMAN, C. A., BECKWITH, W., GIDDIS, M. M. AND KASTIN, A. J. (1974) Melanocyte-stimulating hormone (MSH) and overtraining effects on extradimensional shift (EDS) learning. *Physiol. Behav.*, **13**, 163–166.

SANDMAN, C. A. *et al.*, in preparation-a.

SANDMAN, C. A., BECKWITH, W. E. AND KASTIN, A. J. Effect of early injections of MSH on later adult discrimination learning in male and female rats, in preparation-b.

SANDMAN, C. A., GEORGE, J. M., NOLAN, J. N. AND KASTIN, A. J. (1975) Enhancement of attention in man with ACTH/MSH 4-10. *Physiol. Behav.*, Submitted.

SPIRTES, M. A., KOSTRZEWA, R. M. AND KASTIN, A. J., MSH and MIF-I effects on serotonin levels and synthesis in various rat brain areas. *Pharm. Biochem. Behav.*, Submitted.

STRATTON, L. O. AND KASTIN, A. J. (1973a) Melanocyte-stimulating hormone in learning and extinction of two problems. *Physiol. Behav.*, **10**, 689–692.

STRATTON, L. O., KASTIN, A. J. AND COLEMAN, W. P. (1973b) Activity and dark-preference responses of albino and hooded rats receiving MSH. *Physiol. Behav.*, **11**, 907–909.

STRATTON, L. O. AND KASTIN, A. J. (1974) Avoidance learning at two levels of motivation in rats receiving MSH. *Horm. Behav.*, **5**, 149–155.

STRATTON, L. O. AND KASTIN, A. J. (1974) Increased acquisition of a complex appetitive task after MSH and MIF. *Pharm. Biochem. Behav.*, Submitted.

WEIJNEN, J. A. W. AND SLANGEN, J. L. (1970) Effects of ACTH-analogues on extinction of conditioned behavior. In *Pituitary, Adrenal and the Brain, Progress in Brain Research, Vol. 32*, D. DE WIED AND J. A. W. M. WEIJNEN (Eds.), Elsevier, Amsterdam, pp. 221–235.

WIED, D. DE (1967) Opposite effects of ACTH and glucocorticoids on extinction of conditioned avoidance behavior. In *Proc. 2nd Int. Congr. on Hormonal Steroids, Milan, May, 1966*, Congr. Series, No. 132, L. MARTINI *et al.* (Eds.), Excerpta Medica, Amsterdam, pp. 945–951.

WIED, D. DE (1969) Effects of peptide hormones in behavior. In *Frontiers in Neuroendocrinology*, W. F. GANONG AND L. MARTINI (Eds.), Oxford University Press, Oxford, pp. 97–140.

Modulating Influences of Hormones and Catecholamines on Memory Storage Processes

JAMES L. McGAUGH, PAUL E. GOLD,
RODERICK VAN BUSKIRK AND JOHN HAYCOCK*

Department of Psychobiology, School of Biological Sciences, University of California, Irvine, Calif. 92664 (U.S.A.)

INTRODUCTION

It is now well established that the retention of newly learned responses can be modified by many treatments which affect brain processes if the treatments are administered shortly after training (McGaugh and Herz, 1972). The experimental findings provide strong support for the view that the treatments affect retention by modulating the neural processes involved in storing new information (McGaugh and Dawson, 1972; Gold and McGaugh, 1974). Most of the studies of memory storage modulation have used treatments, such as electrical stimulation of the brain, convulsant drugs, or antibiotics, which have non-specific, widespread, and poorly understood influences on brain function. Such findings suggest that memory storage is influenced perhaps by any alteration in brain function. However, there is extensive recent evidence indicating that some treatments that have profound influences on neural activity have no modulating influences on memory storage. For example, the elicitation of brain seizures with direct electrical stimulation of the brain or convulsant drugs is not a sufficient condition for producing retrograde amnesia in rats and mice (Gold and McGaugh, 1973; Van Buskirk and McGaugh, in press). Further, retention deficits produced by antibiotic drugs such as cycloheximide generally occur only if 85–95% of brain protein synthesis is inhibited (Glassman, 1969).

On the other hand, memory storage can be modulated by treatments which produce no gross alterations in brain functioning. Low doses of stimulants such as strychnine, pentylenetetrazol, and amphetamines administered shortly after training facilitate retention (McGaugh, 1973). Alteration in retention can be produced by low intensity (and sub-seizure) electrical stimulation of some brain regions (Gold et al., 1974).

The fundamental question is, of course, "What kinds of alterations in neuronal activity are effective in influencing memory storage processes?" A general assumption underlying research on this problem is that understanding the neural bases of the modulating influences may provide clues to processes normally involved in memory storage.

---

* NSF Predoctoral Fellow.

References p. 161–162

There is much experimental evidence supporting the general view that retention is influenced by processes associated with the state of arousal elicited by an experience (*cf.* Bloch, 1970; Kety, 1972; Gold and McGaugh, 1974). It may be that substances released during states of arousal, including hormones and catecholamines, have important roles in modulating the storage of recent experiences and that treatments which affect memory do so, at least in part, by influencing neurohumoral agents. The extensive evidence from the work of de Wied and his associates (de Wied, 1974) strongly suggests that hormones can modulate the retention of learned responses. And, the work of several recent studies (Randt *et al.*, 1971; Dismukes and Rake, 1972; Davies *et al.*, 1974) indicates that retention is influenced by treatments which affect catecholamine systems in the brain.

This paper reports some of the recent findings of our laboratory concerning the possible involvement of catecholamines and hormones as modulators of memory storage processes.

Catecholamines and memory storage

In a series of studies we have examined the effects, on retention, of drugs which affect catecholamine metabolism. In all of these experiments the drugs were administered either shortly before or shortly after a brief training session and the animals were subsequently tested for retention of the training experience. In most of our studies the animals, either rats or mice, were trained on a one-trial inhibitory (passive) avoidance task. Animals were placed in a small starting chamber and received a footshock as they entered the second chamber of a straight alley. Retention was assessed by the response latencies on a retention test trial given from 1 to 7 days later. In some studies the animals were first trained to enter the second chamber by rewarding them with water on a series of pretraining trials. In other studies, no pretraining was given. Drug effects on catecholamines were determined in other animals by measuring levels of dopamine (DA) and norepinephrine (NE) (Shellenberger and Gordon, 1971) at various time intervals following administration of the treatments.

Retention in mice was impaired by pretrial administration of several drugs including storage inhibitors (reserpine and Ro4-1284), tyrosine hydroxylase inhibitors (α-methyl-*para*-tyrosine and dipyridyl) and dopamine-*beta*-hydroxylase inhibitors (diethyldithiocarbamate (DDC) and 1-phenyl-3-(2-thiazolyl)-thiourea (U-14,624)). However, when the drugs were administered after training only DDC affected retention. Consequently, we subsequently examined the behavioral effects of DDC in some detail. It is of interest to note that posttrial injections of reserpine did not disrupt retention even at a dose of 5.0 mg/kg which reduced DA and NE by more than 50% within several hours following training. Thus, our results do not confirm those of other studies (Allen *et al.*, 1974) suggesting that reserpine produces retrograde amnesia.

The effects of posttrial injections of DDC on retention in mice (tested 1 week after training) of the inhibitory avoidance response are shown in Figs. 1 and 2. Fig. 1 shows the effect of the DDC dose when the drug was administered immediately after training.

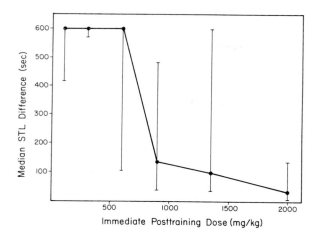

Fig. 1. Dose–response effects of immediate posttraining administration of DDC on inhibitory avoidance retention performance in mice. Mice were trained on a one-trial, step-through, inhibitory avoidance task and injected i.p. with saline or DDC immediately afterwards. Seven days later step-through latencies were assessed. Each point represents the median step-through latency (STL) difference (test minus training latency) for 16 animals. Error bars indicate the interquartile ranges. Animals receiving saline had a value of 600 (347.9–600) sec. (From Van Buskirk *et al.*, in preparation.)

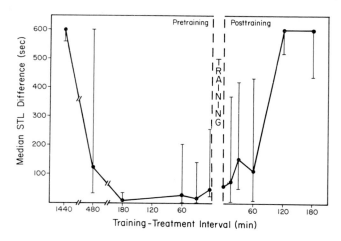

Fig. 2. Effects of training–treatment interval on DDC-induced retention deficits for inhibitory avoidance learning in mice. Different groups of mice received 900 mg/kg i.p. DDC at various times before or after training on a one-trial, step-through, inhibitory avoidance task. Seven days after training, test step-through latencies were assessed. Each point represents the median step-through latency (STL) difference for 16 animals. Error bars indicate the interquartile ranges. Animals receiving saline had a value of 600 (271.8–600) sec. (From Van Buskirk *et al.*, in preparation.)

Impairment of retention was produced by 900 mg/kg. Fig. 2 shows the effect of varying the time, before or after training, of a dose of 900 mg/kg. As is indicated, retention was impaired by injections administered within 8 hr before training and 1 hr following training. The effects of the pretrial injections of DDC (as well as the other drugs discussed above) are difficult to interpret. It might be that the effects

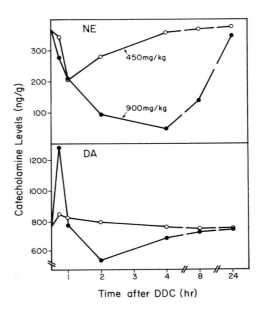

Fig. 3. Effects of DDC on whole brain catecholamine levels in mice. Mice were injected i.p. with either saline, 450 mg/kg DDC, or 900 mg/kg DDC. At various times following injection animals were sacrificed and brain norepinephrine (NE) and dopamine (DA) were assayed according to Shellenberger and Gordon (1971). Each point is the mean of 4 determinations except saline values, represented at the zero time point, which had 8 determinations. Values for the saline-injected animals were 379±3 μg NE/g and 771±32 μg DA/g. (From Haycock *et al.*, in preparation.)

are due to impairment of memory storage. However, when the drugs are administered before training, they may alter the animal's responsiveness to the training experience. The effects of the posttrial injections suggest that DDC impairs memory storage processes.

As Fig. 3 shows, the dose used to affect retention (900 mg/kg) markedly reduces the levels of NE for several hours. Dopamine levels were significantly increased shortly after the DDC injections and are then slightly reduced for about an hour. A dose which does not significantly affect retention (450 mg/kg) only slightly affected levels of norepinephrine and dopamine. Thus, these results are consistent with the interpretation that the retention loss produced by the higher dose of DDC is due to the differential effects of DDC on dopamine and norepinephrine. Further, the findings are generally consistent with those of other studies of the effects of DDC on retention in rats and mice (Randt *et al.*, 1971; Osborne and Kerkut, 1972).

However, the problem is somewhat more complicated. In another study, we examined the effects of DDC on the learning, by mice, of an active avoidance response (2-way shuttle). Mice were given 50 training trials on an automated shuttle box and 50 retraining trials 1 week later. DDC was administered in various doses immediately after training and at a dose of 900 mg/kg at intervals up to 4 hr after training. Retention performance, as indicated by avoidance errors, is shown in Fig. 4. Under these conditions, DDC enhanced retention. The degree of enhancement varied directly with the

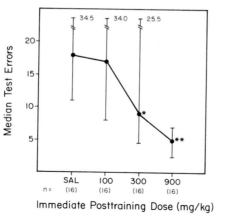

Fig. 4. Dose–response effects of immediate posttraining DDC on retention of an active avoidance response in mice. Mice were trained (50 trials) on a two-way shuttle avoidance task and retrained 7 days later. Immediately after training they were injected with saline or DDC. Each point represents the median number of errors (for 16 animals) on the retraining test. Error bars indicate the interquartile ranges. Mann–Whitney U-test, two-tailed: *, $P < 0.05$; **, $P < 0.02$. (From Haycock *et al.*, in preparation.)

dose and decreased as the interval between training and retention was increased. Thus, with the particular procedures used, DDC administered to mice following training impairs retention of an inhibitory avoidance response and facilitates the retention of an active avoidance response.

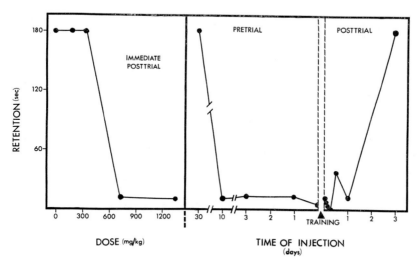

Fig. 5. Effects of DDC dose and time of injection on inhibitory avoidance retention performance in rats. Rats were trained on a one-trial, step-through, inhibitory avoidance task and tested 6 days later. Retention scores are the median-latency differences between testing and training. Left, various doses of DDC were injected immediately following training. Right, 680 mg/kg DDC was administered to rats at various times prior to or after training. (From Van Buskirk *et al.*, in preparation.)

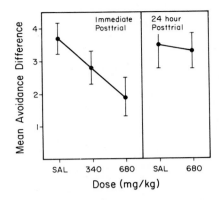

Fig. 6. The effects of posttraining administration of DDC on retention of an active avoidance response in rats. Rats (N = 7–11 per group) received 8 training trials on a one-way shuttle task and 8 retraining trials 3 days later. Saline or DDC (340 or 680 mg/kg) was injected i.p. either immediately after training or 24 hr later. The difference between correct responses on training and retraining is shown as Mean Difference Score. The scores of the group given 900 mg/kg immediately posttraining are significantly lower than the saline controls ($P < 0.01$) and the 450 mg/kg group ($P < 0.05$). The latter group did not differ significantly from the saline groups or the 24 hr DDC delay group. (From Spanis *et al.*, in preparation.)

The findings of several studies using rats are less complex. In rats, posttrial injections of DDC impair retention in three kinds of tasks: inhibitory avoidance, active avoidance, and discrimination learning.

Fig. 5 shows the results of a study of the effects of DDC on inhibitory avoidance learning. The rats were given a single training trial and a retention test trial 6 days later. Retention deficits were produced only at a dose of 680 mg/kg. At this dose, the effects are greater than those seen in mice. Impairing effects are obtained with injections of DDC given within 10 days before training and 1 day after training. Fig. 6 shows the effects of posttraining injections of DDC on the learning of a one-way active avoidance response. The rats were given 8 massed training trials. The rats avoided a footshock by moving from one end of an alley to the other within 10 sec after they were placed in the alley. Immediately after training, animals were then injected with saline or DDC (340 or 680 mg/kg). An additional two groups received either saline or DDC (680 mg/kg) 24 hr later. All animals were given 8 additional training trials 3 days after the original training. Retention is indicated by improvement (mean difference in avoidance scores on training and retraining) in avoidance responses on the retention test. As Fig. 6 indicates, the smallest amount of improvement was found in the rats given 680 mg/kg DDC immediately after the training. The groups given the delayed DDC injections or the lower dose did not differ from the saline-injected controls.

In another experiment, we examined the effects of DDC on discrimination learning. Rats in this study were given 5 massed training trials on a Y-maze visual discrimination task. The animals were trained to escape from footshock by running to an illuminated arm of the maze. They were then injected with DDC either immediately after the training or 2 hr later and given 7 retraining trials 1 week later. As Fig. 7

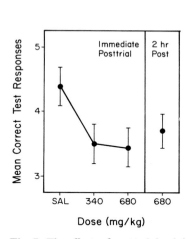

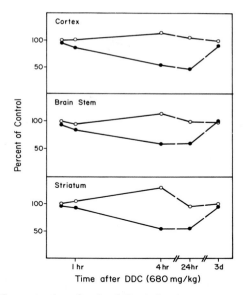

Fig. 7. The effects of posttraining injections of DDC on retention of a visual discrimination response in rats. Rats (N = 16–18 per group) received 5 training trials and 6 retraining trials 1 week later. Three groups received i.p. injections of saline or DDC (340 or 680 mg/kg) immediately after training. The mean number of correct responses made on the 6 retention trials are shown. The scores of both immediate DDC groups are significantly lower than those of the controls ($P < 0.05$). The 2 hr delay group scores did not differ significantly from the controls. (From Spanis *et al.*, in preparation.)

Fig. 8. Effects of DDC on regional catecholamine levels in rats. Rats were injected with either saline or 680 mg/kg DDC. At various times following injection, animals were sacrificed and the cortices (including amygdala), brain stems (pons and medulla), and corpus striatum (including n. accumbens and nucleus of the stria terminalis) were dissected out. Catecholamines were assayed according to Shellenberger and Gordon (1971). Each point represents 4 determinations. (From Van Buskirk *et al.*, in preparation.)

shows, retention was significantly impaired by DDC (at both 340 and 680 mg/kg) if the injections were given immediately after training. The delayed injection was ineffective.

Fig. 8 shows the effects of DDC on levels of dopamine and norepinephrine in rats. Dopamine levels were only slightly affected. Norepinephrine levels were significantly reduced for at least 24 hr following DDC administration.

Overall, these findings are consistent with the hypothesis that the retention deficit produced by DDC may be due to the selective decrease in norepinephrine due to inhibition of dopamine-*beta*-hydroxylase. However, this is only one of several possible interpretations. For example, the fact that DDC chelates metals suggests that the drug may affect retention by influencing other systems which involve metal-requiring enzymes. Further, the chelation of zinc results in the bleaching of sulfide silver (Timm's) staining in the hippocampal mossy fibers (Danscher *et al.*, 1973). Consequently, the interpretation of the effects of DDC on retention in terms of effects on catecholamines must be viewed with reservation. Further experiments are needed to determine which of the many effects of DDC are critical for producing the modulatory influences on memory storage processes. Our findings that retention is not significantly influenced by posttrial injections of several drugs which affect catecholamine metabolism suggest that, at the very least, the overall levels of catecholamines following training are not critical for memory storage. It might well be that memory storage processes

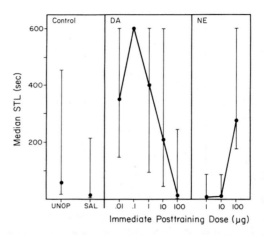

Fig. 9. Dose–response effects of immediate posttraining, i.v. injections of norepinephrine and dopamine on inhibitory avoidance retention performance in mice. Mice were trained on a one-trial, step-through, inhibitory avoidance task. Immediately following training, 1 μl of either saline, norepinephrine (NE) or dopamine (DA) was administered through a unilaterally placed cannula into the ventricles. Twenty-four hours later test step-through latencies were assessed. Points represent the median step-through latency differences (STL, test latencies minus training latencies). Error bars represent the interquartile ranges. Where no error bars are shown, the interquartile ranges smaller than individual point. (From Haycock *et al.*, in preparation.)

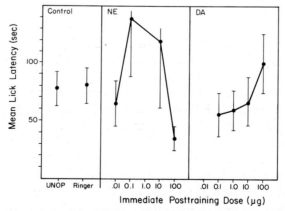

Fig. 10. Dose–response effects of immediate posttraining, i.v. injections of norepinephrine and dopamine on inhibitory avoidance retention performance in water-deprived mice. Mice were first pretrained to lick from a water spout. On training day the mice received a footshock for licking from the spout. Immediately following training, 1 μl of either Ringer's or a given dose of norepinephrine (NE) or dopamine (DA) was administered through a unilaterally placed cannula into the ventricles. Twenty-four hours later latencies to lick were assessed. Points represent mean lick latency differences (testing latencies minus training latencies) $\pm$ S.E.M. (From Haycock *et al.*, in preparation.)

are modulated if the levels of different amines are selectively modified. Knoll (1973) has suggested, for example, that the facilitating effects of amphetamines on learning may be due to an increase in catecholamines combined with a decrease in serotonin.

In other recent experiments, we have attempted to investigate the effects of catechol-amines on learning by administering dopamine and norepinephrine directly into the cerebral ventricles. In these studies, mice were first implanted with ventricular cannulae (unilaterally into the left lateral ventricle). Following recovery from surgery they were then trained on a one-trial inhibitory avoidance task and administered either dopamine or norepinephrine i.v. (1 μl) immediately after training. Both catecholamines significantly enhanced retention, but the effects depended upon the particular training task used. Fig. 9 shows the results of a study in which the animals were simply punished for stepping from one compartment to another and retested the following day. As can be seen the effects varied with the dose administered. The dopamine injections were particularly effective at doses from 0.01 to 1.0 μg. Norepinephrine was less effective with the doses investigated. Fig. 10 shows the results of an experiment in which the animals were first water-deprived and trained to drink at the end of the alley. Then they were given a single footshock while drinking and retested the next day. In this task norepinephrine was more effective than dopamine in enhancing retention. Greatest effects were found with 0.1 μg of norepinephrine.

Thus, these findings considered together with those of our studies of DDC are consistent with the general hypothesis that catecholamines may influence memory storage processes. However, the details of the findings indicate that the effects are quite complex. Modulatory influences are apparently obtained only when the balance between levels of different catecholamines is altered, and the effects seem to depend upon the particular task used.

Hormones and memory storage

In another series of experiments we have investigated the effects, on memory storage, of posttrial injections of several hormones, including epinephrine, norepinephrine, ACTH, and vasopressin. Some of these findings are reported in detail in other papers presented at this meeting (Gold et al., 1975; Van Buskirk et al., 1975) so we will only summarize some of the general findings here. In several studies we have found that retention of inhibitory avoidance as well as discrimination learning is enhanced by posttraining injections of ACTH. Fig. 11 shows the effects of posttrial injections of ACTH on retention of a one-trial inhibitory avoidance task. As is indicated, the effect depends upon the dose of ACTH used. Other findings (Gold and Van Buskirk, in press) indicate that retention is affected by injections of epinephrine. The effect (whether facilitation or impairment) depends upon the intensity of the punishing footshock. Further, the effects can be blocked by adrenergic blocking agents.

Thus, these findings are generally consistent with those of other studies indicating that memory is affected by hormones (de Wied, 1974). It is particularly interesting to note that several different hormones have similar effects on memory. The major

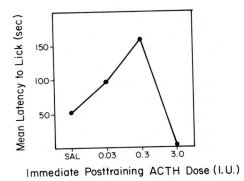

Fig. 11. Effects of posttraining administration of ACTH on retention of an inhibitory avoidance response in rats. Rats were trained with a low footshock in a one-trial inhibitory avoidance task. Immediately after training, rats received injections of either saline or ACTH. Animals which received the 0.3 I.U. dose of ACTH had latencies significantly higher than those of saline controls ($P < 0.02$, two-tailed). Animals which received the high dose (3.0 I.U.) of ACTH had latencies significantly lower than those of the saline control group. (From Gold and Van Buskirk, in preparation.)

question raised by these studies is that concerning the mechanism(s) of action. Do hormones directly modulate CNS processes involved in memory storage, or are their effects on memory due to other influences? It is conceivable that memory storage processes can be modulated by a variety of general chemical changes induced by training experiences. On the other hand, it may be that the hormones have a common basis such as the regulation of norepinephrine biosynthesis. For example, Versteeg's (1973) findings that $ACTH_{4-10}$ produces a significant increase in the turnover of brain norepinephrine are quite interesting in this regard. Whether the effects of ACTH and other hormones on memory are due to influences on catecholamines remains to be determined.

Concluding comments

Twenty-five years have passed since the publication of the first experimental evidence that memory storage processes are modulated by treatments administered after training. Most of the experiments published in the intervening years have attempted to clarify the nature of the modulating influences. The findings of recent studies from several laboratories strongly suggest that we may be coming closer to achieving an understanding of the modulating influences of posttraining treatments on memory storage processes. Further investigation of the influences of alterations in central catecholamines and hormones should continue to provide important clues to the processes involved in memory storage.

ACKNOWLEDGEMENTS

This study was supported by USPHS Research Grants MH 12526, MH 25384 and HD 07981 and Training Grant MH 11095-08.

We thank Curt Spanis, Mark Handwerker, Robert Rose and John Meligeni for their contributions to the research reported in this paper.

REFERENCES

ALLEN, C., ALLEN, B. S. AND RAKE, A. V. (1974) Pharmacological distinctions between "active" and "passive" avoidance memory formation as shown by manipulation of biogenic amine active compounds. *Psychopharmacologia (Berl.)*, **34**, 1–10.

BLOCH, V. (1970) Facts and hypotheses concerning memory consolidation. *Brain Research*, **24**, 561–575.

DANSCHER, G., HAUG, F. M. S. AND FREDENS, K. (1973) Effect of diethyldithiocarbamate (DEDTC) on sulphide silver stained boutons: reversible blocking of Timm's sulphide silver stain for "heavy" metals in DEDTC treated rats (light microscopy). *Exp. Brain Res.*, **16**, 521–532.

DAVIES, J. A., JACKSON, B. AND REDFERN, P. H. (1974) The effect of amantadine, L-Dopa, (+)-amphetamine and apomorphine on the acquisition of the conditioned avoidance response. *Neuropharmacology*, **13**, 199–204.

DISMUKES, R. K. AND RAKE, A. V. (1972) Involvement of biogenic amines in memory formation. *Psychopharmacologia (Berl.)*, **23**, 17–25.

GLASSMAN, E. (1969) The biochemistry of learning: an evaluation of the role of RNA and protein. *Ann. Rev. Biochem.*, **38**, 605–646.

GOLD, P. E. AND MCGAUGH, J. L. (1973) Relationship between amnesia and brain seizure thresholds in rats. *Physiol. Behav.*, **10**, 41–46.

GOLD, P. E. AND MCGAUGH, J. L. (1974) A single-trace, two-process view of memory storage processes. In *Short Term Memory*, D. DEUTSCH AND A. J. DEUTSCH (Eds.), Academic Press, New York, N.Y., pp. 355–376.

GOLD, P. E. AND VAN BUSKIRK, R. Facilitation of time-dependent memory processes with posttrial epinephrine injections. *Behav. Biol.*, in press.

GOLD, P. E. AND VAN BUSKIRK, R. In preparation.

GOLD, P. E., VAN BUSKIRK, R. AND MCGAUGH, J. L. (1975) Effects of hormones on time-dependent memory storage processes. In *Hormones, Homeostasis and the Brain, Progr. in Brain Res.*, Vol. 42, W. H. GISPEN, TJ. B. VAN WIMERSMA GREIDANUS, B. BOHUS AND D. DE WIED (Eds.), Elsevier, Amsterdam, pp. 210–211.

GOLD, P. E., ZORNETZER, S. F. AND MCGAUGH, J. L. (1974) Electrical stimulation of the brain: effects on memory storage. In *Advances in Psychobiology*, Vol. 2, G. NEWTON AND A. RIESEN (Eds.), Wiley-Interscience, New York, N.Y., pp. 64–75.

HAYCOCK, J. W., VAN BUSKIRK, R. AND MCGAUGH, J. L. In preparation.

KETY, S. (1972) Brain catecholamines, affective states, and memory. In *The Chemistry of Mood, Motivation, and Memory*, J. L. MCGAUGH (Ed.), Plenum Press, New York, N.Y., pp. 65–80.

KNOLL, J. (1973) Modulations of learning and retention by amphetamines. In *Brain, Nerves and Synapses*, Vol. 4, *Proc. 5th Int. Congr. Pharmacol.*, F. E. BLOOM AND G. H. ACHESON (Eds.), Karger, Basel, pp. 55–68.

MCGAUGH, J. L. (1973) Drug facilitation of learning and memory. *Ann. Rev. Pharmacol.*, **13**, 229–241.

MCGAUGH, J. L. AND DAWSON, R. G. (1972) Modification of memory storage processes. In *Animal Memory*, W. K. HONIG AND P. H. R. JAMES (Eds.), Academic Press, New York, N.Y., pp. 215–242.

MCGAUGH, J. L. AND HERZ, M. J. (1972) *Memory Consolidation*, Albion Publishing Company, San Francisco, Calif., 204 pp.

OSBORNE, R. H. AND KERKUT, G. A. (1972) Inhibition of noradrenalin biosynthesis and its effects on learning in rats. *Comp. gen. Pharmacol.*, **3**, 359–362.

RANDT, C. T., QUARTERMAIN, D., GOLDSTEIN, M. AND ANAGNOSTE, B. (1971) Norepinephrine biosynthesis inhibition: effects on memory in mice. *Science*, **172**, 498–499.

SHELLENBERGER, M. K. AND GORDON, J. H. (1971) A rapid, simplified procedure for simultaneous assay of norepinephrine, dopamine, and 5-hydroxytryptamine from discrete brain areas. *Analyt. Biochem.*, **39**, 356–372.

SPANIS, C. W., HANDWERKER, M. J., ROSE, R. AND MCGAUGH, J. L. In preparation.

VAN BUSKIRK, R., GOLD, P. E., HAYCOCK, J. W. AND MCGAUGH, J. L. In preparation.

VAN BUSKIRK, R., GOLD, P. E. AND MCGAUGH, J. L. (1975) Mediation of epinephrine effects on memory processes by α- and β-receptors. In *Hormones, Homeostasis and the Brain*, W. H. GISPEN, TJ. B. VAN WIMERSMA GREIDANUS, B. BOHUS AND D. DE WIED (Eds.), Elsevier, Amsterdam, p. 210.

VAN BUSKIRK, R., HAYCOCK, J. W. AND MCGAUGH, J. L., In preparation.

VAN BUSKIRK, R. AND MCGAUGH, J. L. (1974) Pentylenetetrazol-induced retrograde amnesia and brain seizures in mice. *Psychopharmacologia (Berl.)*, in press.

VERSTEEG, D. H. G. (1973) Effect of two ACTH-analogs on noradrenalin metabolism in rat brain. *Brain Research*, **49**, 483–485.

WIED, D. DE (1974) Pituitary–adrenal system hormones and behavior. In *The Neurosciences*, F. O. SCHMITT AND F. G. WORDEN (Eds.), MIT Press, Cambridge, Mass., pp. 653–666.

within 10.0 sec were considered to have no passive avoidance tendency as 10.0 sec is about the longest latency for NoFS–NoCO$_2$ subjects to enter the chamber on the test trial (Rigter, 1973). Rats entering within 10.1–299.9 sec were regarded to display an incomplete passive avoidance tendency. A refusal to enter within 300.0 sec was considered to be a complete passive avoidance response. In the analysis of the results by means of the one-tailed Yates test (Yates, 1948) the three classes received a statistical weighting of 0, 1 and 2, respectively.

Fig. 1 shows that the rats in the FS–NoCO$_2$ group displayed passive avoidance behavior at the test trial: the latencies of this group were higher than those of the NoFS–NoCO$_2$ group ($z = 4.27$, $P < 0.0001$). The rats from the placebo FS–CO$_2$ group, with one exception, failed to show passive avoidance. The FS–CO$_2$ group did not significantly differ from the NoFS–NoCO$_2$ group ($z = 1.03$, $P < 0.05$). It can thus be concluded that the CO$_2$ treatment induced amnesia. Administration of ACTH$_{4-10}$ 1 hr prior to the test trial caused a reduction of amnesia. The extent of this reduction decreased as the interval between the drug treatment and the test trial increased (compared to the placebo FS–CO$_2$ group: 1 hr: $z = 3.44$, $P < 0.001$; 2 hr: $z = 3.37$, $P < 0.001$; 4 hr: $z = 2.72$, $P < 0.001$; 6 hr: $z = 2.34$, $P < 0.01$); when given 8 hr before the test, ACTH$_{4-10}$ was no longer effective ($z = 0.62$, $P > 0.05$). The FS–CO$_2$ group which was treated with ACTH$_{4-10}$ 1 hr prior to the test trial did not significantly differ from the FS–NoCO$_2$ group which is indicative of a complete absence of amnesia. The extent of amnesia increased as the interval between drug treatment and the test trial was prolonged from 2 to 8 hr (2 hr: $z = 2.65$, $P < 0.01$; 4 hr: $z = 2.43$, $P < 0.01$; 6 hr: $z = 3.58$, $P < 0.001$; 8 hr: $z = 4.00$, $P < 0.0001$).

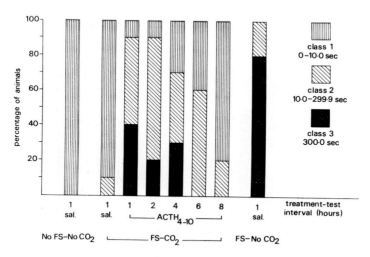

Fig. 1. Time course of the effect of ACTH$_{4-10}$ on CO$_2$-induced amnesia for a one-trial passive avoidance response. The figure shows the latencies of groups of rats (10/group) at the retrieval test. The scores were divided into 3 classes: (1) 0–10.0 sec (no avoidance); (2) 10.1–299.9 sec (incomplete avoidance); and (3) 300.0 sec (complete avoidance). Sal.: 1 ml saline/rat s.c.; 100 μg ACTH$_{4-10}$/rat was injected s.c. either 1, 2, 4, 6 or 8 hr prior to retrieval. FS: footshock; NoFS: no footshock; CO$_2$: CO$_2$ treatment; NoCO$_2$: sham amnesic treatment.

Permanence of the anti-amnesic effect of ACTH$_{4-10}$

Rigter (1973) demonstrated that spontaneous recovery of memory following CO_2-induced amnesia for a passive avoidance response could not be detected even up to 4 weeks after the acquisition trial, provided that the animals were subjected to only one retrieval trial. Therefore, it was deemed of interest to study whether ACTH$_{4-10}$ is able to attenuate amnesia, irrespective of the duration of the acquisition-test interval.

Twelve groups of 10 male Wistar rats weighing 200–220 g were used. Three groups received the NoFS–NoCO$_2$, 6 groups the FS–CO$_2$, and 3 groups the FS–NoCO$_2$ treatment. The animals were subjected to the test trial either 24 hr, 1 week or 2 weeks after the acquisition trial. For each acquisition test interval, 1 NoFS–NoCO$_2$, 2 FS–CO$_2$ and 1 FS–NoCO$_2$ groups were used. All groups were s.c. injected 1 hr prior to the test trial: the NoFS–NoCO$_2$, 1 FS–CO$_2$ and the FS–NoCO$_2$ groups received placebo whereas the second FS–CO$_2$ group was treated with 100 μg/rat.

Fig. 2 shows that the latencies of NoFS–NoCO$_2$ rats were shorter than 10.0 sec irrespective of the duration of the acquisition-test interval. Passive avoidance was present in all FS–NoCO$_2$ groups. The FS–NoCO$_2$ groups did not differ significantly from each other ($z \leqslant 0.52$, $P > 0.05$).

All placebo FS–CO$_2$ groups displayed amnesia (compared to the corresponding FS–NoCO$_2$ groups: 24-hr interval: $z = 4.00$, $P < 0.0001$; 1 week: $z = 3.64$, $P < 0.001$; 2 weeks: $z = 4.02$, $P < 0.0001$). The duration of the acquisition-test interval did not affect the degree of amnesia in these groups ($z \leqslant 0.59$, $P > 0.05$). ACTH$_{4-10}$ caused a reduction of amnesia irrespective of the duration of the acquisition-test interval (compared to the corresponding placebo FS–CO$_2$ groups: 24-hr interval: $z = 2.54$, $P < 0.01$; 1 week: $z = 1.81$, $P < 0.05$; 2 weeks: $z = 1.82$, $P < 0.05$). The ACTH$_{4-10}$-treated FS–CO$_2$ groups did not differ significantly from each other ($z \leqslant 1.01$, $P > 0.05$).

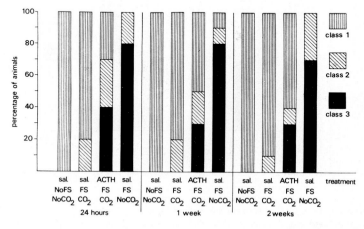

Fig. 2. Permanence of the anti-amnesic effect of ACTH$_{4-10}$. The retrieval test was given either 24 hr, 1 week or 2 weeks after acquisition. Saline or 100 μg ACTH$_{4-10}$/rat were administered 1 hr prior to retrieval. See further the legend to Fig. 1.

DESGLYCINAMIDE–LYSINE VASOPRESSIN

Time course of the anti-amnesic effect of desglycinamide–lysine vasopressin

Several observations suggest that the mechanism whereby lysine vasopressin and
ACTH influence behavior is basically different. Thus, administration of pitressin, a
crude pituitary extract containing vasopressin, inhibits extinction of avoidance
responses whether the treatment is given during acquisition or extinction, whereas
ACTH or ACTH analogues are only effective if given during the extinction period
(de Wied and Bohus, 1966). Furthermore, the effects of a single administration of
lysine vasopressin on extinction or passive avoidance are more enduring than the
effects of ACTH or ACTH analogues (de Wied, 1971; Thompson and de Wied, 1973).
Rigter *et al.* (1974) reported that whereas $ACTH_{4-10}$ attenuated amnesia only when
given prior to retrieval, the vasopressin analogue desglycinamide–lysine vasopressin
antagonized amnesia both when administered 1 hr before acquisition and 1 hr before
retrieval. Desglycinamide–lysine vasopressin (DG–LVP) almost completely lacks the
endocrine effects of vasopressin but exerts the same effects on learning behavior in
rats (de Wied *et al.*, 1972).

The time course of the "pre-acquisition" anti-amnesic effect of DG–LVP was
studied. Ninety male rats, weighing 200–230 g, were used. They were randomly
divided into 1 NoFS–NoCO$_2$, 7 FS–CO$_2$ and 1 FS–NoCO$_2$ groups. Each group
contained 10 rats. A 10 μg/ml solution of DG–LVP was prepared in the same way
as described for $ACTH_{4-10}$. The vehicle was used as placebo. The NoFS–NoCO$_2$,
1 FS–CO$_2$ and the FS–NoCO$_2$ groups were injected s.c. with 1 ml placebo 1 hr prior
to acquisition. Four other FS–CO$_2$ groups were treated s.c. with 10 μg/rat DG–LVP
either 1, 2, 4, 6 hr before acquisition. In addition, 1 FS–CO$_2$ group received DG–LVP

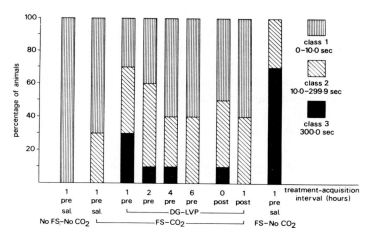

Fig. 3. The effect of "pre-acquisition" treatment with desglycinamide–lysine vasopressin (DG–LVP)
on CO$_2$-induced amnesia for a one-trial passive avoidance response. DG–LVP, 10 μg/rat, was
administered s.c. either prior to acquisition ("pre": 1, 2, 4, or 6 hr) or following acquisition and
application of CO$_2$ ("post": 0 and 1 hr). See further the legend to Fig. 1.

References p. 170–171

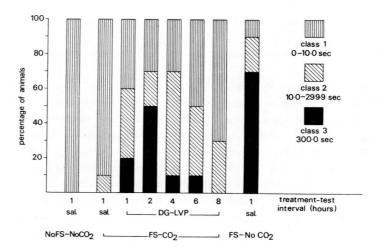

Fig. 4. The effect of "pre-retrieval" treatment with desglycinamide–lysine vasopressin (DG–LVP) on CO_2-induced amnesia for a one-trial passive avoidance response. DG–LVP, 10 µg/rat, was administered s.c. either 1, 2, 4, 6 or 8 hr prior to retrieval. See further the legend to Fig. 1.

immediately following acquisition and amnesic treatment whilst the remaining $FS–CO_2$ group was given DG–LVP 1 hr later.

Fig. 3 shows that DG–LVP administered 1 hr prior to acquisition reduced amnesia ($z = 2.15$, $P < 0.05$), although the reversal of amnesia was not complete (compared to the $FS–NoCO_2$ group: $z = 2.15$, $P < 0.05$). DG–LVP given 2–6 hr before acquisition did not significantly affect amnesia ($z \leqslant 1.51$); similarly, DG–LVP did not significantly influence amnesia if injected 0–1 hr after acquisition and amnesic treatment.

In a subsequent study the time course of the "pre-retrieval" anti-amnesic effect of DG–LVP was examined. Eight groups of 10 male rats were used, *i.e.*, 1 NoFS–$NoCO_2$ group, 6 $FS–CO_2$ groups and 1 $FS–NoCO_2$ group. The NoFS–$NoCO_2$, 1 $FS–CO_2$ and the $FS–NoCO_2$ groups received placebo 1 hr prior to retrieval. The other $FS–CO_2$ groups were treated with 10 µg/rat DG–LVP either 1, 2, 4, 6, or 8 hr prior to retrieval. The retrieval test was given 24 hr after acquisition. The results are seen in Fig. 4. Administration of DG–LVP 1–6 hr prior to retrieval attenuated amnesia (1 hr: $z = 2.34$, $P < 0.001$; 2 hr: $z = 2.88$, $P < 0.01$; 4 hr: $z = 2.65$, $P < 0.01$; 6 hr: $z = 1.95$, $P < 0.05$). However, except for the group which received DG–LVP 2 hr to retrieval, in all these groups some amnesia was present (compared to the $FS–NoCO_2$ group; 1 hr: $z = 2.20$, $P < 0.05$; 2 hr: $z = 0.99$, $P < 0.05$; 4 hr: $z = 2.39$, $P < 0.01$; 6 hr: $z = 2.69$, $P < 0.01$). Administration of DG–LVP 8 hr prior to retrieval did not affect amnesia ($z = 1.12$, $P > 0.05$).

CONCLUSION

Previously, we reported that $ACTH_{4-10}$ attenuates amnesia when given 1 hr prior to the retrieval test but not when administered prior to the acquisition trial. The peptide did not affect locomotor behavior (Rigter *et al.*, 1974; Rigter and van Riezen, 1975). In the present investigation, the time course of the anti-amnesic effect of $ACTH_{4-10}$ was studied. The peptide was able to antagonize CO_2-induced amnesia for a passive avoidance response if given within 8 hr prior to the retrieval test. Administration of $ACTH_{4-10}$ 8 hr prior to retrieval was ineffective. The fact that the anti-amnesic effect of $ACTH_{4-10}$ is only found in temporal contiguity with the retrieval trial suggests that the peptide has a direct action on the process of retrieval. Quinton (1972) designed an experiment in which the retrieval test was given 30 min after injection of the amnesic agent cycloheximide. ACTH was given either 15 min prior to cycloheximide, or interspersed between cycloheximide and the test trial. Only if given after the amnesic treatment, ACTH caused a reduction of amnesia. The present results suggest that it was the temporal contiguity with the retrieval trial and not with the amnesic treatment which was responsible for the anti-amnesic effect.

In the second experiment it was found that amnesia remained present over a 2-week period. Irrespective of the duration of the acquisition-test interval, "pre-retrieval" administration of $ACTH_{4-10}$ resulted in an attenuation of amnesia. This suggests that the anti-amnesic effect of the peptide cannot be ascribed to an interaction with physiological changes induced by the amnesic treatment as such changes presumably wear off within a few days (Nielson, 1968; van Eys *et al.*, 1975).

Taken together, the results indicate that $ACTH_{4-10}$ promotes retrieval. The mechanism of action is unknown. It is possible that some or part of the relevant memory item(s) survive the amnesic treatment and that $ACTH_{4-10}$ facilitates the retrieval of these item(s) at the retrieval test. However, in that case one should expect that weak memory items are subject to forgetting and therefore the retrieval-promoting effect of $ACTH_{4-10}$ would decline over a 2-week period. On the other hand, it is possible that $ACTH_{4-10}$ reverses a disturbance of retrieval induced by amnesic treatments. More data are required to allow a decision between these two explanations.

Previously, we showed that DG–LVP not only antagonizes amnesia when given 1 hr prior to retrieval but also when administered 1 hr prior to acquisition (Rigter *et al.*, 1974). This finding indicates that DG–LVP has a qualitatively different effect to $ACTH_{4-10}$. In the present investigation it was found that the time course of the "pre-acquisition" effect of DG–LVP was much steeper than that of the "pre-retrieval" effect. In keeping with the results for $ACTH_{4-10}$, DG–LVP reduced amnesia when given within 8 hr of the retrieval test. However, "pre-acquisition" administration of DG–LVP was only effective if it took place within 2 hr of the acquisition trial. The finding that this peptide attenuates amnesia when administered within 2 hr of acquisition suggests that this peptide is able to promote memory consolidation either by facilitating the consolidation process or by protecting memory from the adverse effects of the amnesic treatment. It is improbable that the short time course of "pre-acquisition" treatment with DG–LVP is due to an interaction of the peptide with some delayed effect of acquisition and/or amnesic treatment as the administration of DG–LVP immediately following acquisition and amnesic treatment only slightly affected amnesia.

References p. 170–171

The finding that the time course of the "pre-retrieval" effect of DG–LVP and $ACTH_{4-10}$ was similar may indicate that these effects are brought about by the same mechanism. If so, it must be concluded that the anti-amnesic effect of DG–LVP contains two different components.

SUMMARY

The ACTH analogue, $ACTH_{4-10}$, attenuated in rats the carbon dioxide-induced retrograde amnesia for a one-trial step-through passive avoidance response, when administered prior to the retrieval test, but not when given prior to the acquisition. The time course of this anti-amnesic effect was studied. It appeared that $ACTH_{4-10}$ attenuated amnesia if given s.c. within 8 hr prior to retrieval. In a second experiment it was found that amnesia remained present over a 2-week period. Irrespective of the duration of the acquisition-test interval, pre-retrieval administration of $ACTH_{4-10}$ resulted in an attenuation of amnesia.

The vasopressin analogue desglycinamide–lysine vasopressin antagonized carbon dioxide-induced amnesia both when administered prior to acquisition and when given prior to retrieval. The time course of the "pre-acquisition" and the "pre-retrieval" effect was different: the peptide had to be given within 2 hr of acquisition and within 8 hr of retrieval in order to be effective.

REFERENCES

ADER, R., WEIJNEN, J. A. W. M. AND MOLEMAN, P. (1972) Retention of a passive avoidance response as a function of the intensity and duration of electric shock. *Psychon. Sci.*, **26**, 125–128.

BOHUS, B. AND WIED, D. DE (1967) Failure of α-MSH to delay extinction of conditioned avoidance behavior in rats with lesions in the parafascicular nuclei of the thalamus. *Physiol. Behav.*, **2**, 221–223.

EYS, G. VAN, RIGTER, H. AND LEONARD, B. E. (1975) The relationship between time-dependent changes in carbon dioxide-induced amnesia and hippocampal monoamine metabolism in rats. *Pharmacol. Biochem. Behav.*, in press.

FLEXNER, J. B. AND FLEXNER, L. B. (1970) Adrenalectomy and the suppression of memory by puromycin. *Proc. nat. Acad. Sci. (Wash.)*, **66**, 48–52.

LANDE, S., FLEXNER, J. B. AND FLEXNER, L. B. (1972) Effect of corticotrophin and desglycinamide lysine vasopressin on suppression of memory by puromycin. *Proc. nat. Acad. Sci. (Wash.)*, **69**, 558–560.

NIELSON, H. C. (1968) Evidence that electroconvulsive shock alters memory retrieval rather than memory consolidation. *Exp. Neurol.*, **20**, 3–20.

PAOLINO, R. M., QUARTERMAIN, D. AND MILLER, N. E. (1966) Different temporal gradients of retrograde amnesia produced by carbon dioxide anesthesia and electroconvulsive shock. *J. comp. physiol. Psychol.*, **62**, 270–274.

QUINTON, E. (1972) Memory retrieval, reactivation and protein synthesis. Paper presented at the meeting of the Rocky Mountain Psychological Ass.

RIGTER, H. (1973) *Amnesia in de Rat*, Ph. D. Thesis, University of Utrecht.

RIGTER, H. AND VAN RIEZEN, H. (1975) The anti-amnesic effect of $ACTH_{4-10}$: its independence of the nature of the amnesic agent and the behavioural test. *Physiol. Behav.*, in press.

RIGTER, H., VAN RIEZEN, H. AND WIED, D. DE (1974) The effects of ACTH and vasopressin analogues on CO_2-induced retrograde amnesia in rats. *Physiol. Behav.*, **13**, 381–388.

THOMPSON, E. A. AND WIED, D. DE (1973) The relationship between the antidiuretic activity of the rat eye plexus blood and passive avoidance behaviour. *Physiol. Behav.*, **11**, 377–380.

WIED, D. DE (1969) Effects of peptide hormones on behaviour. In *Frontiers in Neuroendocrinology*, W. F. GANONG AND L. MARTINI (Eds.), Oxford University Press, Oxford, pp. 97–140.

WIED, D. DE (1971) Long term effect of vasopressin on maintenance of a conditioned avoidance response in rats. *Nature (Lond.)*, **232**, 58–60.

WIED, D. DE AND BOHUS, B. (1966) Long term and short term effects on retention of a conditioned avoidance response in rats by treatment with long acting pitressin and α-MSH. *Nature (Lond.)*, **212**, 1484–1486.

WIED, D. DE, GREVEN, H. M., LANDE, S. AND WITTER, A. (1972) Dissociation of the behavioural and endocrine effects of lysine vasopressin by tryptic digestion. *Brit. J. Pharmacol.*, **45**, 118–122.

WIMERSMA GREIDANUS, TJ. B. VAN AND WIED, D. DE (1971) Effects of systemic and intracerebral administration of two opposite acting ACTH-related peptides on extinction of conditioned avoidance behavior. *Neuroendocrinology*, **7**, 291–301.

YATES, F. (1948) The analysis of contingency tables with groupings based on quantitative characters. *Biometrika*, **35**, 178–181.

Effects of Lysine-8-Vasopressin on Punishment-Induced Suppression of a Lever-Holding Response

PAUL GARRUD

Department of Experimental Psychology, University of Oxford, South Parks Road, Oxford, OX1 3PS
(Great Britain)

The attempt to find a good psychological explanation of the effects of pituitary and adrenal hormones in behavioral situations has not yet been successful; see for example, de Wied (1974) and Smith (1973). The influence of these substances on punishment has been exclusively studied in one-trial passive avoidance situations, in which the resumption of the punished behavior, after a single presentation of electric shock, is the dependent measure; punished emergence (Levine and Levin, 1970); punished drinking (Anderson *et al.*, 1968; Levine and Jones, 1965; Bohus *et al.*, 1970; Guth *et al.*, 1971; Endröczi, 1972); punished step down (Weiss *et al.*, 1970; Dempsey *et al.*, 1972); punished light avoidance (Korányi *et al.*, 1967; Bohus and Korányi, 1969); punished step through (Bohus *et al.*, 1972; Tamásy *et al.*, 1973). A great number of different peptides and steroids have been tested in these situations, and their employment has contributed a good deal to pharmacological advance. However, the interpretation of changes in performance is unclear, since one could say that the memory of the aversive electric shock had been affected, or alternatively, that the ability of the animal to learn that electric shock will not now occur when it performs the punished behavior, has been altered, or, yet again, that the animal's motivation is different; it is more, or less, fearful as a result of the drug injection. If one could relate these results to ones gained from other types of situation in which such alternative explanations are either supported or do not hold up, then interpretation would be both easier and more easily justified, but the majority of other behavioral situations that have been used with these substances are also ones in which the reinforcement conditions or some other experimental conditions are changed contiguously with the drug treatment; typically, extinction and reversal learning have been used in active avoidance and appetitive situations (Bohus, 1973; Garrud *et al.*, 1974).

For this reason, I decided to investigate the effects of various hormones on performance in a continual punishment situation, of which only vasopressin is reported here.

Experiment 1

Six male albino Wistar rats were food deprived to 85% of their initial body weight

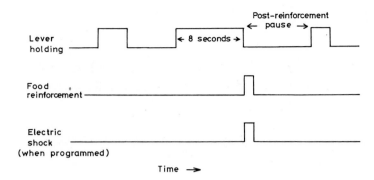

Fig. 1. Experiment 1 procedure.

and then were trained to hold down a lever for progressively longer times in order to obtain a pellet of food. When the animals had begun to learn this task, the procedure was fixed, and subsequently the animals had to hold down the lever for 8 sec, when the food reinforcement, and in the later stages of the experiment, electric shock, were delivered automatically. A similar procedure, though not identical, has been used by Millenson and MacMillan (1975), and by Platt *et al.* (1973). When performance

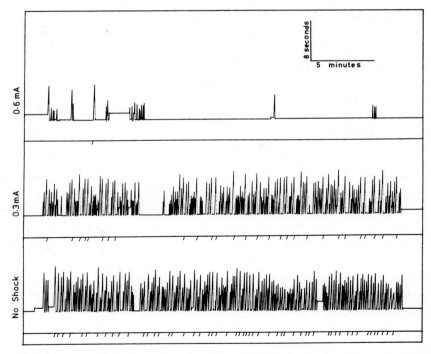

Fig. 2. Cumulative record of the performance of an individual animal under no shock, 0.3 mA shock and 0.6 mA shock conditions. The upper trace pen in each panel steps vertically when the lever is being held down, and it resets to the bottom when the lever is released. The lower trace pen in each panel deflects downwards when reinforcement (or reinforcement + electric shock) is delivered.

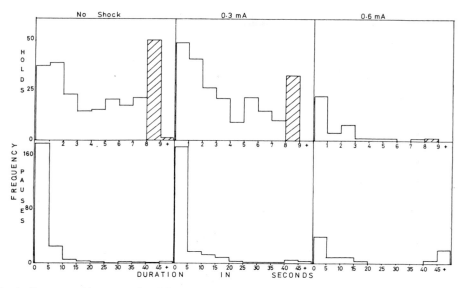

Fig. 3. Frequency histograms for different durations of lever holds (upper panels) and pauses (lower panels), under no shock, 0.3 mA shock and 0.6 mA shock conditions, for the same individual as in Fig. 2.

had stabilized on the schedule, electric shock was introduced and gradually increased until it reached an intensity of 0.3 mA. A graphical representation of the procedure is shown in Fig. 1. Shock duration was 1 sec. The effects of lysine vasopressin (LVP, Postacton, Ferring Läkemedel) were examined on this partially suppressed bar holding performance, and then the shock was gradually increased again to a value of 0.6 mA, and the effect of LVP on this heavily suppressed performance was measured. The 0.3 mA shock used was above the aversion threshold, and elicited flinching; the 0.6 mA shock used was a severely aversive stimulus and elicited running, prancing and vocalization (Myer, 1971).

The behavior patterns produced under no shock, 0.3 mA shock and 0.6 mA shock for one individual animal, are shown in Fig. 2.

Histograms of the duration of bar holds and of the pauses between successive bar holds are shown for the same individual animal in Fig. 3.

The basic pattern of responding that all the animals showed, before shock was introduced, is that the length of the successive holds tends to increase until the animal is reinforced. After reinforcement, the animal tends to pause for several seconds, and then to begin responding again. The first hold after a reinforcement is most often the shortest duration hold. This pattern is repeated. The basic pattern, just described, continues to occur under 0.3 mA shock, and also under 0.6 mA shock except that under the higher shock the pattern of successive holds, becoming longer in duration until a reinforcement is received, does not occur, and there is no relationship between the duration of one bar hold and the duration of the next.

The main effects of the introduction and subsequent increase in electric shock are:

References p. 185–186

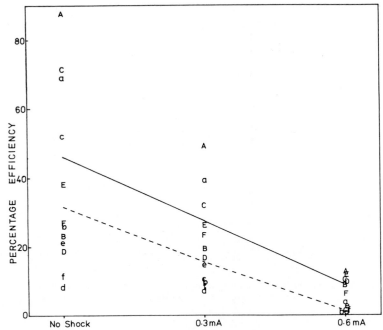

Fig. 4. Percentage efficiency for each individual animal (represented by the letters A–F), and for the group means (represented by the lines), measured in two ways: (i) the ratio of $\dfrac{number\ of\ reinforced\ holds}{total\ number\ of\ holds}$ (lower case letters and broken line), and (ii) the ratio of $\dfrac{total\ duration\ of\ reinforced\ holds}{total\ duration\ of\ all\ holds}$ (upper case letters and solid line): under no shock, 0.3 mA shock and 0.6 mA shock conditions.

(1) The number of reinforced bar holds decreases.
(2) The number of non-reinforced bar holds also goes down.
(3) The relative length of each pause increases.

The reduced rate of reinforcement is common to all 6 animals in the experiment although their individual differences are quite large.

The ratio of number of reinforced holds to total number of holds and the ratio of duration of reinforced holds to total time spent holding in the session are shown in Fig. 4. There is a clear relationship between the intensity of shock and both measures of the relative efficiency with which the animals respond, efficiency decreasing with increasing shock intensity. The figure also shows that this pattern of decreasing efficiency is consistent within all 6 animals, despite their large individual differences.

Fig. 5 shows the pattern of breaks in responding that occur in each session as a function of whether the preceding lever hold was reinforced or not. The increasing length of pauses that occurs with increasing shock intensity (see Fig. 3) is clearly due to increased duration of pausing immediately after the animal has received a shock (and food reinforcement). There is remarkably little effect of the introduction of mild, or intense, electric shock on the pauses that occur after non-reinforced responses.

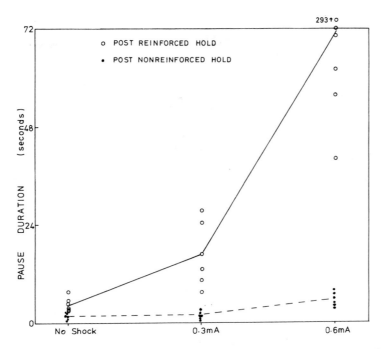

Fig. 5. Post-reinforcement pause duration for individual animals (open symbols) and for group mean (solid line), and post-non-reinforced hold pause duration for individual animals (closed symbols) and for group mean (broken line), under no shock, 0.3 mA shock and 0.6 mA shock conditions.

The punishment of this bar holding response then produces consistent changes in the pattern of behavior shown; the intensity of the punishment also bears a direct relationship to the magnitude of those changes. The effects of the punishment are to produce a decline in the number of contingent responses (*i.e.* 8-sec lever holds). Secondly, punishment also produces a decline in the number of non-contingent responses (*i.e.* lever holds less than 8 sec), but this decline is proportionately less than the decline in contingent responses, and so the animals' performance becomes less efficient, or alternatively, the relative amount of abortive responding increases. Thirdly, punishment produces an immediate post-punishment suppression of responding that is much larger than that produced by the food reinforcement alone.

In order to investigate the effects of a drug in this situation, one must look for changes in the pattern of behavior produced by the punishment, and therefore attention here will principally be paid to the three measures that are profoundly affected by punishment, reinforcement rate, efficiency, and post-reinforcement pausing.

The effects of LVP in a dose of 3 μg were examined on this punished behavior under 0.3 mA shock and under 0.6 mA shock.

Acute administration under 0.3 mA shock conditions produced somewhat variable results, and so chronic treatment with the drug for 5 days was used to examine its

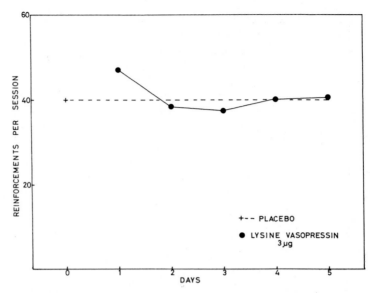

Fig. 6. Effect of chronic treatment with LVP on number of reinforcements obtained in a session under 0.3 mA shock.

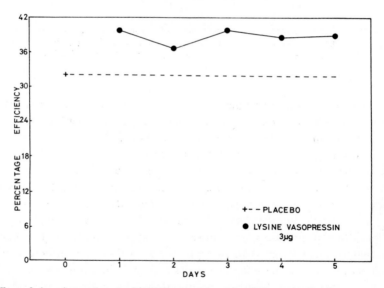

Fig. 7. Effect of chronic treatment with LVP on percentage efficiency (ratio of $\frac{total\ duration\ of\ reinforced\ holds}{total\ duration\ of\ all\ holds} \times 100$) under 0.3 mA shock.

effects. The effect of this treatment on the rate of reinforcement (*i.e.* the number of shocks + food reinforcements received in a session) is shown in Fig. 6.

There is very little change in reinforcement rate with the drug treatment, although there is a significant increase in the number of reinforcements obtained on the first

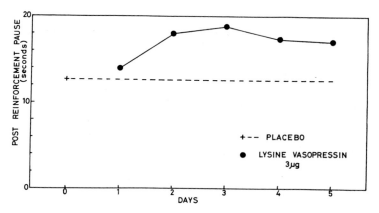

Fig. 8. Effect of chronic treatment with LVP on post-reinforcement pause duration under 0.3 mA shock.

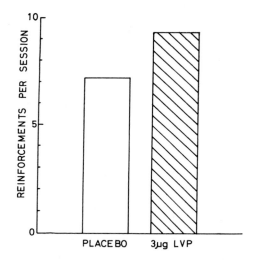

Fig. 9. Effect of acute treatment with LVP on number of reinforcements obtained in a session under 0.6 mA shock.

day of treatment ($P < 0.05$ by sign test). The effect of LVP on the animals' efficiency is shown in Fig. 7. There is a clear and significant increase in efficiency ($P < 0.01$ by matched t-test) as a result of the treatment, and this increase occurs in all 6 animals over all 5 days of treatment (*i.e.* significant increase on every day, $P < 0.05$ by sign test). The effect of chronic treatment with LVP on post-reinforcement pausing is shown in Fig. 8.

Here, there is a lengthening of the mean post-reinforcement pause, that is significant ($P < 0.01$ by matched t-test), and occurs on all 5 days of treatment consistently in all 6 animals.

Chronic administration of LVP under 0.3 mA conditions produced little change in reinforcement rate, but an increase in efficiency and also an increase in post-rein-

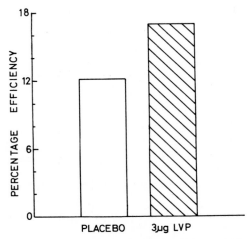

Fig. 10. Effect of acute treatment with LVP on percentage efficiency (ratio of
$$\frac{total\ duration\ of\ reinforced\ holds}{total\ duration\ of\ all\ holds} \times 100)\ \text{under 0.6 mA shock.}$$

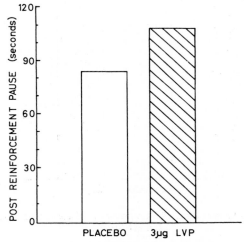

Fig. 11. Effect of acute treatment with LVP on post-reinforcement pause duration under 0.6 mA shock.

forcement pause duration. The effect of acute administration of the same dose (3 μg) of LVP on performance under 0.6 mA conditions was then examined.

The effect of this treatment on the rate of reinforcement is shown in Fig. 9. There is a small increase in the number of reinforcements obtained in a session from 7.1 to 9.4 ($P < 0.05$ by sign test); *i.e.* the animals received slightly more shocks. The effect of LVP on the efficiency of the animals is shown in Fig. 10. There is a significant and substantial increase in efficiency with the acute administration of LVP, that is quite marked (12.0–17.3 %, $P < 0.01$ by matched *t*-test). The effect of LVP on post-reinforcement pausing is shown in Fig. 11.

Again there is a significant increase in the length of the post-reinforcement pause, that is consistent in all 6 animals ($P < 0.05$ by sign test), LVP treatment producing a longer lasting suppression of responding after each electric shock.

Acute treatment with LVP under 0.6 mA shock conditions produced an increase in reinforcement rate, a marked increase in efficiency, and also an increase in post-reinforcement pause length. Probably, the increase in reinforcement rate was a transitory effect, since such an increase in reinforcement rate also occurred under 0.3 mA shock, but only on the first day of treatment.

The effects of LVP on this punished behavior, then, are consistent under two widely different levels of shock: LVP produces increased suppression of responding immediately after a reinforcement (food + electric shock), and also produced an enhanced efficiency of responding; *i.e.* that an animal, when responding, was more likely to produce a criterion response (an 8-sec lever hold) after LVP treatment.

It seemed likely that these two effects were separate and independent results of the treatment with LVP, since introduction, and increased intensity, of electric shock increased the length of post-reinforcement pausing, but decreased the animals' efficiency of responding. However, in situations in which rats receive occasional aversive electric shocks, it is well known that there are likely to be many incidences of the animals' freezing (adopting an immobile posture); this is thought to be an instance of a species-specific defense reaction (Bolles, 1971). It is possible that an increase in efficiency of lever holding might be brought about by an animal freezing while holding the lever down, and indeed there have been reports of lever holding occurring in lever pressing avoidance situations, in which an animal has only to press a lever in order to avoid shock (Barcik and Collins, 1972; Campbell, 1962; Migler, 1963). The gross skeletal activity of the same 6 animals was measured, therefore, when they were responding (*i.e.* holding the lever down) and when they were not responding (*i.e.*

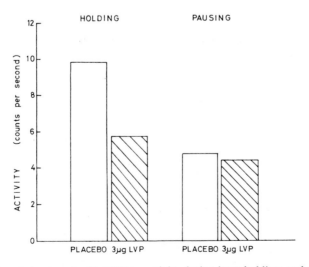

Fig. 12. Effect of acute treatment with LVP on activity during lever holding, and on activity during pauses in lever holding, under 0.6 mA shock.

pausing). The effects of injection of LVP on this activity count were examined. The results of this experiment are shown in Fig. 12. Activity was measured with an ultra-sonic activity monitor. All animals showed higher activity counts when responding than when pausing, in the undrugged condition. Injection of 3 μg LVP did not change the activity of the animals while they were pausing, but it severely reduced their activity while they were responding ($P < 0.01$ by matched t-test). Thus the possibility that both the increased suppression of behavior after a shock and the increased efficiency of responding shown by these animals when treated with LVP are produced by a single action of the drug is strongly supported. The absence of any change in activity while pausing may be due to a floor effect *i.e.* the animals' activity may, already in the undrugged state, reflect more or less total immobility or alternatively, it is possible that the change in activity seen with LVP is specific to those parts of the behavior pattern that are spatially or temporally contiguous with the aversive stimulus. Evidence that this effect of LVP is specific to electric shock-related changes in activity is gained from a further experiment.

Experiment 2

Eight untrained male albino Wistar rats were injected with LVP or saline, when undeprived and subsequently when food deprived, and their activity, when only placed in the apparatus for a 15-min period, was measured in the same way as in experiment 1. The results are shown in Fig. 13.

There was absolutely no alteration in activity in either the non-deprived, or the food-deprived condition with either of the two doses of LVP used, although the food deprivation produced a much higher baseline level of activity.

The effect of LVP in the punishment experiment (experiment 1) was clearly and

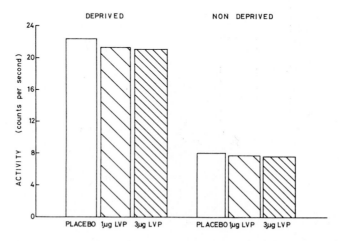

Fig. 13. Effect of two acute doses of LVP on activity during a 15-min period, in deprived and undeprived conditions.

simply to enhance the effects of electric shock and stimuli associated with the electric shock.

The generality of this finding was investigated by examining the effects of LVP in a Conditioned Emotional Response (CER) procedure (Estes and Skinner, 1941).

Experiment 3

Four male hooded Lister rats were trained to press a lever for food reinforcement on a variable interval (VI) 1-min schedule. When their performance had stabilized, pairings of a 30-sec tone as conditioned stimulus (CS), with an unavoidable 0.6 mA electric shock as unconditioned stimulus (US), or a 30-sec light stimulus which was never followed by the electric shock US, were presented while the animals were responding on the VI schedule. Responding during the tone CS that preceded the shock was almost completely suppressed, but after stabilization, baseline responding and responding during the light CS that was never followed by a shock were not suppressed relative to pre-shock levels. The effects of 2 μg LVP on responding during tone CS (CS+), light CS (CS−) and baseline periods are shown in Fig. 14. This dose of LVP significantly suppressed baseline response rate, but had no significant effect on response rate during CS+ or CS−, although the absence of any effect during CS+ periods may be due to a floor effect, as responding was already heavily suppressed. Table I shows the number of responses made in 3 successive 10-sec periods during the CS+ and 3 successive 10-sec periods immediately after the delivery of the shock US.

There was no indication that LVP treatment produced any post-shock suppression in this situation. LVP significantly suppressed baseline response rate in this CER procedure, but did not alter the effects of a shock associated stimulus (CS+), or of a non-shock associated stimulus (CS−). Possibly partial suppression of responding produced by a CS+ paired with 0.3 mA shocks might show an increase with LVP

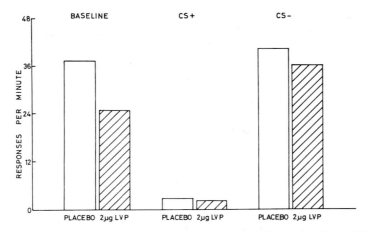

Fig. 14. Effects of acute treatment with LVP on response rate during baseline, CS+ and CS− periods.

TABLE I

EFFECTS OF LVP ON RESPONSE RATE DURING PRE-CS+, CS+, AND POST-CS+ PERIODS IN EXPERIMENT 3

	Successive 10-sec periods									
	Pre-CS+			*CS+*			*Post-CS+*			
	1	*2*	*3*	*4*	*5*	*6*	*7*	*8*	*9*	
Lysine-8-vasopressin	7	11	9	0	1	0	8	9	10	⎫ Number of
Placebo	8	9	11	1	1	0	10	9	9	⎭ responses

treatment, since Weiss *et al.* (1970) reported that pituitary–adrenal hormones had significant effects when conditions promoted mild and generalized effects of aversive stimulation, but not when the conditions promoted strong and specific effects of aversive stimuli.

However, the overall failure to find similar effects of LVP in the CER procedure limits the interpretation of its effects in the punishment procedure.

CONCLUSIONS

It is not possible to draw any general conclusion about the behavioral effects of LVP from these experiments. In a continual punishment procedure (experiment 1), LVP was found to enhance the effects of aversive stimulation; it increased the latency to make the first response after each shock and it increased the amount of freezing that the animals displayed in the situation. It is worth noting that these effects are straight-forward, and directly comparable to those found in one-trial passive avoidance situations; increased latency to respond after a shock (van Wimersma Greidanus *et al.*, 1975) and potentiation of freezing (Bohus, 1975) have both been found with LVP. Although these effects were shown to be specific to an aversive situation (experiment 2), little effect of LVP was found in a CER situation (experiment 3), only generalized suppression of the instrumental baseline occurred as a result of treatment. This result, however, was obtained with only one dose and treatment regimen, and only one set of experimental parameters, and therefore is preliminary.

Extension of experimental work with the peptide LVP, to performance in appetitive tasks, as well as performance on active avoidance schedules, is necessary before any account of its psychological effects can be complete.

SUMMARY

The influence of peptide and steroid hormones on changes in behavior produced by aversive stimulation has been studied most often by the use of one-trial passive avoidance situations, in which the latency to resume the punished behavior is measured.

The effects of lysine-8-vasopressin were investigated, therefore, in a continual punishment situation.

Food-deprived rats were trained to hold down a lever for 8 sec in order to obtain food reward. When they were performing stably on this schedule, electric shock was introduced contingent upon completion of an 8-sec lever hold, being delivered at the same time as the food. Administration of lysine-8-vasopressin prolonged the time taken to make the next response after each shock and increased the efficiency with which the animals performed, consistently under mild and severe levels of punishment. It was found that the increase in efficiency was most probably produced by an increase in the amount of freezing as a defense reaction to the aversive stimulation. There was no change in activity and no evocation of freezing as a result of lysine-8-vasopressin treatment in a non-aversive situation. Comparison with results from a conditioned emotional response experiment suggests that these effects of the peptide are specific to the punishment procedure used. The best description of these results is to say that lysine-8-vasopressin enhanced the effect of electric shock and of stimuli associated with electric shock. Directly comparable results have recently been reported from one-trial passive avoidance experiments.

ACKNOWLEDGEMENTS

The synthetic lysine-8-vasopressin (Postacton) was generously supplied by Ferring AB, P.O.B. 9007, Malmö 9, Sweden.

The author is supported by a Research Studentship from the U. K. Science Research Council.

REFERENCES

ANDERSON, D. C., WINN, W. AND TAM, T. (1968) Adrenocorticotrophic hormone and acquisition of a passive avoidance response: a replication and extension. *J. comp. physiol. Psychol.*, **66**, 497–499.

BARCIK, J. D. AND COLLINS, D. E. (1972) Shock elicited defensive behavior and passive avoidance performance. *Psychonom. Sci.*, **28**, 37–40.

BOHUS, B. (1973) Pituitary–adrenal influences on avoidance and approach behavior of the rat. In *Drug Effects on Neuroendocrine Regulation, Progress in Brain Research, Vol. 39*, E. ZIMMERMANN, W. H. GISPEN, B. H. MARKS AND D. DE WIED (Eds.), Elsevier, Amsterdam, pp. 407–420.

BOHUS, B. (1975) Pituitary peptides and adaptive autonomic responses. In *Hormones, Homeostasis and the Brain, Progress in Brain Research, Vol. 42*, W. H. GISPEN, TJ. B. VAN WIMERSMA GREIDANUS, B. BOHUS AND D. DE WIED (Eds.), Elsevier, Amsterdam, pp. 275–283.

BOHUS, B. AND KORÁNYI, L. (1969) Hormonal conditioning of adaptive behavioural processes. In *Results in Neurophysiology, Neuroendocrinology, Neuropharmacology and Behaviour, Recent Developments of Neurobiology in Hungary, Vol. ii*, K. LISSÁK (Ed.), Akadémiai Kiadó, Budapest, pp. 50–76.

BOHUS, B., GRUBITS, J., KOVÁCS, G. AND LISSÁK, K. (1970) Effect of corticosteroids on passive avoidance behaviour of rats. *Acta physiol. Acad. Sci. hung.*, **38**, 381–391.

BOHUS, B., ADER, R. AND WIED, D. DE (1972) Effects of vasopressin on active and passive avoidance behavior. *Horm. Behav.*, **3**, 1–7.

BOLLES, R. C. (1971) Species-specific defense reactions. In *Aversive Conditioning and Learning*, F. R. BRUSH (Ed.), Academic Press, New York, N.Y., pp. 183–234.

CAMPBELL, S. L. (1962) Lever holding and behavior sequences in shock-escape. *J. comp. physiol. Psychol.*, **55**, 1047–1053.

DEMPSEY, G. L., KASTIN, A. J. AND SCHALLY, A. V. (1972) The effects of MSH on a restricted passive avoidance response. *Horm. Behav.*, **3**, 333–338.

ENDRÖCZI, E. (1972) *Limbic System, Learning and Pituitary–Adrenal Function*, Akadémiai Kiadó, Budapest, pp. 23–79.

ESTES, W. K. AND SKINNER, B. F. (1941) Some quantitative properties of anxiety. *J. exp. Psychol.*, **29**, 390–400.

GARRUD, P., GRAY, J. A. AND WIED, D. DE (1974) Pituitary–adrenal hormones and extinction of rewarded behaviour in the rat. *Physiol. Behav.*, **12**, 109–119.

GUTH, S., SEWARD, J. P. AND LEVINE, S. (1971) Differential manipulation of passive avoidance by exogenous ACTH. *Horm. Behav.*, **2**, 127–138.

KORÁNYI, L., ENDRÖCZI, E., LISSÁK, K. AND SZEPES, E. (1967) The effect of ACTH on behavioral processes motivated by fear in mice. *Physiol. Behav.*, **2**, 439–445.

LEVINE, S. AND JONES, L. E. (1965) Adrenocorticotropic hormone (ACTH) and passive avoidance learning. *J. comp. physiol. Psychol.*, **59**, 357–360.

LEVINE, S. AND LEVIN, R. (1970) Pituitary–adrenal influences on passive avoidance in two inbred strains of mice. *Horm. Behav.*, **1**, 105–110.

MIGLER, B. (1963) Barholding during escape conditioning. *J. exp. Anal. Behav.*, **6**, 65–72.

MILLENSON, J. R. AND MACMILLAN, A. ST. C. (1975) Abortive responding during punishment of bar holding. *Learning and Motivation*, in press.

MYER, J. S. (1971) Some effects of noncontingent aversive stimulation. In *Aversive Conditioning and Learning*, F. R. BRUSH (Ed.), Academic Press, New York, N.Y., pp. 469–536.

PLATT, J. R., KUCH, D. O. AND BITGOOD, S. C. (1973) Rats' lever-press durations as psychophysical judgements of time. *J. exp. Anal. Behav.*, **19**, 239–250.

SMITH, G. P. (1973) Adrenal hormones and emotional behaviour. In *Progress in Physiological Psychology*, Vol. 5, E. STELLAR AND J. M. SPRAGUE (Eds.), Academic Press, New York, N.Y., pp. 299–343.

TAMÁSY, V., KORÁNYI, L., LISSÁK, K. AND JANDALA, M. (1973) Open-field behavior, habituation and passive avoidance learning: effect of ACTH and hydrocortisone on normal and adrenalectomised rats. *Physiol. Behav.*, **10**, 995–1000.

WIED, D. DE (1974) Pituitary–adrenal system hormones and behavior. In *The Neurosciences Third Study Program*, F. O. SCHMITT AND F. G. WORDEN (Eds.), MIT Press, Cambridge, Mass., pp. 653–666.

WEISS, J. M., MCEWEN, B. S., SILVA, M. T. AND KALKUT, M. (1970) Pituitary–adrenal alterations and fear responding. *Amer. J. Physiol.*, **218**, 864–868.

WIMERSMA GREIDANUS, TJ. B. VAN, BOHUS, B. AND WIED, D. DE (1975) The role of vasopressin in memory processes. In *Hormones, Homeostasis and the Brain, Progress in Brain Research*, Vol. 42, W. H. GISPEN, TJ. B. VAN WIMERSMA GREIDANUS, B. BOHUS AND D. DE WIED (Eds.), Elsevier, Amsterdam, pp. 135–141.

A Modulatory Effect of Pituitary Polypeptides on Peripheral Nerve and Muscle

F. L. STRAND AND A. CAYER

Biology Department, New York University, Washington Square, New York, N.Y. 10003 (U.S.A.)

Pituitary polypeptides are implicated in many ways in the modulation of nervous activity. Behavioral studies by de Wied and his colleagues have shown that ACTH (corticotropin) maintains aversely motivated behavior (de Wied, 1966). Comparative studies on the effects of small fragments of the ACTH molecule demonstrate that these behavioral effects are confined to the decapeptide $ACTH_{1-10}$ or the hepta-peptide $ACTH_{4-10}$. As these polypeptide fragments are without endocrine effects (de Wied, 1969a), they must affect nervous activity independent of adrenal cortical mediation.

α-MSH (melanocyte-stimulating hormone) and β-MSH, polypeptides that share the same amino acid sequence as $ACTH_{4-10}$, also affect the performance of a number of behavioral tasks. They increase the resistance to extinction of an active avoidance response (de Wied and Bohus, 1966; de Wied, 1969a and b) and delay extinction of a passive avoidance response (Sandman *et al.*, 1971). The posterior pituitary poly-peptide, lysine vasopressin, is also involved in the modification of behavior. Lysine vasopressin has a long term facilitatory effect on the consolidation of a conditioned avoidance response (de Wied, 1971).

Within the nervous system, ACTH can be shown to activate directly cells in the hypothalamus and midbrain (Steiner *et al.*, 1969; van Delft and Kitay, 1972) and to increase the excitability of spinal cord cells (Nicolov, 1967). These effects are directly opposite to those evoked by the application of adrenal steroids (Feldman *et al.*, 1961; Pfaff *et al.*, 1971). The implantation of $ACTH_{1-10}$ in various brain regions indicates that it exerts its effects within the nervous system (van Wimersma Greidanus and de Wied, 1971). An augmentation of evoked potentials in the spinal cord by β-MSH has been demonstrated by Krivoy and Guillemin (1961) and Kastin *et al.* (1973) have reported changes in electroencephalographic patterns following MSH administration.

Studies on peripheral nerve and skeletal muscle *(in situ)* also indicate an extradrenal effect of pituitary polypeptides, an action which may involve the neuromuscular junction. The administration of 10 mU ACTH increases muscle action potential amplitude and contraction height and delays fatigue in normal, adrenalectomized and hypophysectomized rats. Adrenalectomy alone, with a concomitant increase in

References p. 192–194

endogenous ACTH, also increases these parameters while hypophysectomy has the reverse effect (Strand et al., 1973/74).

As these experiments utilized the natural ACTH molecule it was of interest to determine whether similar results could be obtained with the fragment $ACTH_{4-10}$ and by α-MSH and β-MSH. The 7-D-phenylalanine isomer of $ACTH_{4-10}$ was also used, as the substitution of the D-isomer of phenylalanine in the 7th position reverses the behavioral effects of the L-peptide (Bohus and de Wied, 1966; de Wied and Greven, 1969).

In these experiments, adult male rats weighing from 200 to 300 g were maintained on a 12 hr dark–12 hr light schedule. All experiments were started at 10:00 a.m. Hypophysectomized rats received supplementary glucose and lettuce during the first week after the operation; subsequently they were fed only standard rat chow. Experiments on the operated rats were run approximately 2 weeks after surgery. Completeness of hypophysectomy was checked on autopsy and by histological examination of the adrenals for atrophy.

All rats were prepared for the experiment and maintained under pentobarbital anesthesia (Diabutal, 35–50 mg/kg i.p.). The sciatic nerve was freed carefully and secured within a small plexiglass chamber which contained 2 platinum stimulating electrodes. The stimulus was a rectangular pulse (duration 0.1 msec, frequency 5/sec, strength 2 × maximal). Nerve action potentials (APs) were recorded from electrodes distal to the stimulating chamber and a concentric needle electrode was inserted into the belly of the ipsilateral gastrocnemius muscle for the recording of muscle APs. The APs were photographed at appropriate time intervals from a dual beam oscilloscope and analyzed statistically.

The experimental procedure consisted of sciatic nerve stimulation for 30 min followed by a 10 min rest, after which stimulation was resumed for a further 10 min. Respiration and muscle temperature were recorded throughout to monitor the animal's condition. For further details see Strand et al. (1973/74).

The polypeptides administered were α-MSH (20 μg/kg and 50 μg/kg); β-MSH (20 μg/kg and 50 μg/kg); $ACTH_{4-10}$-7-L-phe (1 μg/kg) and $ACTH_{4-10}$-7-D-phe (1 μg/kg and 10 μg/kg). These were given i.p. to both normal and hypophysectomized rats 5 min before nerve stimulation began. Control groups of normal and hypophysectomized rats received saline injections.

(I) Modulating effect of pituitary polypeptides on muscle action potentials and fatigue

Although all the polypeptides tested, with the exception of $ACTH_{4-10}$-7-D-phe, increase muscle AP amplitude and decrease fatigue in intact and hypophysectomized rats, these effects are more marked in the hypophysectomized animals and there are some time differences. Fig. 1 shows that β-MSH exerts an immediate effect, while the augmentation due to α-MSH and $ACTH_{4-10}$-7-L-phe is seen only after 2 min and becomes more marked as stimulation continues. It is seen again as fatigue sets in during the second stimulation period after rest (Fig. 2). This is interesting in view of the fact that while a single response from a hypophysectomized rat does not differ

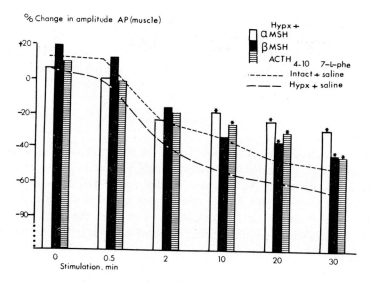

Fig. 1. Change in muscle AP amplitude during indirect stimulation in hypophysectomized (hypx) rats administered α-MSH (20 μg/kg); β-MSH (20 μg/kg); ACTH$_{4-10}$-7-L-phe (1 μg/kg) and ACTH$_{4-10}$-7-D-phe (1 μg/kg and 10 μg/kg). The effects of the D-isomer are essentially the same as the saline treated controls and not shown separately; 8 rats per group. $P < 0.05$ (*) *versus* hypx, saline treated rats. Differences between the polypeptide treated, hypophysectomized rats and the intact controls were not significant.

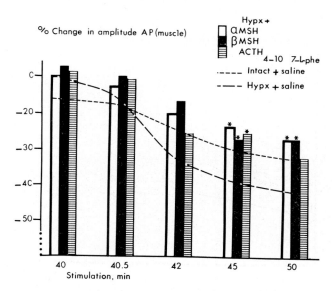

Fig. 2. Effect of rest and subsequent stimulation on muscle AP amplitude in hypophysectomized (hypx) rats administered α-MSH (20 μg/kg); β-MSH (20 μg/kg); ACTH$_{4-10}$-7-L-phe (1 μg/kg) and ACTH$_{4-10}$-7-D-phe (1 μg/kg and 10 μg/kg). The effects of the D-isomer are essentially the same as the saline treated controls and not shown separately; 8 rats per group. $P < 0.05$ (*) *versus* hypx, saline treated rats. Differences between the polypeptide treated, hypophysectomized rats and the intact controls were not significant.

References p. 192–194

from normal, a marked decline in AP amplitude is provoked by repetitive stimulation. Torda and Wolff (1952) correlate this to a decrease in the synthesis of acetylcholine in hypophysectomized rats, reversible by the administration of ACTH. The pituitary polypeptides we tested appear to be most effective during this period of falling response.

(II) Modulating effect of pituitary polypeptides on nerve action potentials and fatigue

In nerve, as in muscle, fatigue is more severe in the hypophysectomized rats and the effectiveness of the polypeptides is correspondingly greater in the operated animals than in the intact controls. $ACTH_{4-10}$-7-L-phe and α-MSH increase nerve AP amplitude and decrease fatigue, effects that appear earlier in nerve than in muscle. Enhancement of AP amplitude is particularly evident in the $ACTH_{4-10}$-7-L-phe treated hypophysectomized animals, being noticeable right at the beginning of the experiment (Fig. 3). β-MSH increases the amplitude of the nerve AP in hypophysectomized animals but this effect is not seen in intact rats (Table I). This supports the suggestion of Krivoy and Zimmermann (1973) that polypeptides raise a lowered response to normal levels or slightly beyond but do not dramatically affect normal parameters. Our experiments also imply that the pituitary polypeptides are modulators of excitability.

There are many possible mechanisms, and combinations of such mechanisms, by which the polypeptides may act peripherally on nerve and muscle. The polypeptide,

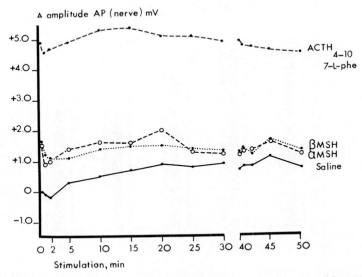

Fig. 3. Difference in amplitude of nerve APs in polypeptide and saline treated hypophysectomized (hypx) rats from intact controls; 30 min stimulation followed by rest and subsequent 10 min stimulation. α-MSH (20 μg/kg), β-MSH (20 μg/kg) and $ACTH_{4-10}$-7-L-phe (1 μg/kg); 8 rats per group. All $ACTH_{4-10}$ values differ from intact, saline treated controls at $P < 0.01$; α-MSH and β-MSH values differ from these controls after 10 min at $P < 0.05$.

TABLE I

AMPLITUDE (mV) OF THE NERVE ACTION POTENTIAL IN INTACT RATS

Results are expressed in means ± S.E.M.; 10 min rest between 30 and 40 min of stimulation.

Stimulation (min)	Saline	α-MSH (20 μg/kg)	β-MSH (20 μg/kg)	ACTH$_{4-10}$ (1 μg/kg)
0	4.48 ± 0.70	6.68 ± 0.69*	4.35 ± 0.60	5.40 ± 0.75
0.5	4.33 ± 0.63	6.38 ± 0.75*	4.37 ± 0.53	4.95 ± 0.73
2	4.24 ± 0.63	6.31 ± 0.74*	4.11 ± 0.50	5.02 ± 0.65
5	3.66 ± 0.46	5.24 ± 0.44*	3.65 ± 0.38	4.62 ± 0.65
10	3.35 ± 0.43	5.56 ± 0.43**	3.45 ± 0.36	4.52 ± 0.57
15	3.0 ± 0.40	5.40 ± 0.43**	3.38 ± 0.38	4.22 ± 0.52*
20	2.73 ± 0.39	5.15 ± 0.47**	3.28 ± 0.30	4.03 ± 0.50*
25	2.78 ± 0.41	5.34 ± 0.45**	3.24 ± 0.34	4.12 ± 0.51*
30	2.74 ± 0.40	4.93 ± 0.48**	3.05 ± 0.34	3.88 ± 0.49*
40	2.6 ± 1.04	4.40 ± 0.34**	3.38 ± 0.56	3.69 ± 0.46*
40.5	2.71 ± 0.41	4.70 ± 0.33**	3.39 ± 0.58	3.93 ± 0.45*
42	2.63 ± 0.36	4.46 ± 0.35**	3.24 ± 0.57	3.84 ± 0.46*
45	2.54 ± 0.32	4.57 ± 0.43**	3.39 ± 0.66	3.68 ± 0.47*
50	2.56 ± 0.37	4.56 ± 0.45**	3.29 ± 0.61	3.71 ± 0.45*

* $P < 0.05$ vs. saline.
** $P < 0.01$ vs. saline.

angiotensin, has both direct effects on smooth muscle cells and indirect effects on its innervation (see review by Nicoll, in press). Angiotensin facilitates ganglionic transmission by increasing the release of acetylcholine from preganglionic nerve terminals (Panisset, 1967). Polypeptides may increase acetylcholine synthesis (Torda and Wolff, 1952) and the synthesis of noradrenaline (Versteeg, 1973).

Direct excitatory effects of various peptides have been demonstrated. Substance P, a polypeptide of the alimentary tract and central nervous system, is capable of depolarizing motoneurons (Otsuka et al., 1972; Konishi and Otsuka, 1974) while lysine vasopressin induces prolonged bursting pacemaker activity in molluscan neurosecretory cells (Barker and Gainer, 1974).

ACTH and its analogs may bind to cell membranes and promote the synthesis of cyclic AMP (Seelig and Sayers, 1972) which plays an important role in both metabolic and synaptic processes in nervous tissue. Singer and Goldberg (1970) suggest a function for cyclic AMP at the neuromuscular junction. It is tempting also to propose cyclic AMP as a mediator for polypeptide action on muscle, for it enhances the release of calcium from the sarcoplasmic reticulum (Entman et al., 1969), restores muscle action potential amplitudes that have been lowered by reserpine or chlorpromazine (Torda, 1974) and activates both muscle glycogenolysis (Schlender et al., 1969) and protein synthesis (Walton et al., 1971). This is a particularly attractive concept as the sarcoplasmic reticulum appears to be a major storehouse for adenyl cyclase (Robison et al., 1971).

The significance of this modulatory role for neurotropic polypeptides lies in the fact that ACTH, MSH and vasopressin all are released by stress. If, as the evidence indicates, they are capable of altering the excitability of both the central and peripheral nervous systems, and, in addition, the excitability of muscle, they can contribute in this manner to the behavioral and physiological adaptations of the organism to stress.

SUMMARY

α-MSH, β-MSH, ACTH$_{4-10}$-7-L-phe and its D-isomer were administered to normal and hypophysectomized rats. These are all pituitary polypeptides, sharing a common amino acid sequence and without adrenocortical stimulating action. ACTH$_{4-10}$-7-L-phe and α-MSH increase the amplitude of sciatic nerve and gastrocnemius muscle action potentials (APs) and decrease fatigue, when measured *in situ* during 30 min of nerve stimulation. β-MSH appears to be effective only in muscle in the intact rat but increases both nerve and muscle APs in the hypophysectomized animals. A similar increase in AP amplitude and decrease in fatigue, due to polypeptide administration, are seen during a second stimulation period after 10 min rest. ACTH$_{4-10}$-7-D-phe has no effect on any of these parameters.

The augmenting action of these polypeptides on AP amplitude is most clearly seen in fatigued animals and particularly in the hypophysectomized, fatigued rat. This suggests that the peptides act as modulators of peripheral excitatory systems, capable of raising a lowered response to normal levels rather than substantially increasing normal parameters.

ACKNOWLEDGEMENTS

Our grateful thanks are due to Dr. David de Wied for advice and ACTH$_{4-10}$-7-L-phe; to Dr. William Krivoy for generous supplies of β-MSH and to N.V. Organon, Oss, The Netherlands, for ACTH$_{4-10}$-7-D-phe. We also thank Ciba Pharmaceutical Company for α-MSH (BA 33761).

This research was performed through partial support from a National Institutes of Health Biomedical Support Grant to New York University.

REFERENCES

BARKER, J. L. AND GAINER, H. (1974) Peptide regulation of bursting pacemaker activity in a molluscan neurosecretory cell. *Science*, **184**, 1371–1372.

BOHUS, B. AND DE WIED, D. (1966) Inhibitory and facilitatory effect of two related peptides on extinction of avoidance behavior. *Science*, **153**, 318–320.

VAN DELFT, A. M. L. AND KITAY, J. I. (1972) Effect of ACTH on single unit activity in the diencephalon of intact and hypophysectomized rats. *Neuroendocrinology*, **9**, 188–196.

ENTMAN, M. L., LEVEY, G. S. AND EPSTEIN, E. S. (1969) Demonstration of adenyl cyclase activity in canine cardiac sarcoplasmic reticulum. *Biochem. biophys. Res. Commun.*, **35**, 728–733.

FELDMAN, S., TODT, J. C. AND PORTER, R. W. (1961) Effect of adrenocortical hormones on evoked potentials in the brain stem. *Neurology (Minneap.)*, **11**, 109–115.

KASTIN, A. J., MILLER, L. H., NOCKTON, R., SANDMAN, C. A., SCHALLY, A. V. AND STRATTON, L. O. (1973) Behavioral aspects of melanocyte-stimulating hormone (MSH). In *Drug Effects on Neuroendocrine Regulation, Progress in Brain Research, Vol. 39*, E. ZIMMERMANN, W. H. GISPEN, B. H. MARKS AND D. DE WIED (Eds.), Elsevier, Amsterdam, pp. 461–470.

KONISHI, S. AND OTSUKA, M. (1974) The effects of substance P and other peptides on spinal neurons of the frog. *Brain Research*, **65**, 397–410.

KRIVOY, W. AND GUILLEMIN, R. (1961) On a possible role of β melanocyte stimulating hormone (β-MSH) in the central nervous system of the mammalia: an effect of β-MSH in the spinal cord of the cat. *Endocrinology*, **69**, 170–175.

KRIVOY, W. AND ZIMMERMANN, E. (1973) A possible role of polypeptides in synaptic transmission. In *Chemical Modulation of Brain Function*, H. C. SABELLI (Ed.), Raven Press, New York, N.Y., pp. 111–121.

NICOLL, R. Peptide receptors in the central nervous system. In *Handbook of Psychopharmacology*, L. L. IVERSEN, S. D. IVERSEN AND S. H. SNYDER (Eds.), Plenum Press, New York, in press.

NICOLOV, N. (1967) Effect of hydrocortisone and ACTH upon the bioelectric activity of spinal cord. *Folia Medica (Plovdiv)*, **9**, 249–255.

OTSUKA, M., KONISHI, S. AND TAKAHASHI, T. (1972) The presence of a motoneuron-depolarizing peptide in bovine dorsal roots of spinal nerves. *Proc. Jap. Acad.*, **48**, 342–346.

PANISSET, J. C. (1967) Effect of angiotensin on the release of acetylcholine from preganglionic and postganglionic nerve endings. *Canad. J. Physiol. Pharmacol.*, **45**, 313–317.

PFAFF, D. W., SILVA, M. T. A. AND WEISS, J. (1971) Telemetered recording of hormone effects on hippocampal neurons. *Science*, **172**, 394–396.

ROBISON, G. A., BUTCHER, R. W. AND SUTHERLAND, E. W. (1971) *Cyclic AMP*, Academic Press, New York, N.Y., p. 159.

SANDMAN, C. A., KASTIN, A. J. AND SCHALLY, A. V. (1971) Behavioral inhibition as modified by melanocyte-stimulating hormone (MSH) and light-dark conditions. *Physiol. Behav.*, **6**, 45–48.

SCHLENDER, K. K., WEI, S. H. AND VILLAR-PALASI, C. (1969) UDP-glucose: glycogen α-4-glucosyltransferase I kinase activity of purified muscle protein kinase. Cyclic nucleotide specificity. *Biochim. biophys. Acta (Amst.)*, **191**, 272–278.

SEELIG, S. AND SAYERS, G. (1972) ACTH$_{1-10}$ and ACTH$_{4-10}$ stimulate cyclic AMP production by isolated adrenal cells. *Fed. Proc.*, **31**, 252.

SINGER, J. J. AND GOLDBERG, A. L. (1970) Cyclic AMP and transmission at the neuromuscular junction. In *Role of Cyclic AMP in Cell Function, Advanc. Biochem. Psychopharmacol., Vol. 3*, P. GREENGARD AND E. COSTA (Eds.), Raven Press, New York, N.Y., pp. 335–348.

STEINER, F. A., RUF, K. AND AKERT, K. (1969) Steroid sensitive neurons in rat brain: anatomical localization and responses to neurohumours and ACTH. *Brain Research*, **12**, 74–85.

STRAND, F. L., STOBOY, H. AND CAYER, A. (1973/74) A possible direct action of ACTH on nerve and muscle. *Neuroendocrinology*, **13**, 1–20.

TORDA, C. AND WOLFF, H. G. (1952) Effect of pituitary hormones, cortisone and adrenalectomy on some aspects of neuromuscular systems and acetylcholine synthesis. *Amer. J. Physiol.*, **169**, 140–149.

TORDA, C. (1974) A potential mechanism for reserpine and chlorpromazine generation of myasthenia gravis-like easy fatigability and parkinsonism involving acetylcholine, dopamine and cyclic AMP. *IRCS* (Research on: Clinical Pharmacology and Therapeutics; Neurology and Neurosurgery, Psychiatry and Clinical Psychology), **2**, 1111.

VERSTEEG, D. H. G. (1973) Effect of two ACTH-analogs on noradrenaline metabolism in rat brain. *Brain Research*, **49**, 483–485.

WALTON, G., GILL, G., ABRASS, I. AND GARREN, L. (1971) Phosphorylation of ribosome-associated protein by an adenosine 3':5'-cyclic monophosphate-dependent protein kinase: Location of the microsomal receptor and protein kinase. *Proc. nat. Acad. Sci. (Wash.)*, **68**, 880–884.

DE WIED, D. (1966) Inhibitory effect of ACTH and related peptides on extinction of conditioned avoidance behaviour in rats. *Proc. Soc. exp. Biol. (N.Y.)*, **122**, 28–32.

DE WIED, D. (1969a) Effects of peptide hormones on behaviour. In *Frontiers of Neuroendocrinology*, W. F. GANONG AND L. MARTINI (Eds.), Oxford University Press, London, pp. 97–140.

DE WIED, D. (1969b) The anterior pituitary and conditioned avoidance behaviour. In *Progress in Endocrinology, Proceedings of the 3rd International Congress of Endocrinology, Mexico, D. F.,*

June 30–July 5, 1968, Excerpta Medica Intern. Congr. Series No. 184, Excerpta Medica, Amsterdam, pp. 310–316.

DE WIED, D. (1971) Long term effect of vasopressin on the maintenance of a conditioned avoidance response in rats. *Nature (Lond.)*, **232**, 58–60.

DE WIED, D. AND BOHUS, B. (1966) Long term and short term effect on retention of a conditioned avoidance response in rats by treatment respectively with long acting pitressin or αMSH. *Nature (Lond.)*, **212**, 1484–1486.

DE WIED, D. AND GREVEN, H. M. (1969) Opposite effect of structural analogues of ACTH on extinction of an avoidance response in rats by replacement of an L-amino acid by a D-isomer. *Proc. Intern. Union of Physiol. Sciences, 7, XXIV International Congress of Physiological Sciences, Washington, August 25–31, 1968*, p. 110.

VAN WIMERSMA GREIDANUS, TJ. B. AND DE WIED, D. (1971) Effects of systemic and intracerebral administration of two opposite acting ACTH-related peptides on extinction of conditioned avoidance behaviour. *Neuroendocrinology*, **7**, 291–301.

Effects of Behaviorally Active ACTH Analogs on Brain Protein Metabolism

M. E. A. REITH, P. SCHOTMAN AND W. H. GISPEN

Division of Molecular Neurobiology, Rudolf Magnus Institute for Pharmacology, and Laboratory of Physiological Chemistry, Medical Faculty, Institute of Molecular Biology, University of Utrecht, Utrecht, De Uithof (The Netherlands)

Removal of the pituitary in rats impairs acquisition of conditioned avoidance behavior in the shuttle box. The poor performance of these rats is restored towards normal by treatment with ACTH (corticotropin) (de Wied, 1964, 1969, 1974). The influence of ACTH on avoidance acquisition is due to an extra target effect, since the rate of acquisition is also normalized by the ACTH fragments $ACTH_{1-10}$ or $ACTH_{4-10}$ which have no detectable corticotropic, systemic or metabolic effects (de Wied, 1969). Under similar conditions the isomer $ACTH_{1-10}$ or $ACTH_{4-10}$ with D-phenylalanine substituted in the 7th position, has no or even a reversing effect on the already deficient avoidance learning in hypophysectomized rats (de Wied *et al.*, 1972). In intact rats extinction of an avoidance response is sensitive to the treatment with ACTH; administration of this hormone during the extinction period markedly delays extinction of a shuttle box (de Wied, 1967) as well as a pole-jumping avoidance response (de Wied, 1974). This effect again is independent of its action on the adrenal cortex, since smaller fragments of ACTH, devoid of corticotropic activity, also increase resistance to extinction. Furthermore, replacement of the phenylalanine residue in position 7 by the D-isomer reverses the effect of ACTH fragments and induces facilitation of extinction (de Wied, 1974). The behavioral effects of these peptides are caused by a direct action on central nervous structures, presumably at the posterior thalamus level (nucleus parafascicularis) as shown by lesion and implantation studies (Bohus and de Wied, 1967; van Wimersma Greidanus and de Wied, 1971; van Wimersma Greidanus *et al.*, 1974).

Previous work suggests that there are neurochemical correlates in the rat brain to the behavioral effect of these neuropeptides (Gispen and Schotman, 1973). It was found that acquisition of avoidance behavior in the shuttle box in hypophysectomized rats treated with $ACTH_{1-10}$ restores the reduced brain stem polysome population in these rats as measured at the end of the training period (Gispen *et al.*, 1970; Gispen and Schotman, 1970; Gispen *et al.*, 1971). Removal of the pituitary also decreases the incorporation of $[^3H]$leucine into brain stem proteins, measured 5 min after injection of the precursor into the diencephalon (Schotman and Gispen, 1974). Treatment of these rats with $ACTH_{1-10}$-7-L-Phe or $ACTH_{4-10}$-7-L-Phe restores leucine incorporation towards normal values (Schotman *et al.*, 1972; Reith *et al.*,

References p. 199–200

1974a). The relationship between the neurochemical and behavioral activities of these ACTH fragments seems rather specific, since the behaviorally inactive sequence $ACTH_{11-24}$ has no effect on the leucine incorporation under similar conditions and the analog $ACTH_{1-10}$-7-D-Phe even further decreases the suppressed incorporation rate in hypophysectomized rats (Schotman *et al.*, 1972). Presumably, these changes in leucine incorporation as found after hypophysectomy and treatment with ACTH fragments reflect alterations in the synthesis of rat brain stem proteins. From a series of experiments on size and metabolism of the precursor pool (Schotman *et al.*, 1972; Reith *et al.*, 1973; Reith *et al.*, 1974b; Schotman *et al.*, 1974) it was concluded that the observed changes in incorporation cannot be accounted for by the effects on the precursor pool. The results with $ACTH_{1-10}$-7-L-Phe or $ACTH_{4-10}$-7-L-Phe on protein synthesis are consistent with those of Reading and Dewar (1971) in intact animals. Rudman *et al.* (1974) studied the effects of melanotropic peptides which share the sequence $ACTH_{4-10}$, on protein synthesis in mouse brain; their observations on the penetration of α-amino isobutyric acid, and the accumulation, the level and incorporation of various amino acids also suggest a stimulatory effect of these peptides on brain protein synthesis.

The data so far do not indicate whether the observed alterations in leucine incorporation are due to a general effect on protein synthesis or to an effect restricted to certain protein species. Previously it was speculated that removal of the pituitary would deplete the rat of pituitary peptides and their breakdown products (Gispen and Schotman, 1973). These peptides (like ACTH fragments) are considered to play a crucial role in avoidance learning of the animal by enhancing the synthesis of certain brain stem proteins. As a result of the lack of these proteins the hypophysectomized rat is unable to store the information necessary to master the task in shuttle box conditioning. Substitution of ACTH-like peptides stimulates the production of such proteins and therefore leads to normal acquisition behavior (Gispen and Schotman, 1973). In subsequent studies on the mechanism of action of these neuropeptides, brain stem proteins were investigated in more detail. Proteins were extracted sequentially with solutions of increasing solubilizing capacity (Grossfeld and Shooter, 1971). By a stepwise treatment with an aqueous buffer, a non-ionic detergent (Triton X-100) and an ionic detergent (SDS), three main protein fractions were obtained. Each fraction was subjected to fractionation on SDS–polyacrylamide gels (Choules and Zimm, 1965; Weber and Osborn, 1969). Both the protein composition and the radioactivity distribution of the gels were determined, the proteins being labeled *in vivo* by a 5-min pulse of $[^3H]$leucine injected into the diencephalon as in the experiments described above (Schotman *et al.*, 1972). The results of this study suggested that hypophysectomy caused an overall decrease in labeling of all protein species, whereas treatment of hypophysectomized rats with $ACTH_{1-10}$-7-L-Phe resulted in a general increase (Reith *et al.*, 1974a; Gispen *et al.*, 1974). These data do not seem to support the view that stimulation of leucine incorporation into proteins by neuropeptides is restricted to certain species of brain stem proteins. In contrast they indicate an influence of the peptide on the mechanism of overall protein synthesis. To substantiate this hypothesis, *in vitro* incorporation of radioactive leucine into

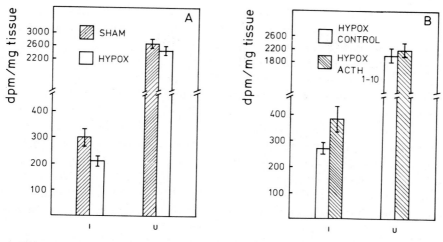

Fig. 1. The *in vitro* uptake (U) and incorporation (I) of [U-^{14}C]leucine in rat brain stem slices. Slices were preincubated for 30 min before adding 1 μCi [^{14}C]leucine and incubation continued for another 30 min. At the end of the incubation, slices were washed three times with ice-cold medium containing unlabeled leucine, each time for 5 min. Results are the mean $\pm$ S.E.M. (vertical bar) for 9 or 10 slices. A: hypophysectomized *versus* sham-operated animals. B: slices, obtained from hypophysectomized rats, incubated with and without 10^{-5} *M* ACTH$_{1-10}$-7-L-Phe.

proteins in slices from the posterior thalamus was studied. Advantages of the *in vitro* system are a controlled supply of the precursor and the possibility to measure precursor uptake simultaneously.

The *in vitro* experiments were carried out 3 weeks after hypophysectomy or sham-operation. The animals were sacrificed by decapitation and a brain stem slice was prepared at about 3400 μm from the frontal zero plane (König and Klippel, 1963) as described elsewhere (Reith *et al.*, 1974c). The slice obtained contained posterior thalamic tissue including the nucleus parafascicularis and weighed approximately 25 mg. This particular brain area was chosen since the nucleus parafascicularis presumably is implicated in the action of ACTH analogs on central nervous structures as pointed out above (van Wimersma Greidanus and de Wied, 1971; van Wimersma Greidanus *et al.*, 1974). After 30 min preincubation, the incorporation of L-[U-^{14}C]-leucine into proteins was measured as described elsewhere (Reith *et al.*, 1974c). The incorporation increased linearly up to at least 60 min after addition of the radio-active precursor. An incorporation period of 30 min was chosen to study the effects of hypophysectomy and ACTH$_{1-10}$-7-L-Phe. Fig. 1A shows the results obtained with slices of hypophysectomized and sham-operated animals. Three weeks after removal of the pituitary, a marked decrease in incorporation was found amounting to approximately 30%. When ACTH$_{1-10}$-7-L-Phe was present in a concentration of 10^{-5} *M* during incubation of slices from hypophysectomized rats, a significant stimulation in incorporation was observed (+ 42%; Fig. 1B). In a first attempt to investigate whether effects on uptake phenomena are involved in these changes in incorporation, an estimation was made of the radioactivity of intracellular amino acid, which has always been considered the source for protein synthesis in brain. Indeed

References p. 199–200

198   M. E. A. REITH *et al.*

Jones and McIlwain (1971) and recently Dunlop *et al.* (1974) have advanced evidence in support of an intracellular precursor pool for protein synthesis in brain slices. To study the intracellular radioactivity, the tissue was transferred to ice-cold medium after the incorporation period and washed during 15 min at $0\,°C$. Under these conditions, extracellular amino acid is removed and amino acid located intracellularly, at least in preparations of rat muscle (Kostyo, 1968; Hider *et al.*, 1971), rat pancreas (van Venrooy *et al.*, 1972) and rat submandibular gland (van Venrooy *et al.*, 1973) is preserved. However, for rat cerebral cortex slices some loss of intracellular amino acid has been reported by Dunlop *et al.* (1974) during a 40-min cold-wash. Nevertheless, using this method, and a less extensive cold-wash of 15 min, we found no indication that the observed changes in incorporation were due to effects on uptake of radioactive precursor into the slices (Fig. 1A and B). No alterations were found in the amount of radioactivity extracted from the tissue during the cold-wash. Therefore, the changes in incorporation most likely reflect changes in protein synthesis. In addition, the alterations found *in vitro* parallel the observations in *in vivo* experiments on the effects of hypophysectomy and $ACTH_{1-10}$-7-L-Phe treatment of hypophysectomized rats (Schotman *et al.*, 1972; Schotman and Gispen, 1974). The *in vitro* data provide further evidence for a direct action of $ACTH_{1-10}$ on central nervous structures, resulting in a change in protein synthesis.

At various levels of brain cell metabolism, effects of treatment with ACTH or its analogs can be monitored. Not only RNA and protein metabolism, but also glucose metabolism (De Kloet and Witter, 1973) and noradrenaline turnover (Versteeg, 1973; Leonard, 1974) seem to be influenced by treatment with N-terminal fragments of ACTH. At present the relationship of the various effects to one another is not clear and further studies are necessary. Nonetheless we have postulated elsewhere that a peptide–brain membrane interaction should be the crucial signal for the brain cell to respond to peptide treatment (Gispen and Schotman, 1973).

SUMMARY

Hypophysectomy was found to interfere with both long-term active avoidance conditioning and brain stem macromolecule metabolism in rats.

Treatment of these rats with $ACTH_{1-10}$-7-L-Phe restored their poor performance in shuttle box conditioning almost to normal levels; conversely, under similar conditions, the analog $ACTH_{1-10}$-7-D-Phe was ineffective or even showed an opposite effect. It appeared that these peptides also affected leucine incorporation into brain stem proteins. In hypophysectomized rats, $ACTH_{1-10}$-7-L-Phe increased the incorporation rate, whereas $ACTH_{1-10}$-7-D-Phe caused an inhibition; the behaviorally neutral $ACTH_{11-24}$ had no effect. These data raised the question as to whether the observed alterations are general effects, or are restricted to a few protein species. Therefore, brain stem proteins were further analyzed, using techniques of sequential extraction and polyacrylamide gel electrophoresis. Hypophysectomy caused a general decrease in labeling of all protein species studied, whereas $ACTH_{1-10}$-7-L-Phe caused an overall increase. These effects might be due to a direct action on the mechanism of protein synthesis, as similar alterations were observed by studying *in vitro* protein synthesis in brain stem slices.

The present data may help to unravel the neurochemical events which underlie the behavioral effect of N-terminal ACTH fragments.

REFERENCES

BOHUS, B. AND DE WIED, D. (1967) Failure of α-MSH to delay extinction of conditioned avoidance behavior in rats with lesions in the parafascicular nuclei of the thalamus. *Physiol. Behav.*, **2**, 221–223.

CHOULES, G. L. AND ZIMM, B. H. (1965) An acrylamide gel soluble in scintillation fluid: its application to electrophoresis at neutral and low pH. *Analyt. Biochem.*, **13**, 336–344.

DE KLOET, E. R. AND WITTER, A. (1973) Metabolism of [U-^{14}C]glucose in rat brain: Effect of ACTH$_{1-10}$. In *Proc. 14th Meeting of Med. Biol. Soc. in The Netherlands, Groningen*, Abstract no. 222.

DUNLOP, D. S., VAN ELDEN, W. AND LAJTHA, A. (1974) Measurements of rates of protein synthesis in rat brain slices. *J. Neurochem.*, **22**, 821–830.

GISPEN, W. H. AND SCHOTMAN, P. (1970) Effect of hypophysectomy and conditioned avoidance behavior on macromolecule metabolism in the brain stem of the rat. In *Pituitary, Adrenal and the Brain, Progress in Brain Research, Vol. 32*, D. DE WIED AND J. A. W. M. WEIJNEN (Eds.), Elsevier, Amsterdam, pp. 236–244.

GISPEN, W. H., DE WIED, D., SCHOTMAN, P. AND JANSZ, H. S. (1970) Effects of hypophysectomy on RNA metabolism in rat brain stem. *J. Neurochem.*, **17**, 751–761.

GISPEN, W. H., DE WIED, D., SCHOTMAN, P. AND JANSZ, H. S. (1971) Brain stem polysomes and avoidance performance of hypophysectomized rats subjected to peptide treatment. *Brain Res.*, **31**, 341–351.

GISPEN, W. H. AND SCHOTMAN, P. (1973) Pituitary–adrenal system, learning and performance: some neurochemical aspects. In *Drug Effects on Neuroendocrine Regulation, Progress in Brain Research, Vol. 39*, E. ZIMMERMANN, W. H. GISPEN, B. H. MARKS AND D. DE WIED (Eds.), Elsevier, Amsterdam, pp. 443–459.

GISPEN, W. H., DE KLOET, E. R., REITH, M. E. A., WIEGANT, V. M. AND SCHOTMAN, P. (1974) Pituitary, peptides and brain function: some neurochemical aspects. *5th Annual Meeting European Brain and Behaviour Society, Rotterdam, September 2–5, 1973, Brain Res.*, **66**, 368–369 (Abstr.).

GROSSFELD, R. M. AND SHOOTER, E. M. (1971) A study of the changes in protein composition of mouse brain during ontogenetic development. *J. Neurochem.*, **18**, 2265–2277.

HIDER, R. C., FERN, E. B. AND LONDON, D. R. (1971) Identification in skeletal muscle of a distinct extracellular pool of amino acids, and its role in protein synthesis. *Biochem. J.*, **121**, 817–827.

JONES, D. A. AND MCILWAIN, H. (1971) Amino acid distribution and incorporation into proteins in isolated, electrically-stimulated cerebral tissues. *J. Neurochem.*, **18**, 41–58.

KÖNIG, J. F. R. AND KLIPPEL, R. A. (1963) *The Rat Brain, a Stereotaxic Atlas*, Krieger Publishing Co., Huntington, p. 25.

KOSTYO, J. L. (1968) Rapid effects of growth hormones on amino acid transport and protein synthesis. *Ann. N.Y. Acad. Sci.*, **148**, 389–407.

LEONARD, B. E. (1974) The effect of two synthetic ACTH analogues on the metabolism of biogenic amines in the rat brain. *Arch. Int. Pharmacol. Ther.*, **207**, 242–253.

READING, H. W. AND DEWAR, A. J. (1971) Effects of ACTH$_{4-10}$ on cerebral RNA and protein metabolism in the rat. *3rd Meeting International Society for Neurochemistry, Budapest*, J. DOMONKOS, A. FONYÓ, I. HUSZÁK AND J. SZENTÁGOTHAI (Eds.), Akadémiai Kaidó, Budapest, p. 199.

REITH, M. E. A., SCHOTMAN, P. AND GISPEN, W. H. (1973) Brain protein metabolism and hypophysectomy, *IRCS Med. Sci.*, (**73-3**) 3-10-6.

REITH, M. E. A., GISPEN, W. H. AND SCHOTMAN, P. (1974a) in preparation.

REITH, M. E. A., GISPEN, W. H. AND SCHOTMAN, P. (1974b) Hypophysectomy and metabolism of brain proteins. In *Central Nervous System, Studies on Metabolic Regulation and Function*, E. GENAZZANI AND H. HERKEN (Eds.), Springer, Berlin, pp. 236–240.

REITH, M. E. A., SCHOTMAN, P. AND GISPEN, W. H. (1974c) Hypophysectomy, ACTH₁₋₁₀ and *in vitro* protein synthesis in rat brain stem slices. *Brain Res.*, **81**, 571–575.

RUDMAN, D. SCOTT, J. W., DEL RIO, A. E., HOUSER, D. H. AND SHEEN, S. (1974) Effect of melanotropic peptides on protein synthesis in mouse brain. *Amer. J. Physiol.*, **226**, 687–692.

SCHOTMAN, P., GISPEN, W. H., JANSZ, H. S. AND DE WIED, D. (1972) Effects of ACTH analogues on macromolecule metabolism in the brain stem of hypophysectomized rats. *Brain Res.*, **46**, 349–362.

SCHOTMAN, P. AND GISPEN, W. H. (1974) Analogues of ACTH, conditioned avoidance behaviour and metabolism of macromolecules in brain of rat. In *Central Nervous System, Studies on Metabolic Regulation and Function*, E. GENAZZANI AND H. HERKEN (Eds.), Springer, Berlin, pp. 231–235.

SCHOTMAN, P., GIPON, L. AND GISPEN, W. H. (1974) Conversion of [4,5-³H]leucine into ³H₂O and tritiated metabolites in rat brain tissue. Comparison of peripheral and intracranial route of administration. *Brain Res.*, **70**, 377–380.

VAN VENROOY, W. J., POORT, C., KRAMER, M. F. AND JANSEN, M. (1972) Relationship between extracellular amino acids and protein synthesis *in vitro* in the rat pancreas. *Europ. J. Biochem.*, **30**, 427–433.

VAN VENROOY, W. J., KUYPER-LENSTRA, A. H. AND KRAMER, M. F. (1973) Interrelationship between amino acid pools and protein synthesis in the rat submandibular gland, *Biochim. biophys. Acta (Amst.)*, **312**, 392–398.

VERSTEEG, D. H. G. (1973) Effect of two ACTH-analogues on noradrenaline metabolism in rat brain. *Brain Res.*, **49**, 483–485.

WEBER, K. AND OSBORN, M. (1969) The reliability of molecular weight determinations by dodecyl-sulfate–polyacrylamide gel electrophoresis. *J. biol. Chem.* **244**, 4406–4412.

DE WIED, D. (1964) Influence of anterior pituitary on avoidance learning and escape behavior. *Amer. J. Physiol.*, **207**, 255–259.

DE WIED, D. (1967) Opposite effects of ACTH and glucocorticosteroids on extinction of conditioned avoidance behavior. In *Proc. of the 2nd Int. Congr. on Hormonal Steroids, Milan, May 1966, Excerpta Medica Int. Congr. Series No. 132*, Excerpta Medica, Amsterdam, pp. 945–951.

DE WIED, D. (1969) Effects of peptide hormones on behaviour. In *Frontiers in Neuroendocrinology*, W. F. GANONG AND L. MARTINI (Eds.), Oxford University Press, New York, N.Y., pp. 97–140.

DE WIED, D., VAN DELFT, A. M. L., GISPEN, W. H., WEIJNEN, J. A. W. M. AND VAN WIMERSMA GREIDANUS, TJ. B. (1972) The role of pituitary–adrenal system hormones in active-avoidance conditioning. In *Hormones and Behavior*, S. LEVINE (Ed.), Academic Press, New York, N.Y., pp. 135–171.

DE WIED, D. (1974) Pituitary–adrenal system hormones and behavior. In *The Neurosciences, Third Study Program*, F. O. SMITT AND F. G. WORDEN (Eds.), Rockefeller Univ. Press, New York, N.Y., pp. 653–666.

VAN WIMERSMA GREIDANUS, TJ. B. AND DE WIED, D. (1971) Effects of systemic and intracerebral administration of two opposite acting ACTH-related peptides on extinction of conditioned avoidance behavior. *Neuroendocrinology*, **7**, 291–301.

VAN WIMERSMA GREIDANUS, TJ. B., BOHUS, B. AND DE WIED, D. (1974) Differential localization of lysine vasopressin and of ACTH₄₋₁₀ on avoidance behavior; a study in rats bearing lesions in the parafascicular nuclei. *Neuroendocrinology*, **14**, 280–288.

Phosphorylation of Proteins from the Brains of Mice Subjected to Short-term Behavioral Experiences

RAMASAMY PERUMAL*, WILLEM HENDRIK GISPEN**, JOHN ERIC WILSON
AND EDWARD GLASSMAN

Division of Chemical Neurobiology, Department of Biochemistry, School of Medicine, The University of North Carolina, Chapel Hill, N. C. 27514 (U.S.A.)

Over the past decade numerous studies have been performed attempting to relate macromolecular events in the central nervous system to learning and memory (see for instance Glassman, 1969; Gispen and Schotman, 1973; Dunn *et al.*, 1974; Rees *et al.*, 1974). Such studies proved to be very difficult and results obtained by different laboratories often appeared to be contradictory. Presumably, such difficulties occur for at least two reasons. First, most of the molecular events taking place in nerve tissue are not yet elucidated, partly because of the limitations of the neurochemical methods available. Second, there are problems concerning the measurement of learning and memory. Since these processes can only be approached indirectly by analyzing the performance of a given subject in a stimulus situation, other factors such as motivation, fatigue etc., may interfere with the observation. Even if an experimental design could be adopted that would selectively deal with learning and memory, the choice of appropriate experimental groups for comparison would be extremely difficult. In active avoidance conditioning, for instance, animals are subjected to stimuli which by themselves may alter brain metabolism (Jakoubek *et al.*, 1972; Gispen and Schotman, 1975; Glassman, 1974; Rees *et al.*, 1974) and these changes may be totally independent of the processes underlying the acquisition of the new behavior. Appropriate behavioral controls, therefore, are key experiments in studies on molecular processes related to learning and memory.

Throughout the literature one can find the idea that plasticity in the central nervous system may be an important mechanism in the acquisition and storage of behavioral experience in the brain (Horn *et al.*, 1973). Previously, it was suggested that one possible mechanism for molecular control of the interneuronal connectivity that could lead to the formation of new neural pathways or networks would be through conformational changes resulting from an altered phosphorylation of synaptic proteins (Glassman *et al.*, 1973). The present paper describes the phosphorylation of proteins

---

* Present address: department of Biochemistry, University of Malaya, Kuala-Lumpur, Malaysia.
** Present address: division of Molecular Neurobiology, Rudolf Magnus Institute for Pharmacology and Laboratory of Physiological Chemistry, Medical Faculty, Institute of Molecular Biology, University of Utrecht, Padualaan 8, Utrecht, De Uithof, The Netherlands.

References p. 206–207

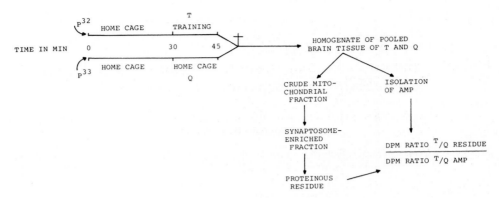

Fig. 1. Experimental design.

obtained from enriched synaptosomal fractions from the brains of mice subjected to short training experiences.

An outline of the experiment is presented in Fig. 1. One of a pair of 6–8-week-old male mice (C57BL/6J from the Jackson Laboratories) was injected intracranially (Adair *et al.*, 1968) with approximately 20 μCi [^{32}P]orthophosphate in 20 μl water, while the other was injected with 20 μCi of carrier-free [^{33}P]orthophosphate from ICN, Irvine, Calif., U.S.A. The mice were coded and placed in their home cages. Twenty-nine minutes after injection one mouse was placed in a jump-box training apparatus and trained as described previously (Zemp *et al.*, 1966). The training lasted 15 min and consisted of about 30 trials. On the average, a mouse made 22 conditioned avoidance responses out of the 30 trials (Fig. 2). The untrained mouse stayed in the home cage during the entire 45 min and will be referred to as Quiet.

At the end of the training, both mice were decapitated after minimal ether anesthetization. The brains were removed and the olfactory bulbs and cerebellum excised. The rest of the brains of both mice were homogenized together at 0–4 °C in 10 ml 0.1 mM

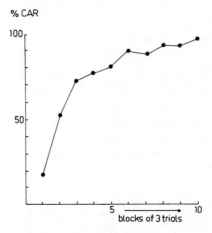

Fig. 2. Mean performance of 6 mice, intracranially injected with radioactive orthophosphate.

sodium phosphate buffer pH 7.6, containing 0.32 M sucrose, and a crude mito-chondrial pellet was isolated from the homogenate. This was suspended and layered on a discontinuous sucrose gradient (0.8 and 1.2 M sucrose), and a synaptosome-enriched fraction was obtained as described by Whittaker (1969). The use of Ficoll–sucrose gradients (Herschman et al., 1972) gave similar results. Electron microscopy confirmed that the preparations used were enriched in intact synaptosomes. The synaptosome-enriched fraction was osmotically shocked in 1 mM (sodium) phosphate, pH 7.6 and frozen overnight. Ice-cold $HClO_4$ was added to a final concentration of 0.25 M. The residue obtained by centrifugation was then washed twice with ice-cold 0.25 M $HClO_4$. Lipids were extracted using acidified 2:1 chloroform–methanol (Bligh and Dyer, 1959). The solid interphase layer was carefully removed and washed twice with ice-cold 0.25 M $HClO_4$, then incubated in 0.25 M $HClO_4$ at 90 °C for 15 min. Following centrifugation, the sediment was washed twice with cold 0.25 M $HClO_4$, and dissolved in Soluene by heating for 2 hr at 50–60 °C. Radioactivity was determined in aliquots from all gradient fractions and extracts. Liquid scintillation counting was performed in a TriCarb Liquid Scintillation Spectrometer Model 3375, using a mixture of toluene–Triton X-100 (2:1, v/v) containing 2,5-diphenyloxazole (PPO, 4 g/l). For each batch of isotope a set of standards quenched to different degrees with different amounts of chloroform was prepared. The correlation between the automatic external standardization and the counting efficiency of the standards was used to compute the disint./min and the ratio of the disint./min in each channel.

The nucleoside monophosphates in 1 ml of the homogenate were separated by means of thin-layer chromatography (Zemp et al., 1966). The nucleotide spots were scraped off, eluted with 0.1 N HCl in scintillation vials, and the radioactivity was determined. The radioisotope ratios of the various brain fractions were corrected for that observed in AMP. The ratio observed in AMP did not differ from that of GMP, UMP or CMP. The radioisotope ratio in AMP was used as a correction factor for the availability of intracellular radioactive phosphate, which varies with the amount of leakage during injection in each brain.

The synaptosome-enriched fraction contained about 27% of the radioactive phosphorus of the total gradient, and about 75% of this radioactivity was acid-soluble. About 18% of the total radioactivity in the synaptosome-enriched fraction was in phospholipid. Almost all of the radioactivity in the final residue was radioactive phosphate covalently bound to proteins (Perumal et al., in prep.). This was shown by the fact that (a) incubation of the residue with alkaline phosphatase rendered over 90% of the radioactivity acid-soluble; (b) RNAse digestion was ineffective in this respect; (c) electrophoresis of tryptic digests revealed radioactivity coincident with ninhydrin positive material; (d) pronase digestion of the residue resulted in the solubilization of 85–95% of the radioactivity; and (e) pronase or HCl hydrolysates contained radioactive phosphoserine and phosphothreonine (Perumal et al. in prep.).

In 14 out of the 15 mouse pairs, the washed acid-insoluble residue from the synaptosome-enriched fraction from the trained mouse contained more radioactive phosphate than the residue from the quiet mouse, as was apparent from the increase in the ratio

$\dfrac{\text{disint./min ratio T/Q residue}}{\text{disint./min ratio T/Q AMP}}$ (see also Fig. 1). The mean relative increase in disint./

min in the residue obtained from trained mice was 34.1%. Although the difference
was variable it occurred very consistently throughout our experiments when training
was involved (Perumal *et al.*, in prep.; Gispen *et al.*, in prep.). Differences in other
fractions obtained during the extraction procedure were much more variable and the

average ratios $\dfrac{\text{disint./min ratio T/Q residue}}{\text{disint./min ratio T/Q AMP}}$ did not differ significantly from 1.00.

Furthermore, it was found that this increased phosphorylation occurred mainly in the
particulate material from the osmotically shocked synaptosome-enriched fraction,
and it was also possible to identify phosphoproteins from isolated membrane fractions
on SDS polyacrylamide gels (Perumal *et al.*, in prep.).

To investigate the time relationship between avoidance conditioning and the increased phosphorylation of proteins of the synaptosome-enriched fraction, 35 pairs
of mice were injected intracranially with [^{32}P]- and [^{33}P]orthophosphate as described
previously. Fifteen minutes after injection, 5 pairs were killed. Three groups of 6 mice
were trained 30 min after injection for periods of 5, 10 or 15 min, respectively. Each
trained mouse and its quiet control were sacrificed immediately after the training
experience. Of the remaining 12 pairs, a mouse of each pair was trained 30 min after
injection for 15 min, and then returned to the home cage. Killing was delayed for
15 min (6 pairs) or 30 min (6 pairs). At the end of the 5 min of training, the mice
avoided at an average level of 50% at the end of 10 min, about 80% and at the end of
15 min, over 90%. In all cases, quiet mice were used for comparison. The brains of all
pairs were processed as described previously.

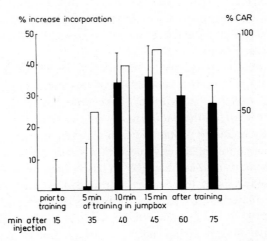

Fig. 3. The percentage increase in phosphate incorporation into proteins from synaptosome-enriched
fractions of brains of trained mice. The open bars represent the mean performance of the trained mice.
The closed bars represent the mean increase in the ratio $\dfrac{\text{disint./min ratio T/Q residue}}{\text{disint./min ratio T/Q AMP}}$. On the horizontal axis the time of killing the mice is indicated.

Fig. 3 shows that before training, and even after 5 min of training no difference exists within the pairs with respect to the neurochemical parameter studied. With further training for 10 or 15 min, however, there is a significant increase in the radioactivity in proteins obtained from synaptosome-enriched fractions; this increase lasts at least 30 min after training. The average ratio of the isotopes in AMP did not differ significantly between the various time points. The data therefore suggest that after a certain amount of training experience an increased phosphorylation of proteins obtained from synaptosome-enriched fractions occurs, lasting beyond the actual period of training.

One would very much like to speculate on the mechanism underlying the altered phosphorylation of these proteins. Many important factors are still unclear, however (*e.g.* what is the phosphate donor? Supposing ATP is the donor, how can one routinely isolate ATP in undegraded form from the same homogenate that is further processed to obtain a synaptosome-enriched fraction? Is one dealing with precursor pool compartmentation and what is the specific activity of these pools? etc.). With respect to the time relationship between avoidance conditioning and the altered phosphorylation, it is clear that a great deal of work needs to be done, before one could even begin to speculate on whether the effect is on synthesis or degradation of phosphoproteins. For this reason we do not speculate on the mechanism even though this is a very important, but at the moment unresolvable, point, but merely refer to an increased amount of radioactive phosphate in the synaptosome-enriched fraction.

The experimental mice were subjected to a variety of behavioral conditions in an attempt to assess the specificity of the observed phenomenon. Such experiments were performed according to Adair *et al.* (1968) and included the following experimental groups for comparison: yoked *versus* quiet and prior-trained-performing *versus* quiet. No significant differences existed with respect to the phosphorylation of the protein fractions of these groups. The ineffectiveness of the yoke procedure is puzzling since in this procedure the mice also underwent a new short-term behavioral experience. Since we do not know what clue(s) in the behavioral experience (jump-box conditioning) trigger(s) the neurochemical response, we are still in a state of collecting data and not fully understanding them. However, it should be noted that the experiments on the effects of various behaviors on uridine incorporation into brain RNA also show that the yoked control does not differ from the quiet control, using the same training apparatus (Zemp *et al.*, 1966; Adair *et al.*, 1968). The ineffectiveness of the yoked and prior-trained performing procedure combined with the finding that the T/Q ratios of the mononucleotides were the same make it highly unlikely that the reported increase in ratio would in fact be due to a decrease in adenyl nucleotide concentration as would occur in rat brain after footshock stress (Dickman *et al.*, 1973). Therefore, it was concluded that the stimulation of the conditioning procedure and the motor activity of the mouse are not responsible for the increased phosphorylation of protein obtained from synaptosome-enriched fractions.

At present the biological significance of this effect is not clear. Recently it has been shown that phosphorylation of synaptosomal membrane protein is c-AMP dependent (Johnson *et al.*, 1971; Johnson *et al.*, 1972; Ueda *et al.*, 1973). It has been claimed that an altered turnover of these proteins in brain tissue could result from electrical stimulation or stimulation by putative transmitter (Heald, 1957, 1962; Trevor and Rodnight, 1965; Jones and Rodnight, 1971; Reddington and Rodnight, 1972). Moreover, a unique type of synaptic transmission involving transmembrane responses to c-AMP has been suggested (Hoffer *et al.*, 1971). A connection between nerve cell activity, c-AMP levels and phosphorylation of synaptic membrane elements has also been postulated (Greengard *et al.*, 1971). The function of brain phosphoproteins has been thought to be linked to ion transport (Wolff and Siegel, 1970; Jones and Rodnight, 1971; Donella *et al.*, 1972). The above cited literature does in fact underscore how little we know of the function of brain phosphoproteins. Notwithstanding this, it may very well be that phosphoproteins are indeed key elements in the brain's response to behavioral experiences, since the phosphorylation of nuclear nonhistone acid-extractable proteins in rat brain is also affected by various behaviors and reminding experiences (Machlus *et al.*, 1974a and b). Further work is in progress to elucidate the role of synaptosomal membrane phosphoproteins with regard to these ideas.

SUMMARY

Proteins of synaptosome-enriched fractions of mouse brain exhibited an increase in the incorporation of radioactive phosphate during 15 min of avoidance conditioning. The increase was initiated between 5 and 10 min of the training and could be detected 30 min beyond the training period.

ACKNOWLEDGEMENTS

This research was supported by grants from the U.S. Public Health Service (MH 18136, NS 07457), the U.S. National Science Foundation (GB 18551), the Ciba–Geigy Corporation and the Dr. Saal van Zwanenbergstichting.

REFERENCES

ADAIR, L. B., WILSON, J. E., ZEMP, J. E. AND GLASSMAN, E. (1968) Brain function and macromolecules. IV: Uridine incorporation into polysomes of mouse brain during different behavioral experiences. *Proc. nat. Acad. Sci. (Wash.)*, **61**, 917–922.

BLIGH, E. G. AND DYER, W. J. (1959) A rapid method of total lipid extraction and purification. *Canad. J. Biochem.*, **37**, 911–917.

DICKMAN, S. H., HARRISON, J. F. AND GROSSER, B. I. (1973) Decrease in adenyl nucleotide concentrations in rat brain components after footshock stress. *Brain Res.*, **53**, 483–487.

DONELLA, A., PINNA, L. A. AND MORET, V. (1972) On the possible role of phosphoproteins as ion carriers. *FEBS Letters*, **26**, 249–251.

DUNN, A., ENTINGH, D., ENTINGH, T., GISPEN, W. H., MACHLUS, B., PERUMAL, R., REES, H. D. AND BROGAN, L. (1974) Biochemical correlates of brief behavioral experiences. In *The Neurosciences, 3rd Study Program*, F. O. SCHMITT AND F. G. WORDEN (Eds.), MIT Press, Cambridge, Mass., pp. 653–666.

GISPEN, W. H. AND SCHOTMAN, P. (1973) Pituitary–adrenal system, learning and performance: some neurochemical aspects. In *Drug Effects on Neuroendocrine Regulation, Progress in Brain Research*,

Vol. 39, E. ZIMMERMANN, W. H. GISPEN, B. MARKS AND D. DE WIED (Eds.), Elsevier, Amsterdam, pp. 443–459.

GISPEN, W. H. AND SCHOTMAN, P. (1975) ACTH and brain RNA: changes in content and labelling of RNA in rat brain stem, submitted.

GLASSMAN, E. (1969) The biochemistry of learning: an evaluation of the role of RNA and protein. *Ann. Rev. Biochem.*, **38**, 605–646.

GLASSMAN, E. (1974) Macromolecules and behavior: a commentary. In *The Neurosciences, 3rd Study Program*, F. O. SCHMITT AND F. G. WORDEN (Eds.), MIT Press, Cambridge, Mass. pp. 667–677.

GLASSMAN, E., GISPEN, W. H., PERUMAL, R., MACHLUS, B. AND WILSON, J. E. (1973) The effect of short experiences on the incorporation of radioactive phosphate into synaptosomal and non-histone acid-extractable nuclear proteins from rat and mouse brain. In *Proceedings 5th International Congress Pharmacology, San Francisco, 1972, Vol. 4*, pp. 14–17.

GREENGARD, P., McAFEE, D. A., SCHORDERET, M. AND KABALAN, J. W. (1971) Cyclic AMP and synaptic transmission. In *Abstracts of the Int. Congr. Physiol. Pharmacol. of cAMP, Milan, Italy*.

HEALD, P. J. (1957) The incorporation of phosphate into cerebral phosphoprotein promoted by electrical impulses. *Biochem. J.*, **66**, 659–663.

HEALD, P. J. (1962) Phosphoprotein metabolism and ion transport in nervous tissue: a suggested connexion. *Nature (Lond.)*, **193**, 451–454.

HERSCHMAN, H. R., COTMAN, C. AND MATHEWS, D. A. (1972) Serological specificities of brain subcellular organelles. I. Antisera to synaptosomal fraction. *J. Immunol.*, **108**, 1362.

HOFFER, B. J., SIGGINS, G. R., OLIVER, A. P. AND BLOOM, F. E. (1971) Cyclic AMP mediation of norepinephrine inhibition in rat cerebellar cortex: A unique class of synaptic responses. *Ann. N.Y. Acad. Sci.*, **185**, 531–549.

HORN, G., ROSE, S. P. R. AND BATESON, P. P. G. (1973) Experiences and plasticity in the central nervous system. *Science*, **181**, 506–514.

JAKOUBEK, B., BUREŠOVA, M., HAJEK, I., ETRYCHOVA, J., PAVLIK, A. AND DEDICOVA, A. (1972) Effect of ACTH on the synthesis of rapidly labelled RNA in the nervous system of mice. *Brain Res.*, **43**, 417–428.

JOHNSON, E. M., MAENO, H. AND GREENGARD, P. (1971) Phosphorylation of endogenous protein of rat brain by cyclic adenosine 3′,5′-monophosphate-dependent protein kinase. *J. biol. Chem.*, **24**, 7731–7739.

JOHNSON, E. M., UEDA, T., MAENO, H. AND GREENGARD, P. (1972) Adenosine 3′, 5′-monophosphate-dependent phosphorylation of a specific protein in synaptic membrane fraction from rat cerebrum. *J. biol. Chem.*, **247**, 5650–5652.

JONES, D. A. AND RODNIGHT, R. (1971) Protein-bound phosphorylation in acid hydrolysates of brain tissue: The determination of [^{32}P]phosphorylserine by ion-exchange chromatography and electrophoresis. *Biochem. J.*, **121**, 597–600.

MACHLUS, B. J., WILSON, J. E. AND GLASSMAN, E. (1974a) Brain phosphoproteins: The effect of short experiences on the phosphorylation of nuclear proteins of rat brain. *Behav. Biol.*, **10**, 43–62.

MACHLUS, B. J., ENTINGH, D., WILSON, J. E. AND GLASSMAN, E. (1974b) Brain phosphoproteins: The effect of various behaviors and reminding experiences on the incorporation of radioactive phosphate into nuclear proteins. *Behav. Biol.*, **10**, 63–73.

REDDINGTON, A. AND RODNIGHT, R. (1972) Effect of putative transmitters and other agents on phosphoprotein turnover in respiring slices of guinea-pig cerebral cortex. *Biochem. J.*, **126**, 14P–15P.

REES, H. D., BROGAN, L. L., ENTINGH, D. J., DUNN, A. J., SHINKMAN, P. G., DAMSTRA-ENTINGH, T., WILSON, J. E. AND GLASSMAN, E. (1974) Effect of sensory stimulation on the uptake and incorporation of radioactive lysine into protein of mouse brain and liver. *Brain Res.*, **68**, 143–156.

TREVOR, A. J. AND RODNIGHT, R. (1965) The subcellular localization of cerebral phosphoproteins sensitive to electrical stimulation. *Biochem. J.*, **95**, 889–896.

UEDA, T., MAENO, H. AND GREENGARD, P. (1973) Regulation of endogenous phosphorylation of specific proteins in synaptic membrane fractions from rat brain by adenosine 3′, 5′-monophosphate. *J. biol. Chem.*, **248**, 8295–8305.

WHITTAKER, V. P. (1969) The synaptosome. In *Handbook of Neurochemistry, Vol. 2*, A. LAJTHA (Ed.), Plenum Press, New York, N.Y., pp. 327–364.

WOLFF, D. J. AND SIEGEL, F. L. (1970) Purification of a calcium binding phosphoprotein from pig brain. *J. biol. Chem.*, **247**, 4180–4185.

ZEMP, J. W., WILSON, J. E., SCHLESINGER, K., BOGGAN, W. O. AND GLASSMAN, E. (1966) Incorporation of uridine into RNA of mouse brain during short-term training experience. *Proc. nat. Acad. Sci. (Wash.)*, **55**, 1423–1431.

Free Communications

Avoidance performance and plasma corticosteroid levels in previously undernourished mice

P. D. Leathwood and M. S. Bush — *Nestlé Products Technical Assistance Co. Ltd., Vevey (Switzerland)*

Mice undernourished in early life showed marked deficits in active avoidance performance as adults. During the first session there was no difference between controls and previously undernourished mice (both groups produced very few conditioned responses). In the second and subsequent sessions performance of the controls was clearly superior[1]. Thus controls appeared to learn more from the first session than did previously undernourished animals, implying a difference between the group in their response to this experience.

The temporal changes in plasma corticosteroid levels after the first 15-min session were similar in the two groups. A peak occurred 15–20 min after the end of the session and resting levels were regained about 2 h later. At 45 and 90 min, however, values for previously undernourished mice were higher than in controls, suggesting that they may recover more slowly from a stressful situation.

1 Leathwood, P. D., Bush, M. S., Berent, C. D., and Mauron, J., *Life Sci.*, 14 (1974) 157–162.

Some effects of $ACTH_{4-10}$ on performance during a continuous reaction task

A. W. K. Gaillard and A. F. Sanders — *Institute for Perception TNO, Soesterberg (The Netherlands)*

Eighteen subjects worked continuously for half an hour in a self-paced reaction task. Half of the subjects were injected with $ACTH_{4-10}$ (30 mg Org OI 63) and the other half with a placebo.

The subjects injected with $ACTH_{4-10}$ showed a larger improvement in reaction time during the experimental session than the placebo group. However, this effect disappeared in a short retest, which was given half an hour after the experimental session.

Thus, the results suggest that $ACTH_{4-10}$ has no effect on learning, but counteracts the build-up of reactive inhibition during the experimental session; that is, the peptide suppresses the decrease in motivation, which usually occurs during continuous performance tasks.

This notion is confirmed by an analysis of extremely long reaction times, which are an indication of "mental fatigue" and "loss of attention" and tend to occur with increasing frequency as a function of time-on-task. An analysis of the reaction time distributions showed that the ACTH group gave relatively few long reaction times. It was concluded that $ACTH_{4-10}$ counteracts the usual decay in performance as a function of time-on-task due to increasing boredom or mental fatigue.

Mediation of epinephrine effects on memory processes by alpha- and beta-receptors

R. B. VAN BUSKIRK, P. E. GOLD AND J. L. MCGAUGH — *Department of Psychobiology, School of Biological Sciences, University of California, Irvine, Calif. 92664 (U.S.A.)*

These studies provide support for a differential role of alpha- and beta-receptors in mediating the memory impairing or facilitating actions of epinephrine. Post-trial injections of epinephrine (0.1 mg/kg) facilitate later retention of inhibitory (passive) avoidance training with weak footshock. The same dose of epinephrine impairs retention of high footshock. The facilitation of retention by post-trial epinephrine was blocked by propranolol (a beta-receptor antagonist); however, propranolol had no effect on the memory impairment produced by epinephrine in the high footshock condition. Conversely, phenoxybenzamine (an alpha-receptor antagonist) blocked the retention impairment produced by epinephrine injected after high footshock, but had no effect on facilitation of retention performance by epinephrine administered after low footshock.

We are interested in the possibility that the epinephrine facilitation or impairment of retention may be due to a direct stimulation of pituitary hormone release that is differentially mediated by alpha- and beta-receptors.

Supported by USPHS Research Grants MH12526, MH25384, MH11095-07 and HD07981.

Effects of hormones on time-dependent memory storage processes

P. E. GOLD, R. B. VAN BUSKIRK AND J. L. MCGAUGH — *Department of Psychobiology, School of Biological Sciences, University of California, Irvine, Calif. 92664 (U.S.A.)*

These experiments provide evidence that hormones can facilitate and impair time-dependent memory processes. In these studies, rats were trained on a one-trial inhibitory (passive) avoidance task with a weak footshock. Immediate post-trial injections (subcutaneous) of epinephrine, norepinephrine, or ACTH facilitated retention performance of the avoidance response as measured 24 h after training. The effectiveness of the treatments in facilitating retention decreased as the time between training and injection was increased. Corticosterone, growth hormone, and vasopressin had no effect on retention under these training conditions. These results suggest that non-specific consequences of a training experience (*e.g.*, hormonal release) may normally modulate memory storage processes in untreated animals.

Post-trial injections of higher doses of epinephrine, norepinephrine, or ACTH impaired later retention. Because release of these hormones is stimulated by many stressful amnestic treatments, *e.g.*, electroconvulsive shock, the findings indicate that, in some cases, hormonal alterations may be involved in the neurobiological mechanisms underlying retrograde amnesia.

Supported by U.S.P.H.S. Research Grants MH12526, MH25384 and HD07981.

Session IV

CENTRAL REGULATION OF HOMEOSTASIS

Chairmen: K. LISSÁK (Pécs, Hungary)
B. BOHUS (Utrecht, The Netherlands)

The Renin–Angiotensin System and Drinking Behavior

JAMES T. FITZSIMONS

The Physiological Laboratory, Cambridge (Great Britain)

During the past 15 years or so it has been established that the renin–angiotensin system has an important part to play in Na homeostasis. Up to now the main interest has been in the renal contribution to Na homeostasis, and there has been a great deal of research on the role of angiotensin in the control of aldosterone secretion and glomerular filtration. Recently it has become increasingly clear that angiotensin also has potent effects on the central nervous system, including stimulation of drinking behavior. Control of water intake is at least as important in the regulation of body fluids as control of excretion so that this new role for the renin–angiotensin system, if substantiated, adds to the system's importance in fluid and electrolyte homeostasis. This paper will deal with the possible contribution that the renin–angiotensin system makes to drinking behavior, and more particularly to drinking caused by extracellular stimuli.

Thirst caused by extracellular depletion

The association of thirst with hemorrhage, vomiting or diarrhea has been known for a very long time. Such thirst cannot be attributable to cellular dehydration, since the fluid lost is essentially isotonic and is derived exclusively from the extracellular compartment. Experimentally a number of procedures which affect the amount or distribution of extracellular fluid may cause drinking.

(1) Reduction in extracellular Na by diet and excessive sweating (McCance, 1936), peritoneal dialysis (Cizek *et al.*, 1951; Huang, 1955; Falk, 1961) or diuresis (Holmes and Cizek, 1951) results in a secondary loss of water from the extracellular space, partly to the exterior but also to the cells which therefore become overhydrated. Despite the cellular overhydration Na depletion is accompanied by increased water intake. This response is quite separate from the increased Na appetite that also results from Na depletion.

(2) Removal of blood is now accepted to be an adequate stimulus to drinking in the rat (Fitzsimons, 1961; Oatley, 1964), and to lower the threshold to cellularly induced thirst in the dog (Kozlowski and Szczepanska-Sadowska, 1975). The amounts of fluid that can be removed in this way are limited by the developing acute anemia which tends to depress drinking behavior. The blood volume is also quickly restored by movement of fluid from the interstitial space. Hypovolemia is therefore small and

References p. 231–233

transient, and since extracellular volume receptors are located in the vascular compartment the resulting drinking behavior is not likely to be striking.

(3) Sequestration of extracellular fluid in the peritoneal cavity (Fitzsimons, 1961) or subcutaneous space (Stricker, 1966) by injecting hyperoncotic colloid causes a functional depletion of the extracellular fluid. In contrast to Na depletion, water and electrolyte in isotonic concentration are removed simultaneously. As in Na depletion there are two behavioral responses, but these are more clearly separated in their time course; an early thirst for water followed by an increased appetite for Na.

(4) The circulatory effects of severe extracellular deficits can be simulated by ligating the abdominal inferior vena cava (Fitzsimons, 1969). Venous return to the heart and therefore cardiac output are reduced and there is a fall in blood pressure. Drinking is increased 1–2 hr after caval occlusion. This and the marked oliguria cause the animal to go into positive fluid balance. Later on as cardiac output and renal function recover a marked preference for Na salts develops.

The renin–angiotensin system and thirst

The mechanisms of extracellularly induced drinking have been much studied in recent years and it now seems highly probable that the renin–angiotensin system is involved in the response to some types of extracellular stimuli. The evidence is as follows.

(1) Many of the stimuli which increase secretion of renin also cause thirst. This may be seen in Table I which gives a list taken from Assaykeen and Ganong (1971) of the principal stimuli that increase renin, together with references to the papers in which these stimuli have been reported to cause thirst. It should be emphasized that the list of renin stimuli has been reproduced in its entirety and unaltered and that it is taken from a work that does not deal with water intake. It will be noted that there are only three stimuli in the whole list for which there have been no reports of thirst.

(2) Drinking to some extracellular stimuli is attenuated or abolished by removal of the endogenous source of renal renin by bilateral nephrectomy, but this reduction does not occur when the animal is made anuric by ureteric ligation. For example, the drinking that follows constriction of the aorta above the renal arteries, constriction of the renal arteries themselves (Fitzsimons, 1969), or injection of the β-adrenergic agonist isoprenaline (Houpt and Epstein, 1971) is entirely abolished by nephrectomy, and drinking in response to caval ligation much reduced (Fitzsimons, 1969). On the other hand, the response to hyperoncotic colloid is unaffected by preliminary nephrectomy (Fitzsimons, 1961). It should be noted that in all those cases where drinking is reduced or abolished by nephrectomy the animal is fully capable of responding normally to a cellular stimulus to thirst.

(3) There is a potent dipsogenic substance in the cortex of the kidney which appears to be identical with renin (Fitzsimons, 1969). Injected into a water-replete animal it causes drinking, especially if the animal has been previously nephrectomized.

(4) Angiotensin II infused intravenously causes the water-replete rat to drink water (Fitzsimons and Simons, 1969). The response is unaffected by adrenalectomy and is greater in the nephrectomized animal.

TABLE I

THE PRINCIPAL STIMULI THAT INCREASE RENIN (Table 3-1, Assaykeen *et al.*, 1971)

References are given to the papers in which these stimuli have been reported to cause thirst. See Fitzsimons (1972) for references not listed in bibliography.

Renin stimulus	Thirst reference
Constriction of aorta or renal artery	Fitzsimons, 1969.
Constriction of inferior vena cava	Fitzsimons, 1969.
Hemorrhage	Wolf, 1958; Fitzsimons, 1961; Oatley, 1964; Kozlowski and Sadowska, 1975.
Dehydration	Wolf, 1958; Adolph, 1967.
Diuretics	
Low sodium diet	McCance, 1936; Holmes and Cizek, 1951; Cizek *et al.*, 1951; Huang, 1955.
Low potassium diet	Smith and Lasater, 1950; Hollander *et al.*, 1957; Fourman and Leeson, 1959.
Adrenal insufficiency	Fitzsimons, 1966.
Exercise	Wolf, 1958.
Upright posture	Wolf, 1958.
Pregnancy	Holmes, 1967.
Cirrhosis with ascites	
Nephrosis	Holmes, 1967.
Heart failure (some cases)	Holmes and Montgomery, 1953; Ramsay *et al.*, 1973.
Malignant hypertension	Brown *et al.*, 1969; Möhring *et al.*, 1975.
Ureteral constriction	Wirth and Fitzsimons (unpublished).
Catecholamines	Zamboni and Siro-Brigiani, 1966; Lehr *et al.*, 1967; Houpt and Epstein, 1971; Setler, 1973.
Stimulation of renal nerves	Meyer *et al.*, 1972.
Stimulation of sympathetic areas in brain	Lehr *et al.*, 1967; Leibowitz, 1971; Fisher, 1973.
Constriction of carotid arteries	
Hypoglycemia	Novin, 1964.

(5) Injection or infusion of angiotensin II into the anterior hypothalamus, preoptic region, septum or cerebral ventricles in doses much smaller than the minimum effective intravenous dose also causes the water-replete animal to drink (Epstein *et al.*, 1970; Severs *et al.*, 1970). The most sensitive region appears to be a periventricular structure, the subfornical organ. Injection of as little as 100 pg angiotensin II into it reliably caused drinking (Simpson and Routtenberg, 1973) (Fig. 1) and its destruction prevented the dipsogenic response to lateral ventricular injections (Phillips *et al.*, 1974).

(6) A variety of mammalian species including the rat, rabbit (Table II), goat (Fig. 2) (Andersson and Eriksson, 1971), cat (Fig. 3) (Sturgeon *et al.*, 1973; Cooling and Day, 1974), dog (Table II) and monkey (Fig. 4) (Setler, 1971; Myers *et al.*, 1973; Sharpe and Swanson, 1974) drink water in response to intracranial angiotensin. The pigeon (Rolls and McFarland, unpublished) and the iguana (Fitzsimons and Kaufman, unpublished) also respond.

(7) Clinically, thirst may be a striking symptom in some patients with chronic

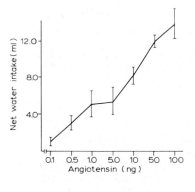

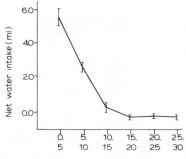

Fig. 1. The top figure shows the increase in water intake above the baseline intake for rats injected with angiotensin into the subfornical organ. The bottom figure gives the net intake as a function of successive 5-min epochs for all doses of angiotensin. Mean values ± S.E. of mean (Simpson and Routtenberg, 1973).

renal failure and malignant hypertension. These patients have a disproportionately high plasma renin in relation to their exchangeable Na and their hypertension, due in part to the hyper-reninemia, cannot be controlled by dialysis (Brown *et al.*, 1971). Bilateral nephrectomy, however, reduces the blood pressure and abolishes the thirst (Brown *et al.*, 1969; Rogers and Kurtzman, 1973). Malignant hypertension with excessive salt loss, hyper-reninemia and high water intake has also been produced in the rat by partial constriction of one renal artery (Möhring *et al.*, 1975). The rat also develops a strong Na appetite after this procedure and if it is allowed to drink saline its condition improves and the plasma renin falls. Though the correlation between plasma renin and water intake is close both clinically and in experimental hypertension, there is the possibility that the diminution in plasma volume resulting from the negative Na balance is at least as important a stimulus to thirst as the increased plasma renin. However, Brown *et al.* (1969) said of their patient that "*Bilateral nephrectomy reduced renin 200-fold and abolished the thirst before changes had occurred in the external balance of sodium and water*" (p. 345).

The hypothesis that the renal renin–angiotensin system plays a role in drinking induced by extracellular stimuli has been described elsewhere (Fitzsimons, 1969,

TABLE II

WATER DRUNK BY (a) RABBITS IN 30 min, AND (b) DOGS IN 2 hr, AND LATENCY OF ONSET OF DRINKING AFTER INTRACRANIAL ANGIOTENSIN OR RENIN

(a) Values from 11 positive sites in 8 rabbits (Findlay, Fitzsimons and Setler, unpublished). (b) Values from 5 dogs with cannulae in lateral ventricle (Fitzsimons, Kozlowski, Szczepanska-Sadowska and Sobocinska, unpublished).

Dose of angiotensin (ng)	N	Positive responses	Latency (min sec)		Water drunk mean ± S.E. of mean (ml)	Significance of increased intake over control
			Mean	Range		
(a)						
0	11	2	15′25″	10′0″–18′45″	0.64 ± 0.54	
10	11	7	8′4″	2′0″–19′0″	9.54 ± 3.12	< 0.02
100	11	9	8′38″	2′0″–20′0″	13.45 ± 3.54	< 0.01
1000	11	8	4′44″	2′0″–20′0″	20.73 ± 6.54	< 0.01
(b)						
0	5	2	27′30″	27′ –28′	7.0 ± 4.4	
50	4	4	26′	10′ –65′	20.0 ± 4.6	> 0.05
500	5	5	11′36″	4′ –33′	175.6 ± 23.6	< 0.001
2500	4	4	7′	2′ –10′	367.7 ± 60.9	< 0.001
5000	4	4	6′52″	3′ –11′	519.5 ± 119.0	< 0.01
10 mU renin	4	4	23′	11′ –55′	339.2 ± 85.2	< 0.01

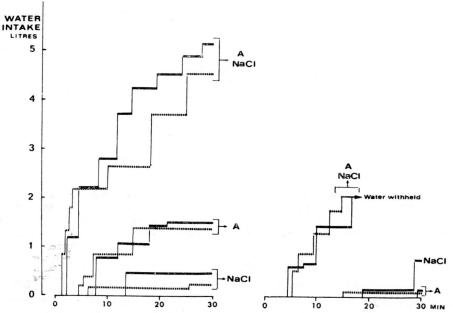

Fig. 2. Drinking by a goat in response to a 30-min infusion of angiotensin alone (A), hypertonic saline alone (NaCl), or both together (A–NaCl), into the third ventricle. Left: two series of infusions in a goat in normal water balance. Angiotensin was given at 2 ng/kg/min and 0.33 M NaCl at 10 μl/min. Right: responses after 100 ml water/kg given by stomach tube 90 min before the infusions. Angiotensin was infused at 1.3 ng/kg/min and 0.5 M NaCl at 10 μl/min (Andersson and Eriksson, 1971).

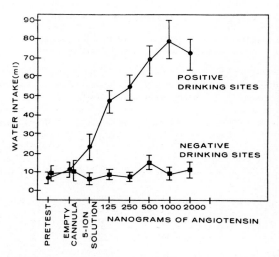

Fig. 3. Drinking elicited by intracranial angiotensin in the cat. 5-Ion solution is a Ringer–Locke's solution. Mean values ± S.E. of mean (Sturgeon *et al.*, 1973).

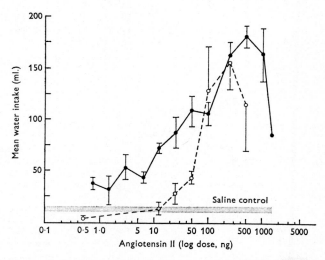

Fig. 4. Dose–response relation to unilateral (○-○) and bilateral (●-●) microinjections of angiotensin II into the septum, anterior hypothalamus and preoptic region of the monkey in normal water balance. Only the first microinjection in a series was plotted. Vertical lines = S.E.M.; number of injections at each dose ranged from 3 to 14 with a mean of 7. (From Sharpe and Swanson, 1974.)

1970b). In brief, an extracellular deficit causes a change in sensory information from stretch receptors in the low-pressure side of the circulation. This altered information, much of it carried in the vagi, activates the neurons in the limbic system concerned in drinking behavior. In addition renin is released reflexly from the kidney and the angiotensin II generated contributes to the drinking behavior by acting directly on these neurons.

It is important to realize that there is a non-hormonal component to extracellular thirst. In many circumstances the deficit that releases renin causes thirst in its own right. Only with stimuli such as aortic or renal artery constriction, or injection of isoprenaline does the non-hormonal component appear to be absent since drinking in response to these stimuli is abolished by nephrectomy.

It is hardly surprising that increases in plasma renin activity are not closely associated with water intake after administration of hyperoncotic colloid, a thirst stimulus unaffected by nephrectomy, or caval ligation, a stimulus partially attenuated by removal of endogenous renin (Leenen and Stricker, 1974). On the other hand, the action of isoprenaline on water intake was found to be closely correlated with its ability to induce renin release (Leenen and McDonald, 1974).

Does circulating angiotensin stimulate brain tissue directly?

The evidence for involvement of the renin–angiotensin system in thirst is, therefore, good and the presumption is that angiotensin II acts directly on sensitive neurons in the limbic system to induce drinking behavior. However, the evidence is also compatible with a hypothesis of peripheral action of angiotensin, "... *the setting in action of a vasoactive system as powerful as the renin–angiotensin system might increase the sensitivity of the vascular stretch receptors to the existing hypovolaemia ...*" (Fitzsimons, 1969, p. 365) (Fig. 5). The fact that drinking can be induced by injecting small amounts of angiotensin directly into the brain does not exclude such a hypothesis. A further complication is the presence of a complete renin–angiotensin system in brain tissue (Fischer-Ferraro *et al.*, 1971; Ganten *et al.*, 1971), which raises the

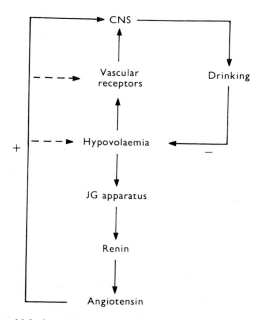

Fig. 5. Possible ways in which the renin–angiotensin system may play a role in drinking caused by extracellular stimuli (Fitzsimons, 1969).

question of a possible neurotransmitter role for cerebral angiotensin quite independent of any role, central or peripheral, for renal renin. It is entirely conceivable that angiotensin formed by renal renin is important in extracellularly induced thirst and that it acts by sensitizing vascular volume receptors to the extracellular deficit; whereas the cerebral renin–angiotensin system is a relatively non-specific neurotransmitter system in neurons concerned with drinking behavior and that this system is set in action by a variety of thirst stimuli, not exclusively extracellular, and perhaps by Na depletion as well.

The main hypothesis, that peripherally generated angiotensin contributes to drinking behavior by acting on thirst neurons in the central nervous system, remains the most attractive. For this hypothesis to be true two conditions must be met. The first is that blood-borne angiotensin should reach dipsogenically sensitive structures in the brain, especially the most sensitive structure, the subfornical organ (Simpson and Routtenberg, 1973). The second is that angiotensin should enhance the effects on drinking of other dipsogenic stimuli.

The subfornical organ is one of several circumventricular structures that lie outside the blood–brain barrier. It is richly vascularized, and so there are excellent *a priori* grounds for supposing that it is accessible to blood-borne hormone. There is also the precedent set by another angiotensin-sensitive circumventricular structure, the area postrema, which is stimulated by blood-borne angiotensin, giving rise to increased sympathetic discharge and a rise in blood pressure (Bickerton and Buckley, 1961; Severs and Daniels-Severs, 1973). We await the outcome of the crucial experiment of what happens to drinking in response to *intravenous* angiotensin after destruction of the subfornical organ.

The subfornical organ is of course exposed to CSF and therefore to substances placed in the cerebral ventricles. The cerebral ventricles are an excellent avenue for the dipsogenic action of angiotensin (Johnson and Epstein, 1975) and it is interesting that the response to *intraventricular* angiotensin is abolished by destruction of the subfornical organ (Phillips *et al.*, 1974). There is suggestive evidence that angiotensin may enter the cerebral ventricles from the blood stream, but it does not penetrate the blood–brain barrier. Volicer and Loew (1971) found radioactive label in the choroid plexuses of the lateral ventricles as well as inside the ventricles themselves, also inside and around the third ventricle, though not in the fourth ventricle, after i.v. injection of [^{14}C]angiotensin. Angiotensin itself or an angiotensin-like peptide has also been found in the CSF of normotensive and hypertensive patients, but unfortunately it is not known whether this peptide is derived from the cerebral renin–angiotensin system or whether it enters the CSF from the blood (Finkielman *et al.*, 1972). Whatever its source, however, increased angiotensin in the CSF would presumably cause drinking.

Whether circulating angiotensin reaches sensitive tissue in the brain through the blood stream, or via the cerebral ventricles after passing through the blood–CSF barrier, or by both routes, is of little consequence to the main hypothesis. What is important is that circulating angiotensin almost certainly reaches sensitive structures in the brain.

Interactions between angiotensin and other stimuli to thirst

The second requirement of the main hypothesis is that systemically administered angiotensin should contribute to the drinking caused by other stimuli to thirst. Infusions of angiotensin II were found to cause additional intake of water in nephrec-tomized rats injected with hypertonic saline (Fig. 6) (Fitzsimons and Simons, 1969). The experiments were performed on nephrectomized rats in order to avoid the complication of the renal response to hypertonic solutions which reduces the amount of water drunk, and also to eliminate endogenous renin secretion, and possible destruction of exogenous angiotensin by the kidney. Infusion of angiotensin also restored the drinking response of the nephrectomized rat subjected to caval ligation to a value similar to that obtained in the uninfused normal animal subjected to caval ligation. In the dog, Kozlowski *et al.* (1972) found that i.v. infusion of angiotensin II at 0.05 μg/min for 1 hr lowered the threshold to drinking in response to i.v. infusion of 5% saline from 4.8 $\pm$ 2.1% cellular dehydration under control conditions to 2.5 $\pm$ 1.3%.

That the site of the interaction between angiotensin and other thirst stimuli is probably in the brain is suggested by the following. In the rat intracranial angiotensin II increased drinking induced by intraperitoneal hypertonic saline (Fig. 7), a cellular stimulus to thirst, or that caused by hyperoncotic colloid, an extracellular stimulus (Fitzsimons, 1970a). Intracranial renin also caused additional drinking in response to hypertonic saline or to a 24-hr period of water deprivation. These results on the rat have been confirmed by Severs *et al.* (1974). In the dog, infusion of angiotensin II

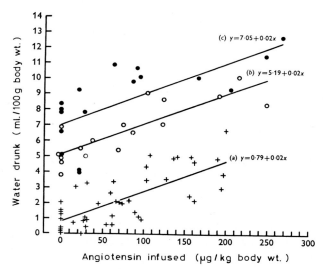

Fig. 6. Regressions of the amount of water drunk in 6 hr on the amount of angiotensin infused in nephrectomized rats after i.v. injection of hypertonic NaCl producing increases in osmotic pressure of (a) 0, (b) 5% and (c) 10%. The three regression lines were parallel but significantly separated one from the other, thus supporting the hypothesis of simple additivity of thirst stimuli (Fitzsimons and Simons, 1969).

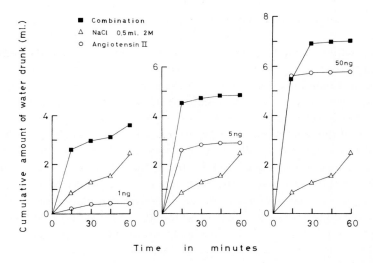

Fig. 7. The mean cumulative amount of water drunk in 1 hr by 6 rats given 1, 5 or 50 pmoles of angiotensin II intracranially, with (■) or without (○) the simultaneous injection of 0.5 ml of 2 *M* NaCl intraperitoneally. Cumulative intake after 2 *M* NaCl alone (△) (Fitzsimons, 1973).

TABLE III

THE EFFECT OF INFUSING ANGIOTENSIN II INTO THE LATERAL CEREBRAL VENTRICLE OF THE DOG ON THE THRESHOLD TO DRINKING IN RESPONSE TO I.V. HYPERTONIC SALINE

The intraventricular infusion was started 6 min before the intravenous infusion of 5% NaCl (4.5 ml/min). Mean values ± S.E. of mean. Number of observations in parentheses (Kozlowski, Fitzsimons, Szczepanska-Sadowska and Sobocinska, unpublished).

Intraventricular infusion	Artificial CSF (75 μl/min)	Angiotensin II (ng/min)			
		3.8	18.8	188	375
Cellular dehydration at the onset of drinking (%)	(10) 3.78 ± 0.43	(7) 2.23 ± 0.14 < 0.02	(10) 2.14 ± 0.33 < 0.01	(7) 2.21 ± 0.39 < 0.05	(3) 1.93 ± 0.64 < 0.1

into the lateral cerebral ventricle at rates of between 3.8 and 375 ng/min lowered the threshold to drinking in response to i.v. infusion of 5% saline (Table III).

Andersson and his colleagues found that angiotensin, dissolved in slightly hypotonic, isotonic or hypertonic NaCl, infused into the third ventricle in the goat, caused thirst (Fig. 2), release of ADH, natriuresis and a rise in blood pressure, the responses being more conspicuous with infusions of angiotensin dissolved in hypertonic (0.25–0.33 *M*) NaCl (Andersson and Eriksson, 1971; Andersson *et al.*, 1972). On the other hand, when angiotensin was dissolved in isotonic or hypertonic solutions of non-electrolytes and infused the effects were much less. Andersson suggested that there is an Na-sensitive system in the vicinity of the third ventricle which may be important in the central control of fluid balance and arterial blood pressure. Angiotensin may stimulate

TABLE IV

WATER DRUNK IN 1 hr AFTER ANGIOTENSIN II DISSOLVED IN DIFFERENT SOLUTIONS INJECTED INTO (a) THE PREOPTIC REGION (1.0 μl), AND (b) THE LATERAL VENTRICLE (10.0 μl) (Fitzsimons, 1973).

Angiotensin (pmoles)	N	Dissolved in			
		0.9% NaCl	1.8% NaCl	5% dextrose	20% sucrose
(a)					
0	7	0	0	0	—
1	9	0.92 ± 0.57	1.39 ± 0.62	0.93 ± 0.41	—
10	7	3.9 ± 1.34	4.27 ± 0.73	3.14 ± 1.0	—
100	7	10.28 ± 1.56	10.23 ± 0.86	8.68 ± 1.62	—
(b)					
0	8	1.86 ± 0.92	—	—	1.04 ± 0.28
10	8	4.32 ± 0.61	—	—	4.35 ± 0.88
100	8	7.76 ± 0.80	—	—	6.29 ± 1.14
0	9	0.12 ± 0.07	0.99 ± 0.34	—	—
10	9	3.0 ± 0.53	3.84 ± 0.93	2.58 ± 0.71	—
100	9	9.6 ± 1.14	7.3 ± 1.65	6.67 ± 0.99	—

these receptors by (1) facilitating the transependymal movement of Na from CSF into brain tissue, (2) sensitizing receptors to the existing Na concentration in brain extracellular fluid, or (3) facilitating entry of Na into receptor cells.

In the rat, however, the dipsogenic effect of angiotensin dissolved in isotonic dextrose, hypertonic sucrose or hypertonic saline and injected into brain tissue or cerebral ventricles was not significantly different from that of angiotensin dissolved in isotonic saline (Table IV) (Fitzsimons, 1973). The fact that intracranial angiotensin augmented the intake of rats made thirsty by injecting hyperoncotic colloid, an extracellular depleting agent that does not affect the extracellular Na concentration, also argues against an Na receptor (Fitzsimons, 1970a). Olsson and Kolmodin (1974) have recently reported that infusion of angiotensin into the carotid artery of the goat potentiates drinking in response to hypertonic saline also infused into the carotid artery. The infusions rates have to be about 15 times the rates used in cerebral ventricular infusions to show potentiation. However, they also found that intracarotid angiotensin enhanced the release of ADH by hypertonic fructose, a result difficult to explain on an Na receptor hypothesis.

The whole question of a specific ependymal Na receptor in the cerebral ventricle concerned in the physiological control of body fluid homeostasis and blood pressure must for the present remain an open one. There is no compelling reason yet to abandon the idea that the osmoreceptor, as elucidated by Gilman, Wolf and Verney, is involved in thirst and ADH release. The drinking and antidiuretic responses to hypertonic solutions given *systemically* can only be explained in terms of a cellular dehydration theory, though there is considerable room for maneuver on where the selectively semipermeable membrane should be located.

Peptide specificity of the angiotensin-sensitive neurons

In some of the earlier experiments on angiotensin-induced drinking in the rat it was an unexpected finding that renin, renin substrate and angiotensin I were as least as effective intracranial dipsogens as angiotensin II (Fitzsimons, 1971). Shortening the octapeptide chain, particularly removal of phenylalanine in position 8, resulted in a loss of dipsogenic activity, and in this respect the structure–activity relationships paralleled those for other biological activities. The discovery of an intrinsic renin–angiotensin system in the central nervous system (Fischer-Ferraro *et al.*, 1971; Ganten *et al.*, 1971) has now provided a possible explanation of how it is that renin, renin substrate and angiotensin I are dipsogenic when it is believed that all other physiological actions of these substances are mediated through angiotensin II. The components of the cerebral system would ensure the local generation of angiotensin II when renin, renin substrate or angiotensin I is injected into the brain. By the use of specific antibodies and peptide antagonists of the renin–angiotensin system it has proved possible to test this explanation (Epstein *et al.*, 1973, 1974). The rationale of the experiment and the antagonists used are shown in Fig. 8. The particular antagonist under study was injected 5–10 min before the dipsogen through the same intracranial cannula and the amount drunk by the rat was compared with the amount drunk after the dipsogen preceded by isotonic saline. The results were as follows. (1) Pepstatin, an inhibitor of the renin–angiotensinogen reaction, significantly reduced renin- and renin substrate-induced drinking but had no significant effect on angiotensin II- and carbachol-induced drinking. (2) The converting enzyme inhibitor, SQ 20881, significantly reduced renin-, renin substrate- and angiotensin I-induced drinking but actually enhanced angiotensin II-induced drinking. This is in agreement with a report by Severs *et al.* (1973) but others (Swanson *et al.*, 1973) found that SQ 20881 did not inhibit angiotensin I-induced drinking. (3) The competitive antagonist of angiotensin II, Sar[1]–Ala[8] angiotensin II, blocked renin-, renin substrate-, angiotensin I- and angiotensin II-induced drinking almost completely without affecting carbachol-

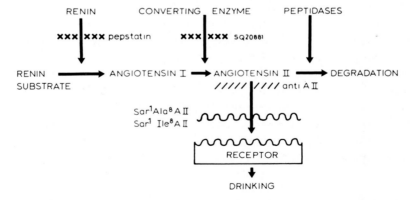

Fig 8. Peptide antagonists and the elucidation of receptors for angiotensin-induced drinking.

induced drinking. (4) Angiotensin II antiserum prevented angiotensin II-induced drinking and attenuated the responses to angiotensin I and renin substrate.

Drinking in response to components of the renin–angiotensin system injected intra-cranially is therefore mainly mediated by local generation of angiotensin II, the intrinsic renin–angiotensin system providing the necessary enzymes to effect the conversion of injected substances to angiotensin II. This of course leaves the questions of what is the physiological function of the cerebral renin–angiotensin system and its relationship to the renal system unanswered.

The relationship between angiotensin-induced drinking and central nervous cholinergic and monoaminergic systems

A further unsolved problem is the relationship between angiotensin and other neuro-transmitter systems in the brain. Angiotensin releases acetylcholine from cerebral cortical tissue (Elie and Panisset, 1970) and cholinergic stimulation of limbic structures

TABLE V

THE AMOUNTS OF WATER DRUNK IN 1 hr AFTER ANGIOTENSIN OR CARBACHOL GIVEN 10–15 AFTER A RECEPTOR BLOCKER

The blocker and dipsogen were given through the same preoptic cannula. Mean values $\pm$ S.E. of mean (Fitzsimons and Setler, 1971, and unpublished).

Receptor blocker (μg)		N	Dipsogen Angiotensin (100 ng)	N	Carbachol (300 ng)
Atropine	0	47	8.3 $\pm$ 0.6	37	8.4 $\pm$ 0.7
	1	12	6.0 $\pm$ 1.7	14	1.2 $\pm$ 1.2*
	10	14	8.3 $\pm$ 1.4	—	—
	100	10	1.8 $\pm$ 1.0*	—	—
Dihydro-	0	8	7.0 $\pm$ 1.2	8	8.2 $\pm$ 1.1
β-erythroidine	10	8	4.6 $\pm$ 1.6	8	6.4 $\pm$ 1.7
Phentolamine	0	14	8.4 $\pm$ 0.9	14	9.8 $\pm$ 1.3
	10	5	10.8 $\pm$ 2.8	5	8.5 $\pm$ 0.9
	20	5	8.9 $\pm$ 1.7	6	3.9 $\pm$ 2.3 (toxic)
	40	5	0.3 $\pm$ 0.3 (toxic)	4	0.8 $\pm$ 0.8 (toxic)
MJ1999	0	7	7.8 $\pm$ 0.9	6	11.4 $\pm$ 2.5
	20	5	8.6 $\pm$ 4.0	6	10.6 $\pm$ 2.4
	40	3	1.1 $\pm$ 1.1 (toxic)	1	toxic
Haloperidol	0	14	8.8 $\pm$ 1.0	7	10.0 $\pm$ 1.8
	2.5	4	3.0 $\pm$ 1.3*	—	—
	5	5	2.8 $\pm$ 1.2*	—	—
	10	5	0.5 $\pm$ 0.3*	7	8.5 $\pm$ 1.4

* $P < 0.05$.

TABLE VI

EFFECTS OF DEPLETION OF CATECHOLAMINES BY 6-HYDROXYDOPAMINE (6-OHDA) ON DRINKING INDUCED
BY ANGIOTENSIN OR CARBACHOL

Mean values ± S.E. of mean (Fitzsimons and Setler, unpublished).

| | | Mean water intake in 1 hr | | | | % Depletion | |
| | | Before 6-OHDA | | After 6-OHDA | | | |
Treatment	N	Angiotensin (100 ng)	Carbachol (300 ng)	Angiotensin (100 ng)	Carbachol (300 ng)	NA	DA
8 μg 6-OHDA (preoptic area)	15	6.2 ± 0.8	7.2 ± 0.9	1.9* ± 0.5	9.6 ± 0.9	preoptc** 46* ± 4	30* ± 5
2 × 250 μg 6-OHDA (intraventricular)	4	8.2 ± 1.2	6.2 ± 1.1	2.2* ± 1.5	6.4 ± 1.3	whole brain 79* ± 4	75* ± 3

* P < 0.05.
** N = 8.
NA, noradrenaline; DA, dopamine.

is a highly effective way of eliciting drinking in the rat. However, blocking cholino-
ceptive sites with atropine abolishes carbachol-induced drinking, but does not affect
angiotensin-induced drinking (Table V) (Fitzsimons and Setler, 1971). There does not,
therefore, appear to be any cholinergic involvement in the angiotensin drinking
response.

On the other hand the evidence for catecholaminergic involvement in the angiotensin response is much stronger. (1) Angiotensin causes release of or interferes with
the reuptake of noradrenaline (Palaic and Khairallah, 1968). (2) There is a close
correlation between the distribution of angiotensin and noradrenaline in different
parts of the brain (Fischer-Ferraro et al., 1971). (3) Angiotensin-induced drinking is
markedly reduced by pretreatment with intracranial 6-hydroxydopamine, which
destroys catecholaminergic nerve terminals, whereas carbachol-induced drinking is
unaffected (Fitzsimons and Setler, unpublished) (Table VI). (4) Neither angiotensin-
induced nor carbachol-induced drinking is significantly reduced by centrally administered α- or β-adrenergic antagonists, but the dopamine antagonist haloperidol
abolishes angiotensin-induced drinking without affecting carbachol-induced drinking
(Fitzsimons and Setler, 1971) (Table V). (5) Noradrenaline attenuates drinking induced
by cellular dehydration and carbachol, but does not affect drinking caused by extracellular thirst stimuli or angiotensin (Setler, 1973). (6) Intraventricular dopamine
(260–520 nmoles) causes some drinking. Preventing the conversion of dopamine to
noradrenaline by inhibiting dopamine β-hydroxylase with FLA-63 depletes the brain
of noradrenaline without affecting dopamine. This treatment produced a marked
decrease in food intake in food-deprived rats and an insignificant increase in water
intake with a consequent increase in the water to food ratio (Table VII) (Setler, 1975).
When L-DOPA was given in addition to FLA-63, the increase in water intake became
highly significant. On the other hand the dopamine antagonist haloperidol inhibited
water intake without affecting the food intake.

TABLE VII

THE EFFECTS OF (1) THE DOPAMINE ANTAGONIST, HALOPERIDOL, (2) THE DOPAMINE β-HYDROXYLASE INHIBITOR, FLA-63, AND (3) FLA-63 PLUS L-DOPA, ON EATING AND DRINKING IN RESPONSE TO OVER-NIGHT DEPRIVATION OF FOOD (Setler, 1975; and Fitzsimons and Setler, unpublished)

	Control	Haloperidol (0.1 mg/kg)	FLA-63 (25 mg/kg)	FLA-63 (25 mg/kg) + L-DOPA (100 mg/kg)
Food (g)	3.5 ± 1.0	—	0.5 ± 0.3*	0*
Water (ml)	3.2 ± 0.8	—	4.5 ± 1.4	7.7 ± 0.6*
Food (g)	7.5 ± 1.2	5.1 ± 1.7	—	—
Water (ml)	5.5 ± 1.0	1.1 ± 0.6*	—	—

* $P < 0.05$ (N = 8).

There therefore appears to be a functional relationship between angiotensin and central catecholaminergic mechanisms, probably dopaminergic, in the control of water intake.

Conclusion

The individual components of the renin–angiotensin system injected systemically or directly into the brain cause a variety of mammals to drink water. The pigeon has been reported to drink in response to intracranial angiotensin, and more recently the iguana has also been found to respond both to systemic and to intracranial angiotensin. The wide phylogenetic distribution of renin–angiotensin-induced drinking is in marked contrast to the restriction of carbachol-induced drinking to one species, the rat. Furthermore in the rat angiotensin, molecule for molecule, is a more potent intracranial dipsogen than carbachol, and unlike carbachol it is also effective when given systemically.

The first experiments implicating angiotensin in thirst led to the suggestion that actual or simulated extracellular fluid deficits activated the renal renin–angiotensin system and that the resulting water intake depended on the action of angiotensin on central thirst neurons as well as altered sensory information reaching these neurons from volume receptors in the low pressure side of the circulation. The relative contributions of hormonal and non-hormonal mechanisms appeared to depend on the particular extracellular thirst stimulus being used. However, despite its efficacy and apparent universality as a dipsogen the possible role of angiotensin in normal fluid balance remains to be elucidated. The scheme illustrated in Fig. 9 should be regarded as a framework for future research.

In view of the sensitivity of diencephalic structures to the dipsogenic action of angiotensin it is reasonable to postulate that circulating angiotensin generated by renal renin reaches the brain and contributes to the drinking response by sensitizing thirst neurons to existing thirst stimuli, but there is still no conclusive evidence that

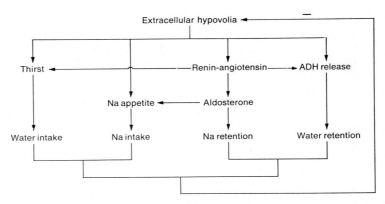

Fig. 9. An outline of some mechanisms concerned in regulating extracellular fluid volume. Note how the kidney may influence intake mechanisms through the renin–angiotensin system and aldosterone.

active blood-borne hormone actually works in this way. We know so little about the peripheral receptors concerned in the non-hormonal component of extracellular thirst mechanisms. We should therefore keep in mind that angiotensin may act on receptors outside the central nervous system.

The question of involvement of renal renin in natural thirst has been further complicated by the discovery of a complete renin–angiotensin system in the brain. The role of this system and its relationship with the renal system are unknown. Is it a peptidergic neurotransmitter system that is concerned with drinking behavior and ADH release in this part of the brain, but with pressor responses elsewhere? Is the stimulation of the receptors of this system by angiotensin generated by renal renin an unusual event occurring in emergencies when large amounts of renal renin are released? Or are both systems directly concerned in the day-to-day regulation of water and sodium? Since angiotensin-induced drinking depends on the integrity of catecholaminergic neurons the role of the renin–angiotensin system (renal or cerebral) may be to transmit information concerning the state of the extracellular fluid to catecholaminergic systems in the brain. The catecholaminergic systems are perhaps less specific in their functions than the renin–angiotensin system, being responsible for aspects of behavior common to a number of regulations. These aspects may well be arousal, non-specific activity, appetitive behavior and the act of ingestion. Activation of the renin–angiotensin system would direct this behavior towards drinking, but other (unknown) systems would turn the behavior towards food or sodium. We are clearly a very long way from understanding all the physiological roles of the renin–angiotensin system(s) nearly 80 years after the discovery of renin by Tigerstedt and Bergman.

SUMMARY

Extracellular dehydration, mimicking the effects of severe extracellular depletion by interfering with the circulation, or administration of β-adrenergic drugs causes drinking in the absence of any loss of cellular water. Drinking in response to such stimuli is in part mediated by the renin–angiotensin system, though there are certainly non-hormonal mechanisms involved as well. Angiotensin may exert its effect through catecholaminergic (perhaps dopaminergic) nervous pathways in the brain. It acts independently of cholinergic mechanisms which may be primarily concerned with cellularly induced thirst. Angiotensin sensitizes thirst neurons to an existing thirst stimulus, the same stimulus that also activated the renin–angiotensin system in the first place. Circulating angiotensin may reach the brain via the blood stream or CSF, or alternatively angiotensin may be generated locally by cerebral iso-renin in response to thirst stimuli.

REFERENCES

ANDERSSON, B. AND ERIKSSON, L. (1971) Conjoint action of sodium and angiotensin on brain mechanism controlling water and salt balances. *Acta physiol. scand.*, **81**, 18–29.

ANDERSSON, B., ERIKSSON, L., FERNÁNDEZ, O., KOLMODIN, C.-G. AND OLTNER, R. (1972) Centrally mediated effects of sodium and angiotensin II on arterial blood pressure and fluid balance. *Acta physiol. scand.*, **85**, 398–407.

ASSAYKEEN, TATIANA A. AND GANONG, W. F. (1971) The sympathetic nervous system and renin secretion. In *Frontiers in Neuroendocrinology*, L. MARTINI AND W. F. GANONG (Eds.), Oxford University Press, New York, N.Y., pp. 67–102.

BICKERTON, R. K. AND BUCKLEY, J. P. (1961) Evidence for a central mechanism in angiotensin-induced hypertension. *Proc. Soc. exp. Biol. (N.Y.)*, **106**, 834–836.

BROWN, J. J., CURTIS, J. R., LEVER, A. F., ROBERTSON, J. I. S., DE WARDENER, H. E. AND WING, A. J. (1969) Plasma renin concentration and the control of blood pressure in patients on maintenance haemodialysis. *Nephron*, **6**, 329–349.

BROWN, J. J., DÜSTERDIECK, G., FRASER, R., LEVER, A. F., ROBERTSON, J. I. S., TREE, M. AND WEIR, R. J. (1971) Hypertension and chronic renal failure. *Brit. med. Bull.* **27**, 128–135.

CIZEK, L. J., SEMPLE, R. E., HUANG, K. C. AND GREGERSEN, M. I. (1951) Effect of extracellular electrolyte depletion on water intake in dogs. *Amer. J. Physiol.*, **164**, 414–422.

COOLING, M. J. AND DAY, M. D. (1974) Drinking in the cat induced by centrally administered angiotensin. *Brit. J. Pharmacol.*, **49**, 150–151P.

ELIE, R. AND PANNISET, J. (1970) Effect of angiotensin and atropine on the spontaneous release of acetylcholine from cat cerebral cortex. *Brain Res.*, **17**, 297–305.

EPSTEIN, A. N., FITZSIMONS, J. T. AND ROLLS, B. J. (1970) Drinking induced by injection of angiotensin into the brain of the rat. *J. Physiol. (Lond.)*, **210**, 457–474.

EPSTEIN, A. N., FITZSIMONS, J. T. AND JOHNSON, A. K. (1973) Prevention by angiotensin II antiserum of drinking induced by intracranial angiotensin. *J. Physiol. (Lond.)*, **230**, 42–43P.

EPSTEIN, A. N., FITZSIMONS, J. T. AND JOHNSON, A. K. (1974) Peptide antagonists of the renin–angiotensin system and the elucidation of receptors for angiotensin-induced drinking. *J. Physiol. (Lond.)*, **238**, 34–35P.

FALK, J. L. (1961) The behavioral regulation of water–electrolyte balance. In *Nebraska Symposium on Motivation*, M. R. JONES (Ed.), University of Nebraska Press, Lincoln, Nebr., pp. 1–33.

FINKIELMAN, S., FISCHER-FERRARO, C., DIAZ, A., GOLDSTEIN, D. J. AND NAHMOD, V. E. (1972) A pressor substance in the cerebrospinal fluid of normotensive and hypertensive patients. *Proc. nat. Acad. Sci. (Wash.)*, **69**, 3341–3344.

FISCHER-FERRARO, C., NAHMOD, V. E., GOLDSTEIN, D. J. AND FINKIELMAN, S. (1971) Angiotensin and renin in rat and dog brain. *J. exp. Med.* **133**, 353–361.

FITZSIMONS, J. T. (1961) Drinking by rats depleted of body fluid without increase in osmotic pressure. *J. Physiol. (Lond.)*, **159**, 297–309.

FITZSIMONS, J. T. (1969) The role of a renal thirst factor in drinking induced by extracellular stimuli. *J. Physiol. (Lond.)*, **201**, 349–368.

FITZSIMONS, J. T. (1970a) Interactions of intracranially administered renin or angiotensin and other thirst stimuli on drinking. *J. Physiol. (Lond.)*, **210**, 152–153P.

FITZSIMONS, J. T. (1970b) The renin–angiotensin system in the control of drinking. In *The Hypothalamus*, L. MARTINI, M. MOTTA AND F. FRASCHINI (Eds.), Academic Press, New York, N.Y., pp. 195–212.

FITZSIMONS, J. T. (1971) The effect on drinking of peptide precursors and of shorter chain peptide fragments of angiotensin II injected into the rat's diencephalon. *J. Physiol. (Lond.)*, **214**, 295–303.

FITZSIMONS, J. T. (1972) Thirst. *Physiol. Rev.*, **52**, 468–561.

FITZSIMONS, J. T. (1973) Angiotensin as a thirst regulating hormone. In *Endocrinology*, R. O. SCOW, F. J. G. EBLING AND I. W. HENDERSON (Eds.), Excerpta Medica, Amsterdam, pp. 711–716.

FITZSIMONS, J. T. AND SETLER, P. E. (1971) Catecholaminergic mechanisms in angiotensin-induced drinking. *J. Physiol. (Lond.)*, **218**, 43–44P.

FITZSIMONS, J. T. AND SIMONS, B. J. (1969) The effect on drinking in the rat of intravenous infusion of angiotensin given alone or in combination with other stimuli of thirst. *J. Physiol. (Lond.)*, **203**, 45–57.

GANTEN, D., MARQUEZ-JULIO, A., GRANGER, P., HAYDUK, K., KARSUNKY, K. P., BOUCHER, R. AND GENEST, J. (1971) Renin in dog brain. *Amer. J. Physiol.*, **221**, 1733–1737.

HOLMES, J. H. AND CIZEK, L. J. (1951) Observations on sodium chloride depletion in the dog. *Amer. J. Physiol.*, **164**, 407–414.

HOUPT, K. A. AND EPSTEIN, A. N. (1971) The complete dependence of beta-adrenergic drinking on the renal dipsogen. *Physiol. Behav.*, **7**, 897–902.

HUANG, K. C. (1955) Effect of salt depletion and fasting on water exchange in the rabbit. *Amer. J. Physiol.*, **181**, 609–615.

JOHNSON, A. K. AND EPSTEIN, A. N. (1975) The cerebral ventricles as the avenue for the dipsogenic action of intracranial angiotensin. *Brain Res.*, **86**, 399–418.

KOZLOWSKI, S., DRZEWIECKI, K. AND ZURAWSKI, W. (1972) Relationship between osmotic reactivity of the thirst mechanism and the angiotensin and aldosterone level in the blood of dogs. *Acta physiol. polon.*, **23**, 369–376.

KOZLOWSKI, S. AND SZCZEPANSKA-SADOWSKA, E. (1975) Mechanisms of hypovolaemic thirst and interactions between hypovolaemia, hyperosmolality and the antidiuretic system. In *Control Mechanisms of Drinking*, G. PETERS, J. T. FITZSIMONS AND L. PETERS-HAEFELI (Eds.), Springer, Berlin, pp. 25–35.

LEENEN, F. H. H. AND MCDONALD, R. H. (1974) The effect of isoproterenol on blood pressure, plasma renin activity, and water intake in rats. *Europ. J. Pharmacol.*, **26**, 129–135.

LEENEN, F. H. AND STRICKER, E. M. (1974) Plasma renin activity and thirst following hypovolemia or caval ligation in rats. *Amer. J. Physiol.*, **226**, 1238–1242.

MCCANCE, R. A. (1936) Experimental sodium chloride deficiency in man. *Proc. roy. Soc. B*, **119**, 245–268.

MÖHRING, J., MÖHRING, B., HAAK, D., LAZAR, J., OSTER, P., SCHÖMIG, A. AND GROSS, F. (1975) Thirst and salt appetite in experimental renal hypertension of rats. In *Control Mechanism of Drinking*, G. PETERS, J. T. FITZSIMONS AND L. PETERS-HAEFELI (Eds.), Springer, Berlin, pp. 155–162.

MYERS, R. D., HALL, G. H. AND RUDY, T. A. (1973) Drinking in the monkey evoked by nicotine or angiotensin II microinjected in hypothalamic and mesencephalic sites. *Pharmacol. Biochem. Behav.*, **1**, 15–22.

OATLEY, K. (1964) Changes of blood volume and osmotic pressure in the production of thirst. *Nature (Lond.)*, **202**, 1341–1342.

OLSSON, K. AND KOLMODIN, R. (1974) Accentuation by angiotensin II of the antidiuretic and dipsogenic responses to intracarotid infusions of NaCl and fructose. *Acta endocr. (Kbh.)*, **75**, 333–341.

PALAIC, D. AND KHAIRALLAH, P. A. (1968) Inhibition of norepinephrine re-uptake by angiotensin in brain. *J. Neurochem.*, **15**, 1195–1202.

PHILLIPS, M. J., LEAVITT, M. AND HOFFMAN, W. (1974) Experiments on angiotensin II and the subfornical organ in the control of thirst. *Fed. Proc.*, **33**, 563.

RAMSAY, D. J., ROLLS, B. J. AND WOOD, R. J. (1973) Increased drinking in dogs during congestive heart failure. *J. Physiol. (Lond.)*, **234**, 48–50P.

ROGERS, P. W. AND KURTZMAN, N. A. (1973) Renal failure, uncontrollable thirst and hyperreninemia. *J. Amer. med. Ass.*, **225**, 1236–1238.

SETLER, P. E. (1971) Drinking induced by injection of angiotensin II into the hypothalamus of the rhesus monkey. *J. Physiol. (Lond.)*, **217**, 59–60P.

SETLER, P. E. (1973) The role of catecholamines in thirst. In *The Neuropsychology of Thirst*, A. N. EPSTEIN, H. R. KISSILEFF AND E. STELLAR (Eds.), Winston, New York, N.Y., pp. 279–291.

SETLER, P. E. (1975) Noradrenergic and dopaminergic influences on thirst. In *Control Mechanisms of Drinking*, G. PETERS, J. T. FITZSIMONS AND L. PETERS-HAEFELI (Eds.), Springer, Berlin, pp. 62–68.

SEVERS, W. B., SUMMY-LONG, J., TAYLOR, J. S. AND CONNOR, J. D. (1970) A central effect of angiotensin: release of pituitary pressor material. *J. Pharmacol. exp. Ther.*, **174**, 27–34.

SEVERS, W. B. AND DANIELS-SEVERS, A. E. (1973) Effects of angiotensin on the central nervous system. *Pharmacol. Rev.*, **25**, 415–449.

SEVERS, W. B., SUMMY-LONG, J. AND DANIELS-SEVERS, E. (1973) Effect of a converting enzyme inhibitor (SQ 20881) on angiotensin-induced drinking. *Proc. Soc. exp. Biol. (N.Y.)*, **142**, 203–204.

SEVERS, W. B., SUMMY-LONG, J. AND DANIELS-SEVERS, A. E. (1974) Angiotensin interaction with thirst mechanisms. *Amer. J. Physiol.*, **226**, 340–344.

SHARPE, L. G. AND SWANSON, L. W. (1974) Drinking induced by injections of angiotensin into forebrain and mid-brain sites of the monkey. *J. Physiol. (Lond.)*, **239**, 595–622.

SIMPSON, J. B. AND ROUTTENBERG, A. (1973) Subfornical organ: site of drinking elicitation by angiotensin II. *Science*, **181**, 1172–1175.

STRICKER, E. M. (1966) Extracellular fluid volume and thirst. *Amer. J. Physiol.*, **211**, 232–238.

STURGEON, R. D., BROPHY, P. D. AND LEVITT, R. A. (1973) Drinking elicited by intracranial microinjection of angiotensin in the cat. *Pharmacol. Biochem. Behav.*, **1**, 353–355.

SWANSON, L. W., MARSHALL, G. R., NEEDLEMAN, P. AND SHARPE, L. G. (1973) Characterisation of central angiotensin II receptors involved in the elicitation of drinking in the rat. *Brain Res.*, **49**, 441–446.

VOLICER, L. AND LOEW, C. G. (1971) Penetration of angiotensin II into the brain. *Neuropharmacology*, **10**, 631–636.

Neurotransmitters and the Regulation of Food Intake

PHILIP TEITELBAUM AND DAVID L. WOLGIN

Psychology Department, University of Illinois, Champaign, Ill. 61820 (U.S.A.)

INTRODUCTION

Nature's abnormalities often provide the clearest insight into normal functions. Perhaps this is why much of the work on the neural regulation of food intake has focussed around two major syndromes of abnormal feeding: hypothalamic hyperphagia (Brobeck *et al.*, 1943) and lateral hypothalamic aphagia (Anand and Brobeck, 1951). With recent advances in techniques for anatomic visualization of monoamine systems in the brain (Andén *et al.*, 1964, 1966), and with the development of methods for selectively destroying catecholamine systems (Ungerstedt, 1971b), there have been very exciting breakthroughs in our understanding of the neurotransmitters involved in these two syndromes. Since the fundamental work of Grossman (1960, 1962), there has been a great deal of work on intracranial application of neurotransmitters to determine their role in normal feeding. However, many methodological problems with this method still exist (Booth, 1972; Routtenberg, 1972; Baile, 1974). Therefore, we will concentrate on the neurotransmitters involved in hyperphagia and aphagia. In what follows, we will try to do 3 things: (1) highlight some major recent advances in our understanding of these syndromes; (2) pinpoint some unresolved issues; and, (3) present some recent findings from our own laboratory and that of others which may indicate lines of thought and work that will prove fruitful in the next few years.

HISTORICAL BACKGROUND

When Fröhlich's syndrome began to be studied in humans, it was thought to be related either to pituitary malfunction or damage to hypothalamus (Erdheim, 1904; Fröhlich, 1940). In work on animals, hypophysectomy was shown not to cause obesity, but subsequent ventromedial hypothalamic damage did (Smith, 1927, 1930; Hetherington and Ranson, 1940). Attention and thinking therefore focused on the hypothalamus.

Brobeck *et al.* (1943) emphasized the overeating as a cause for the obesity produced by ventromedial hypothalamic (VMH) damage. Anand and Brobeck (1951) showed that lateral hypothalamic destruction led to aphagia and death from inanition. Therefore, two systems seemed mainly involved in the control of feeding: a medial satiety system that serves to inhibit an excitatory lateral hypothalamic feeding system. A great deal of behavioral, anatomical and physiological analyses of these syndromes has continued up to the present time (for reviews, see Code, 1967; Morgane, 1969; Stevenson, 1969; Epstein, 1971; Hoebel, 1971) and some of the details will be presented here as they become relevant. But a major change in thinking about the neural control of feeding resulted from the development of anatomical and biochemical methods for correlating brain systems with their neurotransmitters.

In the early 1960s, Swedish neuroanatomists developed the histochemical fluorescence technique for tracing catecholamine pathways in the brain (Falck and Hillarp, 1959; Carlsson et al., 1962a, b). With this method it became possible to trace entire systems from their cells of origin in the hindbrain or midbrain to their sites of action in hypothalamus, basal ganglia, limbic system and cortex (Andén et al., 1966). Their relevance to the aberrations seen in the regulation of food intake was first demonstrated by Ungerstedt (1970, 1971b). He used 6-OHDA (6-hydroxydopamine), a neurotoxin that can selectively destroy brain catecholamine systems (Bloom et al., 1969; Uretsky and Iversen, 1970). Ungerstedt (1970, 1971b) applied 6-OHDA locally to the zona compacta of the substantia nigra, the cells of origin of the dopamine system in the brain. These cells pass through the far-lateral hypothalamus (implicated earlier in aphagia by Morgane, 1961) and medial internal capsule, then through the globus pallidus to end on cells in the caudate putamen. Destruction of these cells produced aphagia and adipsia, whether the 6-OHDA was injected into the substantia nigra, ventral tegmentum or far-lateral hypothalamus. Ungerstedt therefore concluded that the lateral hypothalamic syndrome was caused by destruction of the nigrostriatal bundle, and that the feeding system involved was dopaminergic. (We will return to a more detailed analysis of the lateral hypothalamic syndrome a little later, but for now let us concentrate on hyperphagia.)

Impressed by these findings, Ahlskog and Hoebel (1973) reasoned that other catecholamine systems might be involved in the *inhibition* of food intake. Amphetamine had long been known to inhibit food intake, and is used clinically in the control of obesity (Costa and Garattini, 1970). Its anorexic effect is mediated by catecholamines (Weissman et al., 1966). As shown by Ungerstedt (1971a) and others, the brain noradrenaline systems have their cells of origin in the hindbrain and course rostrally. There are two major divisions of these systems: the ventral noradrenergic bundle originates in the medulla oblongata and pons and projects to the hypothalamus and basal forebrain; the dorsal noradrenergic bundle originates in the locus coeruleus, courses through the lateral hypothalamus and for the most part continues onward to the limbic system and the neocortex. Although they are pretty much intermingled, in the midbrain they separate into a dorsal and a ventral component. Ahlskog and Hoebel (1973) demonstrated that selective destruction of the ventral noradrenergic bundle (VNAB), either electrolytically or with 6-OHDA, produced overeating and obesity. Destruction of the dorsal noradrenergic bundle had no apparent effect on feeding.

Is this the basis of the well-known ventromedial hypothalamic syndrome? As will become clear in the rest of this discussion, to interpret the function of the systems of the brain, one must carefully analyze the behavior they produce, and we believe that the importance of such behavioral analysis has not been sufficiently understood or appreciated. For instance, from an earlier behavioral study of hypothalamic hyperphagia, several things have been clearly demonstrated. Although VMH animals overeat to the point of extreme obesity, they are very finicky. They refuse to eat and will starve for long periods if the food is even slightly unpalatable (Kennedy, 1950; Teitelbaum, 1955). Similarly they will not work hard to obtain food (Miller et al., 1950; Teitelbaum, 1957). Affective responses to contrast seem to be involved. If they become used to eating unpalatable foods or working hard for it preoperatively, then, unlike such animals faced postoperatively with these situations for the first time, they continue to overeat and overwork and gain weight (Singh, 1973, 1974). In addition to being finicky, VMH animals are more sensitive than normal animals to the anorexic action of amphetamine (Stowe and Miller, 1957; Epstein, 1959; Reynolds, 1959).

On the other hand, the VNAB hyperphagic animals are not finicky. They are just like normal animals in their reaction to palatable or unpalatable diets (Ahlskog, 1974; Hoebel, 1974). Furthermore, unlike VMH animals, they are much less sensitive to the anorexic action of amphetamine (Ahlskog, 1974; Ahlskog and Hoebel, 1973). Therefore, the VNAB would appear to be one of the main systems in the brain through which amphetamine exerts its anorexic action. Since the VNAB courses through the medial forebrain bundle in the lateral hypothalamus, its destruction may explain one of the paradoxical effects of lateral hypothalamic damage, i.e., the loss of sensitivity to amphetamine anorexia (Carlisle, 1964; Panksepp and Booth, 1973; Fibiger et al., 1973; Stricker and Zigmond, 1975)*. If the VNAB is the same satiety system demonstrated by Leibowitz in the perifornical region, amphetamine's action on it should be blocked, as she has demonstrated, by beta-adrenergic blocking agents, such as propranolol (Leibowitz, 1970; but see Lehr and Goldman, 1971).

The VNAB animals differ in at least two more ways from VMH animals. Even with relatively complete destruction of the ventral noradrenergic bundle, they do not become as obese as VMH animals (Ahlskog, 1973). Also, unlike the VMH syndrome, their overeating depends on the presence of the pituitary gland. In hypophysectomized animals, destruction of the VNAB does not produce overeating (Ahlskog et al., 1974). Therefore, this experimental form of obesity is new — clearly dependent on noradrenergic function, and different in several respects from VMH obesity. Perhaps the metabolic changes demonstrated recently in VMH animals (Woods et al., 1974) relate to VNAB destruction (Hoebel, 1974). In more recent work, Hoebel and his coworkers (Hoebel, 1974) have found that depletion of serotonin by intraventricular PCPA (para-chlorophenylalanine) also causes overeating and obesity. Furthermore, like VMH rats, serotonin-depleted hyperphagics are still sensitive to the anorexic action of amphetamine. Further behavioral comparisons are obviously needed here.

---

* Since damage to the nigrostriatal bundle also attenuates amphetamine-induced anorexia (Fibiger et al., 1973; Stricker and Zigmond, 1975), there must be a dopaminergic, as well as noradrenergic, basis for amphetamine anorexia. Recent data by Baez (1974) supports this dual mediation hypothesis.

Nigrostriatal aphagia versus the lateral hypothalamic syndrome

We can ask the same question about the nigrostriatal pathway that we asked of the ventral noradrenergic bundle: is the syndrome seen after its destruction based on the same deficits as those produced by lateral hypothalamic damage? Lateral hypothalamic rats recover feeding and drinking in an invariant sequence of stages (stage I — aphagia and adipsia; stage II — anorexia and adipsia; stage III — adipsia with dehydration aphagia; and stage IV — partial recovery; Teitelbaum and Epstein, 1962). If the lesions are large, they never regain some of the controls over thirst that prompt the normal rat to drink (cellular dehydration, Epstein and Teitelbaum, 1964; hypovolemia, Stricker and Wolf, 1967) and so they drink only prandially (when they eat; Epstein and Teitelbaum, 1964). Although they do eat more in the cold, they do not eat more in response to a lowered blood glucose availability produced by 2-deoxy-D-glucose (Kanner and Balagura, 1971; Miselis and Epstein, 1971; Wayner *et al.*, 1971) or by insulin (Epstein and Teitelbaum, 1967). Finally, they are hypersensitive to unpalatable qualities of their food (Teitelbaum and Epstein, 1962). To answer the question posed above, Marshall and Teitelbaum (1973) and, in a more detailed analysis, Marshall *et al.* (1974) repeated Ungerstedt's technique of local application of 6-OHDA to the cell bodies in the zona compacta of the substantia nigra in the rat. Like lateral hypothalamic rats, nigrostriatal-damaged animals became aphagic and adipsic, and had to be kept alive by tube-feeding. They progressed through the same four stages of recovery. Even after they recovered their capacity to eat pellets and drink water, similar regulatory abnormalities persisted. They did not drink normally in response to cellular dehydration or hypovolemia. They did not drink normal quantities of water in the absence of food (which suggests that they drink only in association with eating). They failed to eat in response to 2-deoxy-D-glucose, but they did overeat in a cold environment. But unlike lateral hypothalamic animals, they were not very finicky in response to unpalatable qualities of the food. (Several of these findings have also been reported by Fibiger *et al.*, 1973.) In most respects, therefore, Ungerstedt appears correct in equating 6-OHDA destruction of the nigrostriatal bundle with the lateral hypothalamic syndrome. Marshall *et al.* (1974) found, like Ungerstedt, that telencephalic noradrenaline was depleted as well as striatal dopamine, leaving open a role for norepinephrine in the syndrome (see Stricker and Zigmond, 1975). Because noradrenaline depletion alone (produced by application of 6-OHDA caudal to the substantia nigra) did not produce aphagia, Ungerstedt asserted the essential transmitter to be dopamine in the nigrostriatal pathway.

His conclusions receive considerable support from the work of Zigmond and Stricker (1972, 1973; Stricker and Zigmond, 1974, 1975). In recent studies they have shown that rats treated with desmethylimipramine and pargyline before intraventricular 6-OHDA had 99% depletion of striatal dopamine, while telencephalic norepinephrine was depleted by only 10%. These rats became severely aphagic and adipsic. They progressed through the same stages of recovery as seen in the lateral hypothalamic syndrome. Although in some respects their animals show a further fractionation of the lateral syndrome, some of the same residual deficits were found. Once again, dopamine seems critical.

Points of controversy

If dopamine is the transmitter involved in an excitatory feeding system, one might expect that its local application to feeding systems in the brain would elicit feeding. However, it seems to act only slightly, if at all (Grossman, 1962; Booth, 1968; Slangen and Miller, 1969). In contrast, intracranial norepinephrine in virtually all species tested (except the cat, Myers, 1964) strongly elicits feeding (Grossman, 1962; Booth, 1967; Sharpe and Myers, 1969; Yaksh and Myers, 1972; Baile, 1974; Setler and Smith, 1974). Indeed, Berger *et al.* (1971) report that intraventricular norepinephrine promotes recovery of eating in the lateral hypothalamic syndrome. Dopamine had no effect at all. In more recent work, Ritter *et al.* (1974) report that intraventricular clonidine, an alpha-adrenergic receptor activator, strongly elicits feeding, with a potency 100 times that of norepinephrine. Again, dopamine was ineffective. This reinforces the view that norepinephrine, not dopamine, is the major transmitter in feeding. How can we reconcile this with Ungerstedt's (1971b) and Stricker and Zigmond's (1974, 1975) implication of dopamine as the major transmitter involved? It is interesting that a very similar controversy has arisen with respect to the transmitter involved in self-stimulation. It has long been known that the self-stimulation system overlaps anatomically with regions involved in many regulatory and instinctive behaviors (Olds *et al.*, 1960; Olds and Olds, 1963). In the lateral hypothalamus, hunger enhances self-stimulation whereas satiety inhibits it (Hoebel and Teitelbaum, 1962; Margules and Olds, 1962). Obesity or satiety can shift its quality in the direction of aversiveness (Hoebel and Thompson, 1969). In a recent review, Hoebel (1974) asserts a role for the self-stimulation system in the regulation of food intake. Stein and his coworkers have provided a great deal of evidence for the role of norepinephrine in self-stimulation (Stein, 1968; Ritter and Stein, 1973). Recently, Antelman *et al.* (1972), Roll (1970), and Poschel and Ninteman (1971) have argued that norepinephrine affects arousal, not reward. In support of the role of dopamine in reward, Yokel and Wise (1975) show that when animals self-inject with amphetamine, pimozide (a dopamine blocker) causes the animals to self-inject much more. Therefore the pimozide seems to act in a manner similar to the decrease in reward produced by decreasing the concentration of amphetamine. As is often the case, both transmitters may be found to be involved (Phillips and Fibiger, 1973; German and Bowden, 1974).

In our view, many of the apparent contradictions in the available experimental evidence will not be resolved until we have a better understanding of the behaviors involved in the regulation of food intake. We believe the current conception of feeding is oversimplified. The major idea underlying most studies of the nervous control of feeding is that of homeostasis. The emphasis is on the control of the constancy of the internal environment, not on the controls over behavior. Feeding is conceived of as an all-or-none unitary homeostatic act; switched on or off as an essentially reflexive control system. In response to error signals that body receptors detect, ingestion is

References p. 245–249

turned on till the error is compensated; witness the current emphasis on meal size, frequency and interval (see Le Magnen, 1971; Oatley, 1973). These are appropriate for a control system analysis, but they tend to limit our view of the behaviors involved in eating or drinking.

Our work on the lateral hypothalamic syndrome over the past few years has forced us to broaden our view. First we discovered that the sequence of the stages of recovery seen in the adult lateral hypothalamic rat closely parallels the development of feeding in infancy. By slowing down the rate of development in newborn rats, either by thyroidectomy (Teitelbaum et al., 1969) or by semi-starvation (Cheng et al., 1971), we were able to isolate stages of development of the control of feeding which seemed identical to the stages seen during recovery in the adult. A similar parallel between stages of recovery of the voluntary use of the hand in stroke patients (Twitchell, 1951) and stages of development of the use of the hand in newborn human infants (Twitchell, 1965, 1969, 1970) has independently been demonstrated. With respect to the behavior involved in feeding, we have therefore come to the view that each stage of development or recovery represents a different level of nervous control. Motivated behavior must be integrated hierarchically, as is the nervous system whose action it manifests, in terms of levels of encephalization (Teitelbaum, 1971). The stages of recovery reveal the stages of nervous control involved in transforming eating from the reflexive ingestion seen in the newborn infant to the operant eating seen in the adult.

To attempt to analyze these levels of control, we have recently focussed on the first two stages of the lateral hypothalamic syndrome (stage I: complete aphagia and adipsia; and stage II: anorexia), which are still very poorly understood. Work by Flynn and his collaborators had indicated that the hypothalamus can exert profound effects on sensorimotor integration. MacDonnell and Flynn (1966) and Flynn et al. (1971) located sites in the hypothalamus of the cat, which when electrically stimulated, evoked biting attack on a rat. If the cat's body was restrained during unilateral hypothalamic excitation and the contralateral snout region was touched, then the cat reflexively turned its head toward the touch. Increasing the intensity of hypothalamic excitation caused the sensory field for this reflex to expand posteriorly along the snout. Similarly, touch of the contralateral lip during hypothalamic excitation could elicit jaw opening, and the sight of a mouse in the contralateral visual field could elicit lunging. These reflexive components of the cat's integrated attack were not typically elicited in the absence of hypothalamic excitation or if the stimuli were presented on the cat's ipsilateral side.

Perhaps similar sensorimotor mechanisms are involved in the control of feeding. If so, then lateral hypothalamic damage might result in the loss of such reflexes. As shown in Fig. 1, lateral hypothalamic injury produces severe deficits in orientation to sensory stimuli, a kind of "sensory neglect", which in turn profoundly affects feeding and attack behavior (Ahlskog, 1974)*. After unilateral damage, rats do not use information from the contralateral side of the body either to initiate attack or to accept

---

* An alternative possibility, that deficits in feeding are caused by incidental damage to the trigeminal system, has recently been proposed by Zeigler et al. (1974).

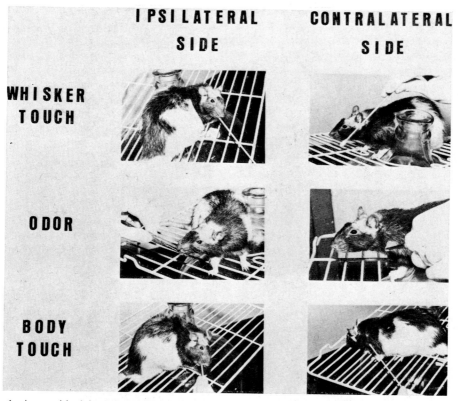

Fig. 1. A rat with right unilateral lateral hypothalamic damage shows precise head orientation and biting to various kinds of stimuli (whisker touch, odor, body touch) on the ipsilateral side (pictures at left) while neglecting the same stimuli presented contralaterally (pictures at right).

food placed there (Marshall *et al.*, 1971; Turner, 1973; Marshall and Teitelbaum, 1974). Furthermore, after bilateral damage, the early stages of recovery from aphagia are correlated with recovery of direct orientation to olfactory and whisker-touch stimuli. A very similar, though slightly less severe form of impairment of sensory orientation is seen in the rat made aphagic by 6-OHDA destruction (Marshall *et al.*, 1974; Stricker and Zigmond, 1974). Therefore, dopamine seems critical for this type of control over feeding as well.

In recent work, John Marshall (1975) has demonstrated the importance of such sensory fields in the control of overeating. Unilateral ventromedial hypothalamic damage leads to exaggerated reactivity to contralateral sensory stimuli (the opposite of sensory neglect) with a consequent preferential overeating of food in the contralateral sensory field. Bilateral damage led to exaggerated sensory orientation on both sides with overeating and obesity. It will be interesting to see whether ventral noradrenergic hyperphagia or serotonin-depletion-induced hyperphagia produces such exaggerated reflexive orientation.

Finally, we will briefly mention our work on the lateral hypothalamic cat. As

References p. 245–249

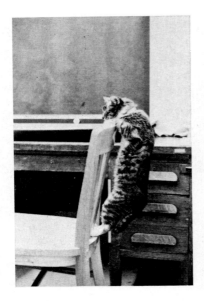
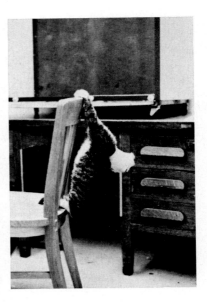
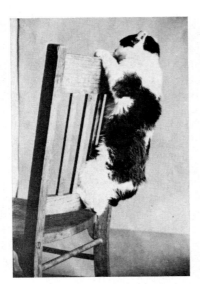
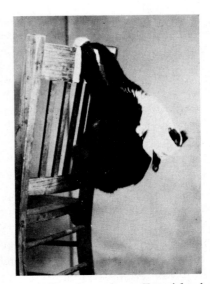

Fig. 2. Top left: cataleptic clinging in lateral hypothalamic undrugged cat. Top right: backfall reaction induced by bandaging head and neck in the same animal. Bottom (from Van Harreveld and Bogen, 1961; copyright, Academic Press): similar phenomena in neurologically intact cat injected with bulbocapnine.

described above, the picture that is beginning to emerge from this work is that the feeding deficits in the early stages of the lateral hypothalamic syndrome are intimately tied to specific sensorimotor impairments. It occurred to us, therefore, that we might gain clearer insight into the nature of the deficits by examining the cat, an animal whose sensorimotor coordination is exquisitely developed.

Wolgin and Teitelbaum (1974) found that, as in the rat, bilateral electrolytic hypothalamic damage produced disruptions of feeding and drinking followed by recovery through the same four stages of aphagia and adipsia, anorexia and adipsia, adipsia with secondary dehydration-aphagia, and partial recovery. Thus, the stages of recovery are intrinsic to the phenomenon and not an artifact of the species used.

The deficits seen in the first two stages are particularly instructive. Like rats, lateral hypothalamic cats typically are somnolent, cataleptic, and akinetic during the stage of complete aphagia. They also show sensory neglect. As shown in Fig. 2 (top), such a cataleptic animal will cling to the back of a chair for long periods of time. A normal cat, by contrast, quickly jumps to the floor. Bulbocapnine also produces such cataleptic clinging (Peters, 1904). In such a drugged cat, bandaging the head yields a slow backfall of the head, inhibiting the grasp, and the animal falls off (Van Harreveld and Bogen, 1961; see Fig. 2, bottom). We have seen the identical reaction in the first day or two postoperatively in lateral hypothalamic damaged cats (Fig. 2, top), without drugs. Because haloperidol, a dopamine blocker, produces the same reaction (DeRyck et al., to be published), it would seem to indicate that in the cat, as in the rat, dopamine

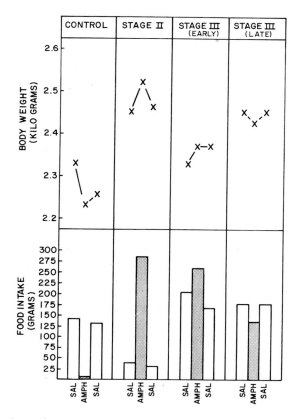

Fig. 3. D-Amphetamine sulfate (2 mg/kg) potentiates feeding in the anorexic cat (stage II) in contrast to its inhibition of food intake in the normal control. With recovery, the anorexigenic effect returns (stage III, early and late).

References p. 245–249

system damage is important in the syndrome (but see Ungerstedt, 1971b). If a painful clamp is applied to the tail (or other forms of stress; see Wagner and Woods, 1950), the catalepsy is overcome and the animal jumps down and runs around briefly.

In this respect, it is interesting that in the totally aphagic cat, the painful clamp on its tail will activate the animal to walk over to palatable food and eat it. Similar phenomena have been seen in 6-OHDA damaged rats (Marshall *et al.*, 1974; Stricker and Zigmond, 1974, 1975). In stage II, when the animal eats, but not enough, vision seems to serve as an activator as well as helping in the localization of food. Such an animal will walk over and eat food if it is placed in the cage, but will not eat if its vision is occluded, even if the food is right under its nose. Later, when smell returns, the phenomenon can be seen more clearly — smell first activates excited searching, and then later in recovery, helps in localization. With the return of smell, a higher level of intake and weight regulation appears to be reached. All of this suggests that activated feeding is another type of control over the act of eating. (Similar ideas, from an alternative point of view, have been expressed by Stricker and Zigmond, 1975.) Because activation also counteracts catalepsy, it is highly likely that the same neural systems (and therefore, the same neurotransmitters) which are involved in counteracting catalepsy may be similarly important in activated feeding.

Finally, as shown in Fig. 3, we found that we could activate feeding and increase body weight dramatically in the anorexic cat by an injection of D-amphetamine sulfate. The same dose given to a normal cat almost totally inhibited food intake and caused a sharp drop in body weight. Similar results have been obtained by Stricker and Zigmond (1975) in rats with electrolytic lesions in the lateral hypothalamus or following intraventricular injections of 6-OHDA. The hyperphagic effect of amphetamine in the lateral hypothalamic animal demonstrates that amphetamine has two effects with respect to feeding: first, its well-known anorexigenic effect, which is usually prepotent; and second, an activating effect on feeding, which is normally inhibited. When the anorexigenic effect is abolished, as with lateral hypothalamic lesions, the activating effect is unmasked. Leibowitz (1970) has shown a similar fractionation of the effects of intra-hypothalamic amphetamine in the neurologically intact rat pretreated with lateral hypothalamic injection of propranolol, a beta-adrenergic blocker. As is also shown in Fig. 3, with recovery, the anorexic action of amphetamine returns, passing through a phase of equal balance between activation and anorexia, where amphetamine seemed to have little effect on eating, to a phase of subnormal anorexia, the effect well-known in lateral hypothalamic animals (Carlisle, 1964; Fibiger *et al.*, 1973; Panksepp and Booth, 1973; Stricker and Zigmond, 1975.) The activational effect of amphetamine may depend on noradrenergic or dopaminergic systems, or both. We are presently attempting to determine the answer by selectively blocking each of them. But the change in amphetamine's apparent effect on feeding behavior reinforces our view that one must consider the stage of recovery that the animal is in, because each stage represents a different level of nervous integration of control over feeding.

In summary then, we believe that new insights into the neurotransmitters involved in the normal regulation of food intake can be achieved by a study of the aberrations in such function produced by brain damage. However, until a detailed behavioral analysis is made of the many levels of nervous control reflected in the many kinds of feeding, we will not fully understand the action of those transmitters.

SUMMARY

The major disturbances in feeding, hypothalamic hyperphagia and lateral hypothalamic aphagia, have recently been tied to specific transmitter systems in the brain. Recent advances along these lines are discussed and several paradoxes are raised. New evidence from behavioral analyses of these syndromes indicates that there are many more levels of control over the act of eating than are presently taken into account. It is suggested that when they are, some of the apparent paradoxes will be resolved.

ACKNOWLEDGEMENTS

This study was supported by USPHS Grant RO1 NS 11671 to Philip Teitelbaum and by a Postdoctoral Fellowship (USPHS 5 TO1 NS 05273) from the Institute of Neurological Sciences, University of Pennsylvania, School of Medicine, to David L. Wolgin.

REFERENCES

AHLSKOG, J. E. (1973) *Brain Norepinephrine and its Involvement in the Regulation of Food Consumption*, Thesis, Princeton University.

AHLSKOG, J. E. (1974) Food intake and amphetamine anorexia after selective forebrain norepinephrine loss. *Brain Research*, 82, 211–240.

AHLSKOG, J. E. AND HOEBEL, B. G. (1973) Overeating and obesity from damage to a noradrenergic system in the brain. *Science*, 182, 166–169.

AHLSKOG, J. E., HOEBEL, B. G. AND BREISCH, S. T. (1974) Hyperphagia following lesions of the noradrenergic pathway is prevented by hypophysectomy. *Fed. Proc.*, 33, 463 (Abstract).

ANAND, B. K. AND BROBECK, J. R. (1951) Hypothalamic control of food intake. *Yale J. Biol. Med.*, 24, 123–140.

ANDÉN, N.-E., CARLSSON, A., DAHLSTRÖM, A., FUXE, K., HILLARP, N. A. AND LARSSON, K. (1964) Demonstration and mapping out of nigro-neostriatal dopamine neurons. *Life Sci.*, 3, 523–530.

ANDÉN, N.-E., DAHLSTRÖM, A., FUXE, K., LARSSON, K., OLSON, L. AND UNGERSTEDT, U. (1966) Ascending monoamine neurons to the telencephalon and diencephalon. *Acta physiol. scand.*, 67, 313–326.

ANTELMAN, S. M., LIPPA, A. S. AND FISHER, A. E. (1972) 6-Hydroxydopamine, noradrenergic reward, and schizophrenia. *Science*, 175, 919–920.

BAEZ, L. A. (1974) Role of catecholamines in the anorectic effects of amphetamine in rats. *Psychopharmacologia (Berl.)*, 35, 91–98.

BAILE, C. A. (1974) Putative neurotransmitters in the hypothalamus and feeding. *Fed. Proc.*, 33, 1166–1175.

BERGER, B. D., WISE, C. D. AND STEIN, L. (1971) Norepinephrine: reversal of anorexia in rats with lateral hypothalamic damage. *Science*, 172, 281–284.

BLOOM, F. E., ALGERI, S., GROPPETTI, A., REVUELTA, A. AND COSTA, E. (1969) Lesions of central norepinephrine terminals with 6-OH-dopamine: biochemistry and fine structure. *Science*, 166, 1284–1286.

BOOTH, D. A. (1967) Localization of the adrenergic feeding system in the rat diencephalon. *Science*, **158**, 515–516.

BOOTH, D. A. (1968) Mechanism of action of norepinephrine in eliciting an eating response on injection into the rat hypothalamus. *J. Pharmacol. exp. Ther.*, **160**, 336–348.

BOOTH, D. A. (1972) Unlearned and learned effects of intrahypothalamic cyclic AMP injection on feeding. *Nature New Biol.*, **237**, 222–224.

BROBECK, J. R., TEPPERMAN, J. AND LONG, C. N. H. (1943) Experimental hypothalamic hyperphagia in the albino rat. *Yale J. Biol. Med.*, **15**, 831–853.

CARLISLE, H. J. (1964) Differential effects of amphetamine on food and water intake in rats with lateral hypothalamic lesions. *J. comp. physiol. Psychol.*, **58**, 47–54.

CARLSSON, A., FALCK, B. AND HILLARP, N. A. (1962a) Cellular localization of brain monoamines. *Acta physiol. scand.*, **56**, **Suppl. 196**, 1–28.

CARLSSON, A., FALCK, B., HILLARP, N. A. AND TORP, A. (1962b) Histochemical localization at the cellular level of hypothalamic noradrenaline. *Acta physiol. scand.*, **54**, 385–386.

CHENG, M. F., ROZIN, P. AND TEITELBAUM, P. (1971) Semi-starvation retards the development of food and water regulations in infant rats. *J. comp. physiol. Psychol.*, **76**, 206–218.

CODE, C. F. (1967) Control of food and water intake. In *Handbook of Physiology, Sect. 6, Alimentary Canal, Vol. 1*, American Physiological Society, Washington, D.C., pp. 319–335.

COSTA, E. AND GARATTINI, S. (Eds.) (1970) *International Symposium on Amphetamines and Related Compounds*, Raven Press, New York.

EPSTEIN, A. N. (1959) Suppression of eating and drinking by amphetamine and other drugs in normal and hyperphagic rats. *J. comp. physiol. Psychol.*, **52**, 37–45.

EPSTEIN, A. N. (1971) The lateral hypothalamic syndrome: its implications for the physiological psychology of hunger and thirst. *Progr. Physiol. Psychol.*, **4**, 263–317.

EPSTEIN, A. N. AND TEITELBAUM, P. (1964) Severe and persistent deficits in thirst produced by lateral hypothalamic damage. In *Thirst in the Regulation of Body Water*, M. J. WAYNER (Ed.), Macmillan (Pergamon), New York, N.Y., pp. 395–406.

EPSTEIN, A. N. AND TEITELBAUM, P. (1967) Specific loss of the hypoglycemic control of feeding in recovered lateral rats. *Amer. J. Physiol.*, **213**, 1159–1167.

ERDHEIM, J. (1904) Über Hypophysenganggeschwulste und Hirncholesteatome. *S. B. Akad. Wiss. Wien*, Abt. III, **113**, 537–726.

FALCK, B. AND HILLARP, S. A. (1959) On the cellular localization of catecholamines in the brain. *Acta anat. (Basel)*, **38**, 277–279.

FIBIGER, H. C., ZIS, A. P. AND MCGEER, E. G. (1973) Feeding and drinking deficits after 6-hydroxydopamine administration in the rat: similarities to the lateral hypothalamic syndrome. *Brain Research*, **55**, 135–148.

FLYNN, J. P., EDWARDS, S. B. AND BANDLER, R. J. (1971) Changes in sensory and motor systems during centrally elicited attack. *Behav. Sci.*, **16**, 1–19.

FRÖHLICH, A. (1940) Ein Fall von Tumor der Hypophysis cerebri ohne Akromegalie (transl. by H. Bruch). *Res. Publ. Ass. Res. nerv. ment. Dis.*, **20**, xvi–xxviii.

GERMAN, D. C. AND BOWDEN, D. M. (1974) Catecholamine systems as the neural substrate for intracranial self-stimulation: a hypothesis. *Brain Research*, **73**, 381–419.

GROSSMAN, S. P. (1960) Eating or drinking elicited by direct adrenergic stimulation of the hypothalamus. *Science*, **132**, 301–302.

GROSSMAN, S. P. (1962) Direct adrenergic and cholinergic stimulation of hypothalamic mechanisms. *Amer. J. Physiol.*, **202**, 872–882.

HETHERINGTON, A. W. AND RANSON, S. W. (1940) Hypothalamic lesions and adiposity in the rat. *Anat. Rec.*, **78**, 149–172.

HOEBEL, B. G. (1971) Feeding: neural control of intake. *Ann. Rev. Physiol.*, **33**, 533–568.

HOEBEL, B. G. (1974) Brain reward and aversion systems in the control of feeding and sexual behavior. In *Nebraska Symp. on Motivation*, M. R. JONES (Ed.), Univ. of Nebraska Press, Lincoln, Nebr., in press.

HOEBEL, B. G. AND TEITELBAUM, P. (1962) Hypothalamic control of feeding and self-stimulation. *Science*, **135**, 375–377.

HOEBEL, B. G. AND THOMPSON, R. D. (1969) Aversion to lateral hypothalamic stimulation caused by intragastric feeding or obesity. *J. comp. physiol. Psychol.*, **68**, 536–543.

KANNER, M. AND BALAGURA, S. (1971) Loss of feeding response to 2-deoxy-D-glucose by recovered lateral hypothalamic rats. *Amer. Zool.*, **11**, 624.

KENNEDY, G. C. (1950) The hypothalamic control of food intake in rats. *Proc. roy. Soc. B*, **137**, 535–549.

KISSILEFF, H. R. (1969) Food associated drinking in the rat. *J. comp. physiol. Psychol.*, **67**, 284–300.

LEHR, D. AND GOLDMAN, W. (1971) Sympathetic regulation of fluid balance and food intake by reciprocal activity of α- and β-adrenergically coded hypothalamic centers. *Proc. int. Union Physiol. Sci.*, **9**, 341.

LEIBOWITZ, S. F. (1970) Amphetamine's anorexic *versus* hunger-inducing effects mediated respectively by hypothalamic beta- *versus* alpha-adrenergic receptors. *Proc. 78th Ann. Conv. APA*, pp. 813–814.

LE MAGNEN, J. (1971) Advances in studies on the physiological control and regulation of food intake. In *Progress in Physiological Psychology, Vol. 4*, E. STELLAR AND J. M. SPRAGUE (Eds.), Academic Press, New York, N.Y., pp. 203–261.

MACDONNELL, M. F. AND FLYNN, J. P. (1966) Control of sensory fields by stimulation of hypothalamus. *Science*, **152**, 1406–1408.

MARGULES, D. L. AND OLDS, J. (1962) Identical "feeding" and "rewarding" systems in the lateral hypothalamus of rats. *Science*, **135**, 374–375.

MARSHALL, J. F. (1975) Increased orientation to sensory stimuli following medial hypothalamic damage in rats. *Brain Research*, **86**, 373–387.

MARSHALL, J. F. AND TEITELBAUM, P. (1973) A comparison of the eating in response to hypothalamic and glucoprivic challenges after nigral 6-hydroxydopamine and lateral hypothalamic electrolytic lesions in rats. *Brain Research*, **55**, 229–233.

MARSHALL, J. F. AND TEITELBAUM, P. (1974) Further analysis of sensory inattention following lateral hypothalamic damage in rats. *J. comp. physiol. Psychol.*, **86**, 375–395.

MARSHALL, J. F., RICHARDSON, J. S. AND TEITELBAUM, P. (1974) Nigrostriatal bundle damage and the lateral hypothalamic syndrome. *J. comp. physiol. Psychol.*, **87**, 808–830.

MARSHALL, J. F., TURNER, B. H. AND TEITELBAUM, P. (1971) Sensory neglect produced by lateral hypothalamic damage. *Science*, **174**, 523–525.

MILLER, N. E., BAILEY, C. J. AND STEVENSON, J. A. F. (1950) Decreased "hunger" but increased food intake resulting from hypothalamic lesions. *Science*, **112**, 256–259.

MISELIS, R. R. AND EPSTEIN, A. N. (1971) Preoptic–hypothalamic mediation of feeding induced by cerebral glucoprivation. *Amer. Zool.*, **11**, 624.

MORGANE, P. J. (1961) Alterations in feeding and drinking behavior of rats with lesions in globi pallidi. *Amer. J. Physiol.*, **201**, 420–428.

MORGANE, P. J. (1969) Neural regulation of food and water intake. *Ann. N. Y. Acad. Sci.*, **157**, 531–1216.

MYERS, R. D. (1964) Emotional and autonomic responses following hypothalamic chemical stimulation. *Canad. J. Psychol.*, **18**, 6–14.

OATLEY, K. (1973) Simulation and theory of thirst. In *The Neuropsychology of Thirst*, A. N. EPSTEIN, H. R. KISSILEFF AND E. STELLAR (Eds.), Winston, Washington, D. C., pp. 199–223.

OLDS, J., TRAVIS, R. P. AND SCHWING, R. C. (1960) Topographic organization of hypothalamic self-stimulation functions. *J. comp. physiol. Psychol.*, **31**, 23–32.

OLDS, M. E. AND OLDS, J. (1963) Approach–avoidance analysis of rat diencephalon. *J. comp. Neurol.*, **120**, 259–295.

PANKSEPP, J. AND BOOTH, D. A. (1973) Tolerance in the depression of intake when amphetamine is added to the rat's food. *Psychopharmacologia (Berl.)*, **29**, 45–54.

PETERS, F. (1904) Pharmakologische Untersuchen über Corydalisalkaloide. *Naunyn-Schmiedeberg's Arch. exp. Path. Pharmak.*, **51**, 130–174.

PHILLIPS, A. G. AND FIBIGER, H. C. (1973) Dopaminergic and noradrenergic substrates of positive reinforcement: differential effects of D- and L-amphetamine. *Science*, **179**, 575–577.

POSCHEL, B. P. H. AND NINTEMAN, F. W. (1971) Intracranial reward and the forebrain's serotonergic mechanism: studies employing *para*-chlorphenylalanine and *para*-chloramphetamine. *Physiol. Behav.*, **7**, 39–46.

REYNOLDS, R. W. (1959) The effect of amphetamine on food intake in normal and hypothalamic hyperphagic rats. *J. comp. physiol. Psychol.*, **52**, 682–684.

RITTER, S. AND STEIN, L. (1973) Self-stimulation of noradrenergic cell group (A6) in locus coeruleus of rats. *J. comp. physiol. Psychol.*, **85**, 443–452.

RITTER, S., WISE, C. D. AND STEIN, L. (1975) Neurochemical regulation of feeding in the rat: facilitation by α-noradrenergic, but not dopaminergic, receptor stimulants. *J. comp. physiol. Psychol.*, in press.

ROLL, S. K. (1970) Intracranial self-stimulation and wakefulness: effect of manipulating ambient brain catecholamines. *Science*, **168**, 1370–1372.

ROUTTENBERG, A. (1972) Intracranial chemical injection and behavior: a critical review. *Behav. Biol.*, **7**, 601–641.

SETLER, P. E. AND SMITH, G. P. (1974) Increased food intake elicited by adrenergic stimulation of the diencephalon in rhesus monkeys. *Brain Research*, **65**, 459–473.

SHARPE, L. G. AND MYERS, R. D. (1969) Feeding and drinking following stimulation of the diencephalon of the monkey with amines and other substances. *Exp. Brain Res.*, **8**, 295–310.

SINGH, D. (1973) Effects of preoperative training on food-motivated behavior of hypothalamic hyperphagic rats. *J. comp. physiol. Psychol.*, **84**, 47–52.

SINGH, D. (1974) Role of preoperative experience on reaction to quinine taste in hypothalamic hyperphagic rats. *J. comp. physiol. Psychol.*, **86**, 674–678.

SLANGEN, J. L. AND MILLER, N. E. (1969) Pharmacological tests for the function of hypothalamic norepinephrine in eating behavior. *Physiol. Behav.*, **4**, 543–552.

SMITH, P. E. (1927) The disabilities caused by hypophysectomy and their repair. *J. Amer. med. Ass.*, **88**, 158–161.

SMITH, P. E. (1930) Hypophysectomy and a replacement therapy in the rat. *Amer. J. Anat.*, **45**, 205–273.

STEIN, L. (1968) Chemistry of reward and punishment. In *Pharmacology: A Review of Progress, 1957–1967*, D. H. EFRON (Ed.), Public Health Service No. 1836, U.S. Government Printing Office, Washington, D. C., pp. 105–123.

STEVENSON, J. A. F. (1969) Neural control of food and water intake. In *The Hypothalamus*, W. HAYMAKER, E. ANDERSON AND W. J. H. NAUTA (Eds.), Thomas, Springfield, Ill., pp. 524–621.

STOWE, F. R. AND MILLER, A. T. (1957) The effect of amphetamine on food intake in rats with hypothalamic hyperphagia. *Experientia (Basel)*, **13**, 114–115.

STRICKER, E. M. AND WOLF, G. (1967) The effects of hypovolemia on drinking in rats with lateral hypothalamic damage. *Proc. Soc. exp. Biol. (N.Y.)*, **124**, 816–820.

STRICKER, E. M. AND ZIGMOND, M. J. (1974) Effects on homeostasis of intraventricular injections of 6-hydroxydopamine in rats. *J. comp. physiol. Psychol.*, **86**, 973–994.

STRICKER, E. M. AND ZIGMOND, M. J. (1975) Recovery of function following damage to central catecholamine-containing neurons: a neurochemical model for the lateral hypothalamic syndrome. *Progr. Physiol. Psychol.*, in press.

TEITELBAUM, P. (1955) Sensory control of hypothalamic hyperphagia. *J. comp. physiol. Psychol.*, **48**, 156–163.

TEITELBAUM, P. (1957) Random and food-directed activity in hyperphagic and normal rats. *J. comp. physiol. Psychol.*, **50**, 486–490.

TEITELBAUM, P. (1971) The encephalization of hunger. In *Progress in Physiological Psychology*, Vol. 4, E. STELLAR AND J. M. SPRAGUE (Eds.), Academic Press, New York, N.Y., pp. 319–350.

TEITELBAUM, P., CHENG, M. F. AND ROZIN, P. (1969) Development of feeding parallels its recovery after hypothalamic damage. *J. comp. physiol. Psychol.*, **67**, 430–441.

TEITELBAUM, P. AND EPSTEIN, A. N. (1962) The lateral hypothalamic syndrome: recovery of feeding and drinking after lateral hypothalamic lesions. *Psychol. Rev.*, **69**, 74–90.

TURNER, B. H. (1973) A sensorimotor syndrome produced by lesions of the amygdala and lateral hypothalamus. *J. comp. physiol. Psychol.*, **82**, 37–47.

TWITCHELL, T. E. (1951) The restoration of motor function following hemiplegia in men. *Brain*, **74**, 443–480.

TWITCHELL, T. E. (1965) The automatic grasping responses of infants. *Neuropsychologia*, **3**, 247–259.

TWITCHELL, T. E. (1969) Early development of avoiding and grasping reactions. In *Modern Neurology*, S. LOCKE (Ed.), Little, Brown, Boston, Mass., pp. 333–345.

TWITCHELL, T. E. (1970) Reflex mechanisms and the development of prehension. In *Mechanisms of Motor Skill Development*, K. J. CONNOLLY (Ed.), Academic Press, London, pp. 25–38.

UNGERSTEDT, U. (1970) Is interruption of the nigrostriatal dopamine system producing the "lateral hypothalamus syndrome"? *Acta physiol. scand.*, **80**, 35A–36A.

UNGERSTEDT, U. (1971a) Stereotaxic mapping of the monoamine pathways in the rat brain. *Acta physiol. scand.*, **Suppl. 367**, 1–48.

UNGERSTEDT, U. (1971b) Adipsia and aphagia after 6-hydroxydopamine induced degeneration of the nigro-striatal dopamine system. *Acta physiol. scand.*, **Suppl. 367**, 95–122.

URETSKY, N. J. AND IVERSEN, L. L. (1970) Effects of 6-hydroxydopamine on catecholamine containing neurones in the rat brain. *J. Neurochem.*, **17**, 269–278.

VAN HARREVELD, A. AND BOGEN, J. E. (1961) The clinging position of the bulbocapninized cat. *Exp. Neurol.*, **4**, 241–261.

WAGNER, H. N. AND WOODS, J. W. (1950) Interruption of bulbocapnine catalepsy in rats by environmental stress. *Arch. Neurol. Psychiat. (Chic.)*, **64**, 720–725.

WAYNER, M. J., COTT, A., MILLNER, J. AND TARTAGLIONE, R. (1971) Loss of 2-deoxy-D-glucose induced eating in recovered lateral rats. *Physiol. Behav.*, **7**, 881–884.

WEISSMAN, A., KOE, B. K. AND TENEN, S. S. (1966) Anti-amphetamine effects following inhibition of tyrosine hydroxylase. *J. Pharmacol. exp. Ther.*, **51**, 339–353.

WOLGIN, D. L. AND TEITELBAUM, P. (1974) *The Role of Activation and Sensory Stimuli in the Recovery of Feeding Following Lateral Hypothalamic Lesions in the Cat.* Paper presented at the Eastern Psychological Association meetings, Philadelphia.

WOODS, S. C., DECKE, E. AND VASSELLI, J. R. (1974) Metabolic hormones and regulation of body weight. *Psychol. Rev.*, **81**, 26–43.

YAKSH, T. L. AND MYERS, R. D. (1972) Hypothalamic "coding" in the unanesthetized monkey of noradrenergic sites mediating feeding and thermoregulation. *Physiol. Behav.*, **8**, 251–257.

YOKEL, R. A. AND WISE, R. (1975) Increased lever pressing for amphetamine after pimozide in rats: implications for a dopamine theory of reward. *Science*, in press.

ZEIGLER, H. P., MARWINE, A. AND KARTEN, H. J. (1974) *The Trigeminal System and the "Lateral Hypothalamic" Syndrome in the Rat.* Paper presented at the Eastern Psychological Association meeting, Philadelphia.

ZIGMOND, M. J. AND STRICKER, E. M. (1972) Deficits in feeding behavior after intraventricular injection of 6-hydroxydopamine in rats. *Science*, **177**, 1211–1214.

ZIGMOND, M. J. AND STRICKER, E. M. (1973) Recovery of feeding and drinking by rats after intraventricular 6-hydroxydopamine or lateral hypothalamic lesions. *Science*, **182**, 717–719.

Neurotransmitters and Temperature Regulation

PETER LOMAX AND MARTIN DAVID GREEN

Department of Pharmacology, School of Medicine and the Brain Research Institute, University of California, Los Angeles, Calif. 90024 (U.S.A.)

The demonstration of relatively high concentrations of amines in the hypothalamus, coupled with the elucidation of the role of this region of the brain in regulating body temperature have suggested that these amines might play an important role as neurotransmitters in thermoregulation. Over the past decade or so there has been a considerable body of research aimed at resolving these questions and several recent symposia have adequately reviewed this work (Bligh and Moore, 1972; Schönbaum and Lomax, 1973; Lomax *et al.*, 1975). It is not possible, at the present time, to construct any unified view or general theory of the function of neurotransmitters in thermoregulatory mechanisms; although integrative models have frequently been proposed, such as those of Bligh (1972) or Myers (1975), these more often represent special cases arising from the author's own research rather than a synthesis of all available data.

Many attempts have been made to describe the thermoregulatory system in terms of cybernetic models of varying complexity (Hardy, 1972). The next step in the analysis of the system has been to propose neuronal networks to replace the black boxes, based on experimental evidences (Hensel, 1973). One of the major controversies concerns the nature of the reference point of the controller — the presence or absence of a temperature independent reference signal. Two major models can be derived: one in which the controlled temperature is compared to a reference value (the "set-point") and appropriate responses are activated to correct any deviation of the controlled temperature from the reference; alternatively, two types of sensors can be postulated, responding to a deviation above or below the controlled temperature, the feedbacks from these are compared and appropriate responses to correct the load error are set in motion (Mitchell *et al.*, 1972; Horowitz, 1975; Houdas and Guieu, 1975). Schematic illustrations of these alterations are seen in Fig. 1. Whatever the detailed nature of the controller, or its precise anatomical location, the net effect of its activity will be integrated to increase or decrease the frequency of firing of the thermoregulatory effector neurons. Whether or not an individual neuron does fire at any instant is a function of its membrane potential and this, in turn, will depend on the actions of excitatory and inhibitory influences on it.

It is in this last respect that the major problems arise in relation to the role of the various neurotransmitters in that one cannot define the exact point in the neuronal loop at which the amine is acting in most studies. Thus, modification of neuro-

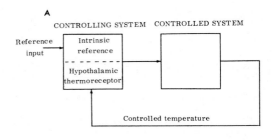

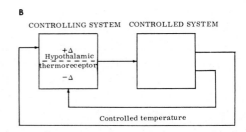

Fig. 1. Proposed models of thermoregulatory control systems. In A the controlled temperature is compared to an intrinsic "set" temperature and appropriate physiological mechanisms are activated to compensate for any difference between these. Various inputs can adjust the "set" level to maintain thermal equilibrium in the face of varying environmental thermal loads. In B separate temperature sensors are activated depending on whether the various peripheral receptors are above or below a fixed temperature. Thermoregulatory mechanisms are activated on the basis of the integrated analysis of these inputs.

transmitter release may disturb the thermoregulatory system: (a) by changing neuronal input; (b) by altering the function of the central thermostats; (c) by attenuating normal effector functions of the system. Furthermore, in many species, especially in man, the major thermoregulatory responses to alterations in environmental temperature are behavioral and these may be markedly altered following manipulation of central neurotransmitter activity. These problems are compounded by the fact that many of the thermoregulatory responses (such as panting, salivation, shivering, vasomotor activity) represent secondary functions of the systems involved so that even though activation of a system might be appropriate in order to regulate body temperature it must be inhibited in order to fulfill a primary function.

Measured responses

It becomes apparent, from consideration of normal thermoregulation that there are many ways in which changes in neurotransmitter activity could modify the function of the central controlling systems or the responses mediated by the centers in the central nervous system. The magnitude of any ensuing change in body temperature will be determined by the degree to which the system is able to compensate for the disturbance. Alternatively, the duration and degree of neurotransmitter action may be

Of the several neuroamines discussed one might conclude that in the case of norepinephrine, 5-HT and acetylcholine the data for assigning a neurotransmitter role is most compelling while histamine and dopamine, in the words of Feldberg (1975), "although not yet admitted to the Club, are knocking at the door". Clearly a considerable amount of further research in this fascinating field is needed and will undoubtedly aid in unravelling the complexities of the central nervous system in general.

SUMMARY

The elucidation of the role of the rostral hypothalamus as a central controller for maintaining body temperature, coupled with the demonstration that this part of the brain contains relatively high concentrations of most of the monoamines that have been suggested as putative central neurotransmitters, has inevitably led to a considerable body of research implicating these monoamines as being intimately concerned with thermoregulation. It is often difficult to separate physiological from pharmacological effects in these several studies. Modification of neurotransmitter release may disturb the thermoregulatory system: (a) by changing neuronal input; (b) by altering the function of the central thermostats; (c) by attenuating normal effector functions of the system. In many species, especially in man, the major thermoregulatory responses to alterations in environmental temperature are behavioral and there is considerable evidence that these responses can also account for body temperature changes following manipulation of central neurotransmitter activity. The current status of the role of monoaminergic neurons in the central nervous system in regulating body temperature is reviewed with particular emphasis on the relevant techniques of investigation.

REFERENCES

BAIRD, J. AND LANG, W. J. (1973) Temperature responses in the rat and cat to cholinomimetic drugs injected into the cerebral ventricles. *Europ. J. Pharmacol.*, **21**, 203–211.

BECKMAN, A. L. (1970) Effect of intrahypothalamic norepinephrine on thermoregulatory responses in the rat. *Amer. J. Physiol.*, **218**, 1596–1604.

BLIGH, J. (1972) Neuronal models of mammalian temperature regulation. In *Essays on Temperature Regulation*, J. BLIGH AND R. MOORE (Eds.), North Holland, Amsterdam, pp. 105–120.

BLIGH, J. AND MOORE, R. (Eds.) (1972) *Essays on Temperature Regulation*. North Holland, Amsterdam, 190 pp.

BOULANT, J. A. AND BIGNALL, K. E. (1973) Hypothalamic neuronal responses to peripheral and deep-body temperatures. *Amer. J. Physiol.*, **225**, 1371–1374.

BREZENOFF, H. E. AND LOMAX, P. (1970) Temperature changes following microinjection of histamine into the thermoregulatory centers of the rat. *Experientia (Basel)*, **26**, 51–52.

BRIMBLECOMBE, R. W. (1973) Effects of cholinomimetic and cholinolytic drugs on body temperature. In *The Pharmacology of Thermoregulation*, E. SCHÖNBAUM AND P. LOMAX (Eds.), Karger, Basel, pp. 182–193.

EISENMAN, J. S. (1972) Unit activity studies of thermoresponsive neurons. In *Essays on Temperature Regulation*, J. BLIGH AND R. MOORE (Eds.), North Holland, Amsterdam, pp. 55–70.

FELDBERG, W. AND MYERS, R. D. (1964) Effects on temperature of amines injected into the cerebral ventricles. A new concept of temperature regulation. *J. Physiol. (Lond.)*, **173**, 226–237.

FELDBERG, W. (1975) Summing up of symposium. In *Temperature Regulation and Drug Action*, P. LOMAX, E. SCHÖNBAUM AND J. JACOB (Eds.), Karger, Basel, pp. 393–395.

FORD, D. M., HELLON, R. F. AND LUFF, R. H. (1973) Cholinergic pathways in the brain stem subserving thermoregulatory mechanisms in the cat. *J. Physiol. (Lond.)*, **231**, 34–35P.

FRENS, J. (1975) Thermoregulation set point changes during lipopolysaccharide fever. In *Temperature Regulation and Drug Action*, P. LOMAX, E. SCHÖNBAUM AND J. JACOB (Eds.), Karger, Basel, pp. 59–64.

HARDY, J. D. (1972) Models of temperature regulation. In *Essays on Temperature Regulation*, J. BLIGH AND R. MOORE (Eds.), North Holland, Amsterdam, pp. 163–186.

HAYWARD, J. N. (1975) The thalamus and thermoregulation. In *Temperature Regulation and Drug Action*, P. LOMAX, E. SCHÖNBAUM AND J. JACOB (Eds.), Karger, Basel, pp. 22–31.

HELLON, R. (1972) Central transmitters and thermoregulation. In *Essays on Temperature Regulation*, J. BLIGH AND R. MOORE (Eds.), North Holland, Amsterdam, pp. 71–86.

HELLON, R. F. AND MISRA, N. K. (1973a) Neurons in the dorsal horn of the rat responding to scrotal skin temperature changes. *J. Physiol. (Lond.)*, **232**, 375–388.

HELLON, R. F. AND MISRA, N. K. (1973b) Neurones in the ventrobasal complex of the rat thalamus responding to scrotal skin temperature changes. *J. Physiol. (Lond.)*, **232**, 389–399.

HELLON, R. F., MISRA, N. K. AND PROVINS, K. A. (1973) Neurones in the somatosensory cortex of the rat responding to scrotal skin temperature changes. *J. Physiol. (Lond.)*, **232**, 401–411.

HENSEL, H. (1973) Neural processes in thermoregulation. *Physiol. Rev.*, **53**, 948–1017.

HORI, T. AND NAKAYAMA, T. (1973) Effects of biogenic amines on central thermoresponsive neurones in the rabbit. *J. Physiol. (Lond.)*, **232**, 71–85.

HORITA, A. AND QUOCK, R. M. (1975) Dopaminergic mechanisms in drug-induced temperature effects. In *Temperature Regulation and Drug Action*, P. LOMAX, E. SCHÖNBAUM AND J. JACOB (Eds.), Karger, Basel, pp. 75–84.

HOROWITZ, J. M. (1975) Neural models on temperature regulation for cold stressed animals. In *Temperature Regulation and Drug Action*, P. LOMAX, E. SCHÖNBAUM AND J. JACOB (Eds.), Karger, Basel, pp. 1–10.

HOUDAS, Y. AND GUIEU, J.-D. (1975) Physical models of human thermoregulation. In *Temperature Regulation and Drug Action*, P. LOMAX, E. SCHÖNBAUM AND J. JACOB (Eds.), Karger, Basel.

JELL, R. M. (1973) Responses of hypothalamic neurones to local temperature and to acetylcholine, noradrenaline and 5-hydroxytryptamine. *Brain Res.*, **55**, 123–134.

JOHNSON, K. G. AND SMITH, C. A. (1973) The nature of the thermoregulatory sensitivity to cholinomimetic drugs in the cerebral ventricles of sheep. *J. Physiol. (Lond.)*, **236**, 31–32P.

KENNEDY, M. S. AND BURKS, T. F. (1974) Dopamine receptors in the central thermoregulatory mechanism of the cat. *Neuropharmacology*, **13**, 119–128.

KIRKPATRICK, W. E. AND LOMAX, P. (1970) Temperature changes following iontophoretic injection of acetylcholine into the rostral hypothalamus of the rat. *Neuropharmacology*, **9**, 195–202.

KNOX, G. V., CAMPBELL, C. AND LOMAX, P. (1973a) Cutaneous temperature and unit activity in the hypothalamic thermoregulatory centers. *Exp. Neurol.*, **40**, 717–730.

KNOX, G. V., CAMPBELL, C. AND LOMAX, P. (1973b) The effects of acetylcholine and nicotine on unit activity in the hypothalamic thermoregulatory centers of the rat. *Brain Research*, **51**, 215–223.

LOMAX, P., SCHÖNBAUM, E. AND JACOB, J. (Eds.) (1975) *Temperature Regulation and Drug Action*, Karger, Basel.

LOMAX, P. AND GREEN, M. D. (1975) Histamine and temperature regulation. In *Temperature Regulation and Drug Action*, P. LOMAX, E. SCHÖNBAUM AND J. JACOB (Eds.), Karger, Basel, pp. 85–94.

MEETER, E. AND WOLTHUIS, O. L. (1968) The effects of cholinesterase inhibitors on the body temperature of the rat. *Europ. J. Pharmacol.*, **4**, 18–24.

MEETER, E. (1973) Investigation of the rapid recovery of rat thermoregulation from soman poisoning. *Europ. J. Pharmacol.*, **24**, 105–107.

MITCHELL, D., ATKINS, A. R. AND WYNDHAM, C. H. (1972) Mathematical and physical models of thermoregulation. In *Essays on Temperature Regulation*, J. BLIGH AND R. MOORE (Eds.), North Holland, Amsterdam, pp. 37–54.

MURAKAMI, N. (1973) Effects of iontophoretic application of 5-hydroxytryptamine, noradrenaline and acetylcholine upon hypothalamic temperature-sensitive neurones in rats. *Jap. J. Physiol.*, **23**, 435–446.

MYERS, R. D. (1975) An integrative model of monoamine and ionic mechanisms in the hypothalamic control of body temperature. In *Temperature Regulation and Drug Action*, P. LOMAX, E. SCHÖNBAUM AND J. JACOB (Eds.), Karger, Basel, pp. 32–42.

NUTIK, S. L. (1973) Convergence of cutaneous and preoptic region thermal afferents on posterior hypothalamic neurons. *J. Neurophysiol.*, **36**, 250–257.

PRZEWLOCKA, B. AND KALUZA, J. (1973) The effect of intraventricularly administered noradrenaline and dopamine on the body temperature of the rat. *Pol. J. Pharmacol. Pharm.*, **25**, 345–355.

REIGLE, T. G. AND WOLF, H. H. (1974) Potential neurotransmitters and receptor mechanisms involved in the central control of body temperature in golden hamsters. *J. Pharmacol.*, **189**, 97–109.

SATINOFF, E. AND CANTOR, A. (1975) Intraventricular norepinephrine and thermoregulation in rats. In *Temperature Regulation and Drug Action*, P. LOMAX, E. SCHÖNBAUM AND J. JACOB (Eds.), Karger, Basel, pp. 103–110.

SCHÖNBAUM, E. AND LOMAX, P. (Eds.) (1973) *The Pharmacology of Thermoregulation*, Karger, Basel.

SCHWARTZ, J. C., JULIEN, C., FÉGER, J. AND GARBARG, M. (1974) Histaminergic pathway in rat brain evidenced by hypothalamic lesions. *Fed. Proc.* **33**, 285.

SNYDER, S. H. AND TAYLOR, K. M. (1972) Histamine in the brain: a neurotransmitter? In *Perspectives in Neuropharmacology*, S. H. SNYDER (Ed.), Oxford University Press, London, pp. 43–73.

Limbic Structures and Behavior: Endocrine Correlates

H. URSIN, G. D. COOVER, C. KØHLER, M. DERYCK, T. SAGVOLDEN AND S. LEVINE*

Institutes of Physiology and Psychology, University of Bergen, Bergen (Norway) and *Department of Psychiatry, Stanford University, Stanford, Calif. 94305 (U.S.A.)

Limbic structures exert profound influences on many types of behavior and are necessary for normal behavior. Following lesions in limbic structures many tasks become difficult or impossible to solve and the memory of previously learned material may also be impaired (Kaada, 1960; Ursin, 1972). The close anatomical relationship between limbic structures and the hypothalamus is evident by changes in autonomic and endocrine processes. This may represent primary changes in regulatory mechanisms, however, it may also be secondary to psychological changes. External stimuli will not have the same effect if there are profound changes in perception, motivation and the problem-solving capacity of the remaining brain. Finally, changes in hormone levels may act back on the brain via nervous feedback or directly on brain cells (de Wied, 1974).

The present review will not attempt to cover the whole field of endocrine correlates to behavior changes following manipulations of limbic structures. In a series of experiments we have tried to elucidate some of these problems by studying the changes in plasma corticosterone in the rat during two-way active avoidance learning. We have studied normal rats as well as rats with lesions in three different limbic structures: the amygdala complex, the cingulate cortex and the septal area. Plasma corticosteroids most probably have no direct effect on avoidance behavior (de Wied, 1974). The avoidance procedure we used did not last more than 10–15 min; the corticosterone does not even reach the peak value until 20 min after a given stressor has been applied (Davidson *et al.*, 1968). In our studies plasma corticosterone has been used as an indicator of the central state of the individual during avoidance training. High levels of corticosterone will be regarded as indicative of preceding high levels of "fear", "activation" or motivation. The fact that ACTH (corticotropin) itself has an influence on consolidation of avoidance behavior (de Wied, 1974) does not affect this assumption.

This report deals only with results from two-way active avoidance acquisition. Limbic structures are known to influence acquisition of active as well as passive avoidance tasks (McCleary, 1966), but there is a high degree of specificity in this control. Lesions producing changes in passive avoidance may not change active avoidance and *vice versa* (McCleary, 1966; Ursin, 1972). The two-way active avoidance task we have studied is particularly interesting since limbic lesions may impair as well as improve performance in this task. Lesions in the amygdala as well as in the cingulate

References p. 273–274

cortex impair this behavior, while lesions in the septal area and in the hippocampus improve performance in this task (McCleary, 1966). Therefore, many factors must be involved in this type of behavior, both from a neuro-anatomical and a psychological point of view. The endocrine correlates of the behavior in this task might elucidate which psychological mechanisms really are involved.

Two distinct sets of hypotheses have been forwarded to explain the reduced learning in two-way active avoidance. The poor performance may be due to a reduced motivational state. If that is the case, corticosteroid levels would be expected to be lower during the early phases of learning. On the other hand, if the reason for the poor performance is reduced problem-solving ability, no change in motivational level should be expected, and, accordingly, the corticosteroid levels during the initial phases of learning should be as in normals. A simple measurement of corticosterone, therefore, should distinguish between these two hypotheses.

The improved performance in rats with septal lesions may also be explained in terms of changed motivation or reactivity. Again, it is possible to measure the postulated changes in internal state by measuring the endocrine correlates. During active avoidance learning there is a reduction in the emotional state as learning proceeds. Many authors have commented upon the reduced "fear" or arousal level during avoidance learning and the apparent "nonchalance" of well-practiced avoiders (Solomon and Wynne, 1954; Rescorla and Solomon, 1967; Maier *et al.*, 1969).

If this is so, one should expect corticosterone levels to be lower in animals that are performing well in a two-way active avoidance situation. We have studied this in normal rats. We have found such a reduction. This phenomenon is an important aspect of the regulation of avoidance behavior and the effects of adequate behavior on physiological processes. It turned out that this dimension must be taken into account when endocrine correlates of behavior are to be discussed.

(1) Plasma corticosterone levels during two-way active avoidance learning in normal rats

Coover *et al.* (1973a) have observed 17 male Möll–Wistar rats during acquisition of a two-way shuttle box task. The rats were studied for 20 sessions, one session per day, each consisting of 10 trials with a 60 sec intertrial interval. Plasma samples for corticosterone assay (Glick *et al.*, 1964) were taken from the rats following four of the sessions: session 1, session 6 or 7, session 16 or 17, and a forced-extinction session (see Fig. 1). Three basal samples were also taken in the course of the experiment. The first basal sample was taken 2 weeks prior to the avoidance session, the second was taken immediately before session 6 or 7, and the third sample was taken before session 16 or 17. A balanced design of basal and postsession blood samplings was used around sessions 6 and 7 and sessions 16 and 17.

The basal samples were taken by quietly entering the animal room and removing the rat to be sampled. This rat was anesthetized by quickly placing it into a cylindrical Plexiglass jar containing cotton soaked in ether. Within 1 min the rat was anesthetized, and within another 0.5–1.5 min a blood sample had been drawn from the surgically

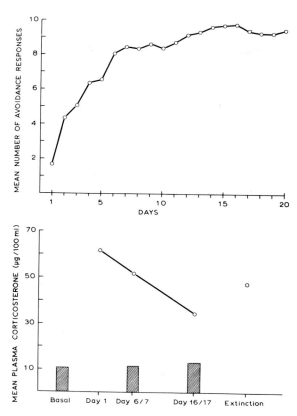

Fig. 1. Active avoidance in normal rats. Top diagram: mean learning curve for 17 normal rats in a two-way active avoidance situation. Lower diagram: mean plasma corticosterone values during avoidance learning in the same 17 normal rats. Shaded bars indicate basal levels.

exposed jugular vein. This is rapid enough so that the total procedure does not significantly affect the plasma corticosterone concentration of the sample obtained (Davidson *et al.*, 1968). Post-avoidance-session sampling was carried out in the same manner, the subject being placed in the ether jar 20 min after introduction to the avoidance apparatus. This necessitated returning the subject to its cage following the avoidance session until the required 20 min from stimulus onset had passed; the sessions lasted only 10–11 min.

There was a significant, but moderate drop (16%) in mean plasma corticosterone level from the initial stage (session 1) to the acquisition phase (session 6 or 7). The number of shocks and the shock duration time was greatly reduced in this period. Since the drop was so small, the shocks are probably not the most important event for the corticosterone increase. In addition, the number of shocks and the corticosterone increases did not correlate within sessions. Our interpretation is that the conditioned stimulus has now become the signal for shocks presumably through a classical conditioning process. This process has been referred to as "factor 1" in the various

References p. 273–274

formulations of the two-factor theory of avoidance (Rescorla and Solomon, 1967).

The most marked reduction in corticosterone output was found in the time from avoidance sessions 6 or 7 to sessions 16 or 17. During this time the rats stabilized their avoidance behavior. Corresponding to this period there is a decrease in the internal state indicative of arousal or "fear". There were also behavioral indications of decreased arousal: bolus droppings declined while there was an increase in sniffing and grooming behavior. It should be noted that the corticosterone response does not decline all the way to basal levels. It is hard to conceive of avoidance behavior occurring without any arousal at all. Even if there is a clear drop in corticosterone levels, and even if the animal appears behaviorally to be minimally aroused, there has to be a minimal level of activation for the animal to perform the proper response.

In conclusion there appear to be three phases in avoidance learning that would have three different endocrine correlates. When the aversive stimulation is high, there is a high level of arousal as indicated by high levels of plasma corticosterone. When acquisition of the avoidance response is occurring, and the aversive stimulation is becoming predictable, there is also a heightened arousal, but less so than in the initial phase. This response is now due to a classical conditioning procedure and corresponds with factor 1 in the two-factor theory of avoidance. However, a third stage occurs when the situation is becoming highly predictable and the animal is coping with the task. The arousal is then decreased, and the physiological response indicative of arousal also decreases. These bodily processes reflect the second factor in the two-factor theory of avoidance.

Our results confirm previous findings that predictability of electric shock (Seligman and Meyer, 1970) and availability of avoidance response (Weiss, 1968) reduce the amount of stomach ulceration, independent of the amount of the aversive stimulation. When an avoidance response has been acquired, the situation itself becomes less stressful or less activating.

This interpretation is further supported by the extinction data. A marked increase in pituitary–adrenal activity over previously stabilized values occurred during the forced-extinction procedure, both when the response was prevented and when it was punished (Fig. 1). Defecation also increased. When the predictability and the control that the rats had acquired no longer existed, the pituitary–adrenal activity again increased. Marked increases in pituitary–adrenal activity have also been observed following extinction of an ongoing appetitive response (Coover *et al.*, 1971). Expectancy of the reinforcement schedule seems to be a decisive factor for corticosterone levels during operant conditioning. Goldman *et al.* (1973) demonstrated an increase in corticosterone response when the frequency of reinforcement suddenly became less than that obtained during training. On the other hand, if the reinforcement frequency was suddenly greater than expected, there was a reduction in the corticosterone level.

The resulting model for pituitary–adrenal activation stresses the cognitive factors in addition to the physical values of the stimuli. In particular, it seems to be important for this activation whether or not an animal develops an expectancy of coping with a situation and whether or not this expectancy is being met.

(2) Corticosterone levels during two-way active avoidance learning in rats with baso-lateral amygdala lesions

It has long been known that amygdala lesions produce avoidance deficits and changes in emotional behavior in a variety of species. It has been discussed whether these changes are due to a motivational change or to a more specific loss of the ability to solve avoidance problems. The corticosterone level in plasma should discriminate between these two main hypotheses. If the motivational state is reduced, there should be a decrement in the corticosterone response also. If it is the problem-solving ability that is changed, the activation should be as intense in the lesioned rats as in normals at the early phases of avoidance learning, and higher than in normals during the later stages, due to the inability to cope with the situation.

Small basolateral lesions in 15 rats produced deficits in two-way active avoidance learning and passive avoidance learning as compared to 15 operated, non-lesioned controls (Coover *et al.*, 1973b). The behavioral situation was the same as that reported

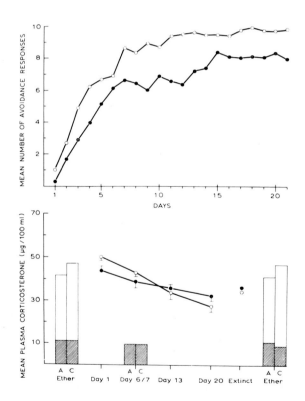

Fig. 2. Top diagram: mean learning curve for 15 rats with amygdala lesions (filled circles) compared with the learning curve for 15 controls (open circles). Lower diagram: mean plasma corticosterone values during avoidance learning in the same rats. Shaded bars indicate basal levels; open bars, ether-stress samples. Standard error of the mean is indicated for mean values by a vertical bar.

above, and the blood-sampling procedure also followed the same principles. The results are evident from Fig. 2.

The deficit in the two-way active avoidance task was accompanied by poor escape behavior during the first trial and persistent long avoidance latencies. In the intertrial intervals there was less "freezing" than in the normal rat. In the open field the rats with amygdala lesions showed less immobility than normal rats. Passive avoidance was also defective. A general deficit in fear, therefore, is a sufficient explanation for all the behavioral differences observed. This is confirmed by the analysis of the plasma corticosteroids. Corticosterone did not rise as high in animals with amygdala lesions as in the normals during their first active-avoidance session.

The findings did not support a general decline in pituitary–adrenal responses or a general decline in arousal. After stabilization of the avoidance response the amygdala lesioned rats exhibited as much arousal or more arousal than normals according to the measurement of plasma corticosterone. Also, there was no effect of these lesions on the basal corticosterone levels. This is in agreement with previous findings in rats. The stress response is present, but it is delayed in its peak time (Knigge, 1961). According to the present data this delay may be due to the psychological factors of the stressors used rather than any primary change in the endocrinological system. Lesions affecting the medial structures of the amygdala complex produce a rise in basal corticosteroids in deer mice (Eleftheriou *et al.*, 1966), but our lesions did not affect the medial nucleus. Amygdala stimulation produces a rapid corticosteroid secretion in a variety of species (Matheson *et al.*, 1971). Comparison with behavioral data resulting from such stimulation suggests that the increases may be secondary to emotional responses (Setekleiv *et al.*, 1961).

(3) Corticosterone levels during avoidance learning in rats with lesions in the cingulate cortex

Coover *et al.* (1974) have also studied plasma corticosterone levels in rats with cingulate lesions. Lesions in the cingulate cortex have produced deficits in two-way active avoidance (Kaada, 1960; McCleary, 1966; Thomas *et al.*, 1968). However, in the 19 rats with bilateral electrolytic lesions in this area we studied, there was no deficit in the two-way active avoidance learning. The learning curve was indistinguishable from that of the control group. There was no change in the basal plasma corticosterone levels or the ether stress values. However, after attaining 90% performance levels, the lesioned rats did not exhibit the diminished pituitary–adrenal response to the avoidance situation to the same degree as the operated controls (Fig. 3). Also, there was not the normal degree of decrease in "freezing" behavior in the intertrial period. The behavioral and the endocrine indications of less fear reduction in rats with this lesion suggest that there is a disruption of the mechanism of reinforcement for instrumental responses. While the amygdala lesions seem to affect the first factor in two-factor theory, the cingulate lesions may disrupt the second process of instrumental learning.

The disruption of the mechanism of reinforcement of instrumental responses, if

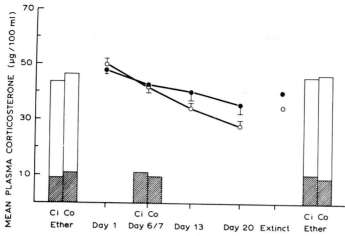

Fig. 3. Mean plasma corticosterone values for 12 rats with cingulate lesions (filled circles) compared with 15 controls (open circles). The learning curve was identical for the lesioned and the control group. Shaded bars indicate basal levels; open bars, ether-stress samples. Standard error of the mean is indicated for mean values by a vertical bar.

severe enough, should cause poor two-way avoidance learning. This has been the finding of many previous cingulate lesion studies using rats (Thomas and Slotnick, 1962; Kimble and Gostnell, 1968). It is possible that our lesions are not deep enough or do not affect the whole responsive area.

An alternative explanation is that the endocrine response to the first session was limited by a ceiling effect, thus masking an increment in fear response, arousal, or the endocrine response. However, the plasma corticosterone levels following session 6/7 were not maximal and there was no difference between groups on that day. In addition, if the animals with cingulate lesions had equally reduced their fear through instrumental responding, from an initial higher level, an increase in hormone response to the extinction session would be expected. The only alteration in hormone level found in the present study was secondary to a defect in fear reduction via instrumental responding. It should be stressed that our hypothesis does not propose any direct effect of cingulate damage on unconditioned responses to pain or in conditioning of fear, or in the direct control of the endocrine system.

There is also evidence of disruption by cingulate damage of reinforcement mechanisms in appetitive situations. Glass et al. (1969) found that rats with large medial cortical lesions failed to run slower following non-reinforced trials in a runway. This suggests a disruption of the behavioral effects of non-reinforcement. This may be a frontal cortex phenomenon, since the frontal cortex in the rat is located on the medial surface (see Divac, 1971).

(4) Plasma corticosterone levels during active avoidance learning in rats with septal lesions

In a still unpublished study, DeRyck, Köhler, Levine and Ursin have studied the

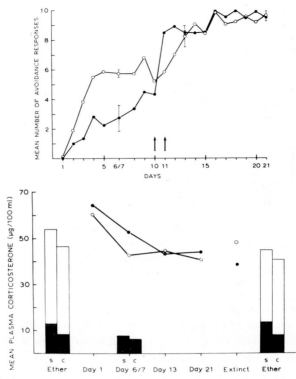

Fig. 4. Top diagram: mean learning curve for ± 10 rats with septal lesions (filled circles) compared with the learning curve for 9 controls (open circles). Lower diagram: mean plasma corticosterone values during avoidance learning in the same rats. Black bars indicate basal levels; open bars, ether-stress samples. Standard error of the mean is indicated for mean values by a vertical bar. The septals performed poorly as compared with controls in the first part of the experiment when a hinged door was placed between the two compartments. The arrow indicates shaping and removal of the door.

changes in plasma corticosterone levels during active avoidance learning in two groups of rats with septal lesions. In the first experiment subtotal bilateral septal lesions were produced electrolytically in 10 rats and 9 rats were sham operated. In the second experiment, 9 rats were operated in the septum; 7 were sham operated.

Previous reports have suggested a change in pituitary–adrenal activity following septal lesions (Usher *et al.*, 1967; Endröczi and Nyakas, 1971). We found no systematic change in basal levels or in ether stress samples. There was a tendency toward higher values for septal groups, this reached significance only for one of the basal samples. We tend to disregard this as due to chance. In another experiment, Sagvolden, Levine and Ursin studied basal values in 27 septals and 32 controls. The mean values were 9.11 and 9.13 (μg/100 ml), respectively. Also in the ether stress samples there were no significant differences, as the means were 49.8 and 50.9, respectively. The septals, however, did not behave identically to the normals in either of the two experiments, and, accordingly, the plasma corticosterone levels after avoidance sessions differ.

In the first experiment, the two compartments of the two way active avoidance box

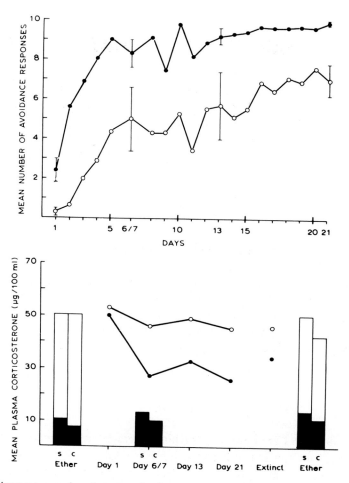

Fig. 5. Top diagram: mean learning curve for 9 rats with septal lesions (filled circles) compared with the learning curve for 7 controls (open circles). Lower diagram: mean plasma corticosterone values during avoidance learning in the same rats. In this experiment there was no door between the two compartments, and the septal lesioned rats showed superior performance compared with controls.

were separated by a hinged Plexiglass door. In the second experiment this door was removed. The situation with the hinged door turned out to be a more difficult situation for the septal lesioned rats than for the normals. There was no difference in the corticosterone levels after the first session, indicating that the effects of the shocks, the novelty of the situation and other factors on day 1 were similar for both groups. They differed in their ability to solve the problem. On day 6 the normal group avoided more than the septal lesioned rats. The door was removed, and both groups now learned the problem quickly. In this case, there was no significant difference between normal and septal lesioned rats in their steroid levels.

When there was no door between the two compartments, the septal lesioned rats showed the improved performance that has been described in this situation by many authors (King, 1958; Lubar and Numan, 1973). The corticosterone levels again followed the performance of the rats. There was a fast and significant drop in corticosterone for the septal group, in accordance with their superior performance as compared with their controls.

In these two experiments we observed even more clearly than in the previous experiments that it is the performance of the rats that is the decisive factor affecting the corticosteroid level. When the situation favors problem solving by septal lesioned rats, they learn fast and drop fast in plasma corticosteroids. When the odds are against this particular type of problem-solving, they learn more slowly and do not show the fast drop in plasma corticosteroids.

CONCLUSION

The main point in this paper is that in rats with limbic lesions the corticosterone levels change in accordance with changes in motivation, reinforcement effect, or problem-solving ability. Without measuring a reliable indicator of the internal state of the rat, it is difficult to decide which psychological mechanisms are involved. For all the groups we have studied the corticosterone response does not depend in any simple "physical" way on the external situation such as shock levels. A very important factor is how the rat behaves, or, more accurately, how the rat perceives and solves the problem.

SUMMARY

Many limbic structures are necessary for normal emotional behavior and avoidance learning. Several anatomical and psychological mechanisms are involved. Plasma corticosterone levels following an avoidance session may differentiate between avoidance deficits. Basolateral amygdala lesions in rats reduced two-way active avoidance learning. There were behavioral indications of less "fear", and the plasma corticosterone levels were lower than in normals following the first day of avoidance training. Basal levels and post-ether-stress levels were not changed. Rats with small lesions in the cingulate cortex showed normal avoidance learning but not the normal decrement in plasma corticosterone observed in intact rats when an avoidance habit is overtrained. It is possible that the avoidance deficit observed in rats with large cingulate lesions is due to a loss of the "fear"-reducing effect of adequate behavior. Rats with septal lesions also showed no change in basal levels, post-ether-stress levels or post-session levels of corticosterone on day 1. Later post-session samples depended on performance.

ACKNOWLEDGEMENTS

The experiments reported in this review were supported in part by Research Grant

NICHHD-02881 from the National Institutes of Health, Grant NGL-05-020-326 from the National Aeronautics and Space Administration, Foundations' Fund for Research in Psychiatry, ONR Contract N 00014-67-A-0112-0005 and the Norwegian Research Council for Science and the Humanities.

REFERENCES

COOVER, G. D., GOLDMAN, L. AND LEVINE, S. (1971) Plasma corticosterone increases produced by extinction of operant behavior in rats. *Physiol. Behav.*, **6**, 261–263.

COOVER, G. D., URSIN, H. AND LEVINE, S. (1973a) Plasma-corticosterone levels during active-avoidance learning in rats. *J. comp. physiol. Psychol.*, **82**, 170–174.

COOVER, G. D., URSIN, H. AND LEVINE, S. (1973b) Corticosterone and avoidance in rats with baso-lateral amygdala lesions. *J. comp. physiol. Psychol.*, **85**, 111–122.

COOVER, G. D., URSIN, H. AND LEVINE, S. (1974) Corticosterone levels during avoidance learning in rats with cingulate lesions suggest an instrumental reinforcement deficit. *J. comp. physiol. Psychol.*, **87**, 970–977.

DAVIDSON, J. M., JONES, L. E. AND LEVINE, S. (1968) Feedback regulation of adrenocorticotropin secretion in "basal" and "stress" conditions: Acute and chronic effects of intrahypothalamic corticoid implantation. *Endocrinology*, **82**, 655–663.

DIVAC, I. (1971) Frontal lobe system and spatial reversal in the rat. *Neuropsychologia (Berl.)*, **9**, 175–183.

ELEFTHERIOU, B. E., ZOLOVICK, A. J. AND PEARSE, R. (1966) Effect of amygdaloid lesions on pituitary–adrenal axis in the deermouse. *Proc. Soc. exp. Biol. (N.Y.)*, **122**, 1259–1262.

ENDRÖCZI, E. AND NYAKAS, C. (1971) Effect of septal lesion on exploratory activity, passive avoidance learning and pituitary–adrenal function in the rat. *Acta physiol. Acad. Sci. hung.*, **39**, 351–360.

GLASS, D. H., ISON, J. R. AND THOMAS, G. J. (1969) Anterior limbic cortex and partial reinforcement effects on acquisition and extinction of a runway response in rats. *J. comp. physiol. Psychol.*, **69**, 17–24.

GLICK, D., VON REDLICH, D. AND LEVINE, S. (1964) Fluorometric determination of corticosterone and cortisol in 0.02–0.05 milliliters of plasma or submilligram samples of adrenal tissue. *Endocrinology*, **74**, 653–655.

GOLDMAN, L., COOVER, G. D. AND LEVINE, S. (1973) Bidirectional effects of reinforcement shifts on pituitary–adrenal activity. *Physiol. Behav.*, **10**, 209–214.

KAADA, B. R. (1960) Cingulate, posterior orbital, anterior insular and temporal polar cortex. In *Handbook of Physiology, Vol. 2*, J. FIELD, H. W. MAGOUN AND V. E. HALL (Eds.), Amer. Physiol. Soc., Washington, D.C., pp. 1345–1372.

KIMBLE, D. P. AND GOSTNELL, D. (1968) Role of cingulate cortex in shock avoidance behavior of rats. *J. comp. physiol. Psychol.*, **65**, 290–294.

KING, F. A. (1958) Effects of septal and amygdaloid lesions on emotional behavior and conditioned avoidance responses in the rat. *J. nerv. ment. Dis.*, **126**, 57–63.

KNIGGE, K. (1961) Adrenocortical response to stress in rats with lesions in hippocampus and amygdala. *Proc. Soc. exp. Biol. (N.Y.)*, **108**, 18–21.

LUBAR, J. F. AND NUMAN, R. (1973) Behavioral and physiological studies of septal function and related medial cortical structures. *Behav. Biol.*, **8**, 1–25.

MAIER, S. F., SELIGMAN, M. E. P. AND SOLOMON, R. L. (1969) Pavlovian fear conditioning and learned helplessness: Effects on escape and avoidance behavior of (a) the CS–US contingency and (b) the independence of the US and voluntary responding. In *Punishment and Aversive Behavior*, B. A. CAMPBELL AND R. M. CHURCH (Eds.), Appleton-Century-Crofts, New York, N.Y., pp. 299–342.

MATHESON, G., BRANCH, B. AND TAYLOR, A. (1971) Effects of amygdaloid stimulation on pituitary–adrenal activity in conscious cats. *Brain Res.*, **32**, 151–168.

McCLEARY, R. A. (1966) Response-modulating functions of the limbic system: initiation and suppression. In *Progress in Physiological Psychology*, E. STELLAR AND J. M. SPRAGUE (Eds.), Academic Press, New York, N.Y., pp. 209–272.

RESCORLA, R. A. AND SOLOMON, R. L. (1967) Two-process learning theory: relationships between Pavlovian conditioning and instrumental learning. *Psychol. Rev.*, **74**, 151–182.

SELIGMAN, M. AND MEYER, B. (1970) Chronic fear and ulcers in rats as a function of the unpredictability of safety. *J. comp. physiol. Psychol.*, **73**, 202–207.

SETEKLEIV, J., SKAUG, O. E. AND KAADA, B. R. (1961) Increase of plasma 17-hydroxycorticosteroids by cerebral cortical and amygdaloid stimulation in the cat. *J. Endocr.*, **22**, 119–127.

SOLOMON, R. L. AND WYNNE, L. (1954) Traumatic avoidance learning: The principles of anxiety conservation and partial irreversibility. *Psychol. Rev.*, **61**, 353–385.

THOMAS, G. J. AND SLOTNICK, B. (1962) Effects of lesions in the cingulum on maze learning and avoidance conditioning in the rat. *J. comp. physiol. Psychol.*, **55**, 1085–1091.

THOMAS, G. J., HOSTETTER, G. AND BARKER, D. J. (1968) Behavioral functions of the limbic system. In *Progress in Physiological Psychology*, *Vol. 2*, E. STELLAR AND J. M. SPRAGUE (Eds.), Academic Press, New York, N.Y., pp. 229–311.

URSIN, H. (1972) Limbic control of emotional behavior. In *Psychosurgery*, E. HITCHCOCK, L. LAITINEN AND K. VAERNET (Eds.), Thomas, Springfield, Ill., pp. 34–45.

USHER, D. R., KASPER, P. AND BIRMINGHAM, M. K. (1967) Comparison of pituitary–adrenal function in rats lesioned in different areas of the limbic system and hypothalamus. *Neuroendocrinology*, **2**, 157–174.

WEISS, J. M. (1968) Effects of coping responses on stress. *J. comp. physiol. Psychol.*, **65**, 251–260.

DE WIED, D. (1974) Pituitary–adrenal system hormones and behavior. In *The Neurosciences*, F. O. SCHMITT AND F. G. WORDEN (Eds.), MIT Press, Cambridge, Mass., pp. 653–666.

Pituitary Peptides and Adaptive Autonomic Responses

BÉLA BOHUS

Rudolf Magnus Institute for Pharmacology, Medical Faculty, University of Utrecht, Vondellaan 6, Utrecht (The Netherlands)

INTRODUCTION

The organism's adaptation to the dynamically changing environment requires a chain of behavioral, autonomic, endocrine and metabolic responses in order to preserve homeostasis. The organization of this repertoire of adaptive responses is ensured by integrative central nervous mechanisms. However, hormonal systems also represent a special integrative role in adaptive processes. It is well recognized that stimuli which provoke changes in emotionality leading to fear, anxiety, disappointment, etc. are among the most potent of all stimuli affecting the release of pituitary–adrenal system or intermediate (MSH, melanocyte-stimulating hormone) or posterior pituitary hormones (vasopressin) (Mason, 1968; Levine *et al.*, 1972; Sandman *et al.*, 1973; Thompson and de Wied, 1973). However, abundant evidence is available suggesting that the release of these pituitary hormones is not only a concomitant of emotional behavior but, in turn, the brain may serve as a target organ of the peptide hormones. The central effects of these peptides then result in modification of adaptive behavior like avoidance, approach or even aggressive and sexual responses (de Wied, 1969; de Wied *et al.*, 1972a, 1974; Brain, 1972; Bohus, 1973, 1974a; Kastin *et al.*, 1973; Garrud *et al.*, 1974).

Although numerous aspects of the behavioral influence of these pituitary hormones have been investigated in detail, very little is known about the effects of these peptides on physiological responses related to emotion and behavioral adaptation. The relations of emotional behavior and cardiovascular system responses (Harris and Brady, 1974; Smith, 1974) suggest that the analysis of the cardiovascular effects of pituitary peptides in relation to emotional behavior may provide information about the role of these peptides in physiological adaptation. Furthermore, a psychophysiological approach may promote a better understanding of the psychological mechanisms involved in the behavioral action of pituitary peptide hormones.

The present paper describes experiments concerning the role of some pituitary peptides in cardiovascular adaptation. The influence of $ACTH_{4-10}$ (ACTH = corticotropin), lysine-8-vasopressin (LVP) and desglycinamide–lysine-8-vasopressin (DG–LVP) on heart rate during extinction of a classically conditioned emotional response and during retention of a passive avoidance response has been studied in the rat. $ACTH_{4-10}$ peptide is practically devoid of adrenocorticotropic activity but contains the behaviorally active sequence of the ACTH molecule (de Wied, 1969). DG–LVP was isolated from hog pituitaries and like LVP (Bohus *et al.*, 1973) is able to restore the deficient learning behavior of hypophysectomized rats (Lande *et al.*, 1973). The behavioral activity of DG–LVP is more or less of a similar magnitude while pressor, antidiuretic and oxytocic activities are about a hundred times less than that of synthetic LVP (de Wied *et al.*, 1972b). Although the behavioral effects of $ACTH_{4-10}$ and vasopressin-like peptides are seemingly very similar, the mechanisms through which they act are different. ACTH or ACTH-like peptides have a short-term effect on processes related to motivation while vasopressin-like peptides bear a long-term effect on behavior probably influencing memory processes (de Wied, 1969, 1971; Bohus *et al.*, 1973).

Pituitary peptides and heart rate changes during classical conditioning

A number of observations suggested that resistance to extinction of conditioned avoidance responses increases when ACTH or vasopressin-like peptides are administered during the extinction period in intact rats (de Wied, 1969). In order to investigate whether the influence of these peptides is only restricted to affect instrumental behavior or more generalized and involves physiological responses, extinction of a classically conditioned cardiac response was studied during the administration of $ACTH_{4-10}$ and LVP. Classical conditioning in the freely moving rat consisted of 3 acquisition and 3 extinction sessions with 12 trials each. A partial reinforcement schedule was applied during the acquisition period: 5 sec presentation of the conditioned stimulus (CS) was randomly followed by an unavoidable footshock (0.5 mA

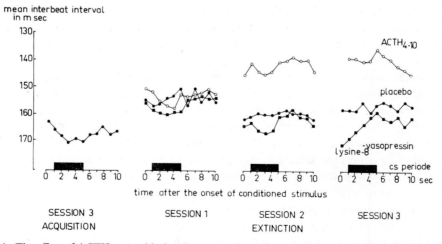

Fig. 1. The effect of ACTH4–10 and lysine-8-vasopressin on the extinction of a classically conditioned cardiac response in the rat. Heart rate is expressed as the mean interbeat interval in msec during the last acquisition and 3 subsequent extinction sessions. ACTH4–10 (20 µg/rat) and lysine-8-vasopressin (1 µg/rat) were administered 1 hr prior to each extinction session. "O" values represent mean interbeat intervals during a 5 sec period preceding the onset of the conditioned stimulus. 10-10 observations per point.

for 1 sec) as unconditioned stimulus. Non-reinforced trials were given during the extinction period. The electrocardiogram of the rats was recorded through wire leads from transcutaneous electrodes and the heart rate was determined by off-line measurement of interbeat intervals with the aid of a PDP 8/I computer. Changes in heart rate during the presentation of the CS indicated the development and retention of the conditioned cardiac response.

Classical conditioning in the free-moving rat results in development of a conditioned bradycardia as indicated by the increase in mean interbeat intervals during the CS presentation (Fig. 1). Heart rate returns to the pre-CS level within a few seconds when the CS is terminated in the non-reinforced trials. Extinction training results in a gradual disappearance of the conditioned cardiac response in the control rats. No significant changes were observed during the presentation of the CS when compared to the heart rate scored during the pre-CS period. Administration of $ACTH_{4-10}$ or LVP 1 hr before each extinction session, however, leads to a delay of extinction of the conditioned cardiac response. The form of the conditioned cardiac response, however, considerably alters as the extinction training progresses. The bradycardiac response which developed during the acquisition period is shifted into a tachycardiac response. Heart rate becomes accelerated after the onset of the CS especially during the third extinction session.

These observations clearly indicate that both $ACTH_{4-10}$ and LVP delay extinction of a classically conditioned cardiac response. Therefore, pituitary peptides do not only affect instrumental but also acquired autonomic responses. If one considers that the conditioned cardiac response is an autonomic correlate of classically conditioned fear, the present observations raise the question as to whether the behavioral effects of these peptides are mediated through an influence on classically conditioned fear. According to the two-factor theory advanced by Mowrer (1947) and more recently summarized by Rescorla and Solomon (1967) avoidance learning involves (a) classical conditioning of fear by CS–UCS pairings, and (b) instrumental conditioning established through reinforcement due to fear extinction. King and de Wied (1974), in fact, demonstrated that LVP can influence avoidance behavior through affecting classical fear conditioning. They observed that rats which received LVP prior to a classical fear conditioning which preceded instrumental conditioning displayed facilitated acquisition and resistance to extinction of a conditioned avoidance response without further peptide administration. However, they also noted that the instrumental response is a more effective substrate for mediating long-term effects of LVP on extinction behavior than the classically conditioned response. Unfortunately, similar observations with ACTH or ACTH-like peptides are lacking. Indirect evidence seems to suggest that it is unlikely that $ACTH_{4-10}$ affects avoidance behavior through classically conditioned fear. It was found that both LVP and $ACTH_{4-10}$ facilitated avoidance learning of hypophysectomized rats but cessation of treatment resulted in a deterioration of performance in $ACTH_{4-10}$ but not in LVP-treated rats (Bohus et al., 1973).

The form of the conditioned cardiac response appeared to be shifted from bradycardia to tachycardia during the extinction training in peptide-treated rats. Biphasic

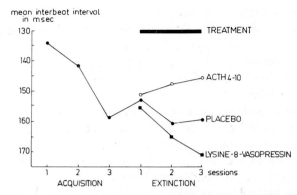

Fig. 2. Changes in generalized heart rate response of rats during acquisition and extinction of a classically conditioned cardiac response: effects of pituitary peptides administered during the extinction period. Each point represents the mean heart rate expressed in interbeat intervals and measured during 5 sec periods preceding the onset of the conditioned stimulus. 10-10 observations per point.

variation in the form of the conditioned cardiac response over successive trials of conditioning in the rat was reported by McDonald *et al.* (1963) and by Black and Black (1967). These authors observed that a decelerative response which appeared during the early trials shifted into an accelerative one during later trials. The fact that the shift in the form of the cardiac response in rats treated with pituitary peptides appeared in the absence of reinforcement suggests that both $ACTH_{4-10}$ and LVP preserve a state which resembles the continuation of the reinforcement. A similar effect may account for the resistance to extinction of conditioned instrumental responses as well.

The absolute heart rate of the classically conditioned rats appears to differ during the peptide treatments. As shown in Fig. 2, heart rate of the rats between the trials as indicated by the mean interbeat intervals of the 5 sec pre-CS periods progressively decreases during the acquisition period when a partial reinforcement schedule is used. Extinction training of this duration does not substantially affect the generalized bradycardia in the control rats. Heart rate of the rats treated with $ACTH_{4-10}$, however, substantially increases while further bradycardia is observed in LVP-treated rats. A number of observations suggests that a generalized bradycardia develops regularly if the presentation of the CS is only partially followed by an UCS during classical conditioning in the rat (Fitzgerald *et al.*, 1966; Caul and Miller, 1968). Accordingly, the present experiments suggest that pituitary peptides differentially affect the cardiac response accompanying conditioned emotionality change.

This finding raises the question as to whether the differential effect of LVP and $ACTH_{4-10}$ on heart rate is specifically coupled with the classical conditioning paradigm and, therefore, indicates different generalized emotional (arousal) state or the peptides influence heart rate without a specific relation to the learning paradigm. Control experiments indicate that pseudo-conditioning (unrelated presentation of CS and UCS), non-signaled presentation of the UCS in a random order or presentation of the CS without the UCS (sensitization training) produce specific heart rate changes, the administration of the peptides fails to affect these cardiac patterns. Heart rate of non-conditioned rats remains also unaffected by $ACTH_{4-10}$ or LVP given 1 hr prior to the observation. Accordingly, the influence of peptides on heart rate appeared to be specifically related to conditioning dependent generalized emotional responses. The tachycardia of $ACTH_{4-10}$-treated rats and bradycardia as observed in rats given LVP may, therefore, represent a different central activity state. If this were true, identical effects of the peptides on the cardiac response may develop through different central mechanisms. Based upon behavioral studies it has been suggested that ACTH and ACTH-like peptides affect behavior by increasing the motivational value of conditioned and unconditioned stimuli while vasopressin-like peptides influence memory processes (Bohus, 1973; de Wied et al., 1974). Accordingly, the generalized cardiac response as differentially affected by the peptides may indicate an increased conditioning-related arousal in $ACTH_{4-10}$-treated rats and a facilitated specific fear in animals given LVP. However, in the absence of stringent control of reinforcement variables and a quantitative measure of behavior in the classical conditioning situation this conclusion may be premature. Therefore, the influence of these peptides on autonomic adaptation was further analyzed by concurrent measurement of behavioral performance and the cardiac response in the rat.

Pituitary peptides and cardiac responses accompanying passive avoidance behavior

The relations between autonomic and behavioral responses have long provided a major source for studying emotional behavior. Cardiovascular changes, particularly heart rate alterations have been viewed as subjects of influences of psychological processes underlying behavior. Besides psychological factors such as motivation, attention, etc. somatic activity involved in a particular behavior as well as baroreceptor reflex regulation of the cardiovascular activity modulate autonomic responses during emotional behavior. Accordingly, a precise control of both autonomic and behavioral responses by concurrent measurements seemed to be an essential requirement in analyzing the observed peptide effects. Passive avoidance behavior of the rat in a step-through situation appeared to be determined by the intensity of the shock punishment and the retention interval (Ader et al., 1972). Heart rate changes accompanying passive avoidance were similarly affected by the same variables (Bohus, 1974b). Furthermore, both ACTH-like peptides and vasopressin and its analogs did improve passive avoidance behavior in this situation (Ader and de Wied, 1972; Bohus et al., 1972; Greven and de Wied, 1973). Accordingly, the influence of $ACTH_{4-10}$ and DG–LVP on heart rate changes accompanying passive avoidance behavior was studied in the rat. DG–LVP was used in these experiments in order to omit any direct circulatory effects (de Wied et al., 1972b).

The passive avoidance behavior was studied in a step-through situation as described by Ader et al. (1972). The rats were pretrained to enter a large dark compartment from a lit elevated platform. On the fourth of these trials, immediately after entering the dark, they received an inescapable footshock. The retention of the passive avoidance response was then studied 24 hr later, the electrocardiogram was recorded

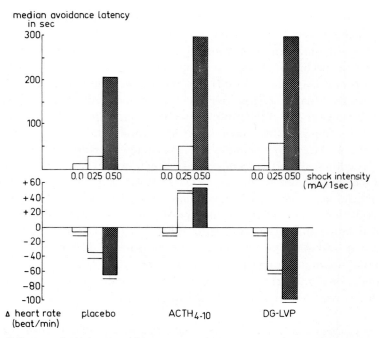

Fig. 3. The influence of pituitary peptides on passive avoidance behavior and heart rate changes accompanying passive avoidance in rats tested 24 hr after a single learning trial. ACTH$_{4-10}$ (15 μg/rat) and desglycinamide–lysine-8-vasopressin (DG–LVP, 0.5 μg/rat) were administered 60 min prior to the 24 hr retention test. $\triangle$ heart rate values represent the mean difference between the heart rate during the retention test and the pre-shock trials in the same rat. Shock intensity values indicate the punishment level of each learning trial. The columns represent the mean or median of 12-12 observations.

with the aid of telemetry and the heart rate was determined through off-line analysis by a PDP-8/I computer (Bohus, 1974b).

Fig. 3 summarizes passive avoidance behavior and heart rate changes of the rat treated with ACTH$_{4-10}$ or DG–LVP prior to the retention trial. One-trial learning results in a shock-intensity related increase in latency to reenter the shock compartment. Heart rate of rats during passive avoidance decreases when compared to heart rate scores during the pretraining. The rate of this bradycardiac response also depends upon the intensity of the shock. Administration of both ACTH$_{4-10}$ and DG–LVP results in a significant increase in avoidance latencies depending upon the shock intensity. Cardiac responses accompanying the facilitated avoidance behavior are, however, differentially affected. Heart rate of the rats treated with ACTH$_{4-10}$ appears to increase during passive avoidance when compared to the pre-shock trials. Unlike avoidance latency, this tachycardiac response does not depend on the shock intensity. On the other hand, a bradycardia accompanies passive avoidance in rats receiving DG–LVP. The rate of bradycardia is dependent on the shock intensity and, similarly to the behavior, facilitated by this peptide. The heart rate of non-shocked rats is not affected by these peptides.

These experiments demonstrate that the pituitary neuropeptides $ACTH_{4-10}$ and DG–LVP influence autonomic adaptive responses but in contrast to their identical effect on behavior, heart rate is differentially affected. Accordingly, the seemingly identical behavioral effect of these peptides is not reflected in their autonomic influence. It may be, therefore, that different brain functions are affected depending upon treatment with ACTH- or vasopressin-like peptides. Specific fear elicited by the punishment in the shock compartment is accompanied by bradycardia while tachycardia may be coupled with generalized arousal (Bohus, 1974b). Therefore, the present observations favor the hypothesis that vasopressin-like peptides affect specific fear responses while ACTH-like peptides facilitate arousal. In fact, it has been suggested that both specific response inhibition and suppressed approach tendency due to generalized emotional arousal may lead to passive avoidance behavior (Spevack and Suboski, 1969; Barcik, 1972). Thus, the heart rate response may differentiate between mechanisms responsible for the improved passive avoidance in peptide-treated rats.

GENERAL CONCLUSIONS

Pituitary neuropeptides related to ACTH or vasopressin profoundly influence adaptive behavior. Despite identical effects on behavior their influences on brain functions involve different mechanisms. Vasopressin-like peptides affect long-term memory functions while ACTH and ACTH analogs influence motivational processes but in a short-term manner (Bohus, 1973; de Wied *et al.*, 1972b, 1974). These peptides also profoundly influence adaptive autonomic processes. First of all, these two classes of peptides delay extinction of a classically conditioned cardiac response. The central role of classical conditioning processes in the adaptation of cardiovascular function to environmental and internal demands has always been accepted since Pavlov and Sherrington. Secondly, the peptides affect heart rate changes which accompany emotional behavior. An important feature of the cardiac effects of these peptides is their conditioning dependent specificity. Their influence of heart rate appears solely in situations where certain learning paradigms are involved as in classical conditioning or in passive avoidance behavior. These influences of ACTH- and vasopressin-like peptides on heart rate changes related to emotional behavior are, however, differential. The dichotomy between behavioral and autonomic effects may reflect their action on different mechanisms: arousal related to motivation *vs.* specific memory functions. This suggestion is in accordance with the formerly mentioned behavioral hypothesis and assumes a primary effect of peptides on psychological mechanisms controlling cardiovascular functions. The observation that both peptides suppress pressor responses elicited by hypothalamic or brain stem stimulation (Bohus, 1974c) seems to provide an alternative hypothesis: pituitary peptides may affect mechanisms related to the control of behavior and cardiovascular function concurrently but separately. Although the mechanism of action of the autonomic effects of these peptides is not clear, one might suggest that neuropeptides play a role in the physiological or pathophysiological regulation of cardiovascular responses related to environmental stress.

References p. 282–283

SUMMARY

The behaviorally active neuropeptides $ACTH_{4-10}$ and lysine-8-vasopressin significantly delay extinction of a classically conditioned cardiac response. However, the cardiovascular consequence of the generalized emotional response which typically develops during classical conditioning is differentially affected by these two peptides. $ACTH_{4-10}$ treatment leads to an increase in heart rate while bradycardia is observed in LVP-treated rats in the intertrial periods during the extinction training. The heart rate of non- or pseudo-conditioned rats is not affected by these peptides.

Administration of both $ACTH_{4-10}$ and desglycinamide–lysine-8-vasopressin facilitates passive avoidance behavior. The heart rate changes which accompany this behavior are, however, differentially affected by these two peptides. Bradycardia as seen in control rats is further facilitated by DG–LVP. Improved passive avoidance behavior after $ACTH_{4-10}$ administration is, however, associated with tachycardia. It is suggested that the differential heart rate response related to emotional behavior may reflect the effect of $ACTH_{4-10}$ on motivation processes while vasopressin-like peptides affect specific memory functions. However, a direct, differential influence on central cardiovascular control systems cannot be excluded.

ACKNOWLEDGEMENTS

The author is indebted to Drs. J. L. Slangen and J. M. van Ree for their help in the computer analysis of the heart rate data. A grant from the Dr. Saal van Zwanenberg-stichting provided the means for the basic instrumentation used in the present experiments.

REFERENCES

ADER, R. AND DE WIED, D. (1972) Effects of lysine vasopressin on passive avoidance learning. *Psychon. Sci.*, **29**, 46–48.

ADER, R., WEIJNEN, J. A. W. M. AND MOLEMAN, P. (1972) Retention of a passive avoidance response as a function of the intensity and duration of electric shock. *Psychon. Sci.*, **26**, 125–128.

BARCIK, J. D. (1972) Step-down passive avoidance: CER or specific avoidance? *Psychon. Sci.*, **27**, 27–28.

BLACK, R. W. AND BLACK, P. E. (1967) Heart rate conditioning as a function of interstimulus interval in rats. *Psychon. Sci.*, **8**, 219–220.

BOHUS, B. (1973) Pituitary–adrenal influences on avoidance and approach behavior of the rat. In *Drug Effects on Neuroendocrine Regulation, Progress in Brain Research, Vol. 39*, E. ZIMMERMANN, W. H. GISPEN, B. H. MARKS AND D. DE WIED (Eds.), Elsevier, Amsterdam, pp. 407–420.

BOHUS, B. (1974a) ACTH, ACTH-like peptides and the sexual behavior of the male rat. In *Rivista di Farmacologia e Terapia 5, vi P, First Int. Symp. on Pharmacology of Sexual Behavior, Forte Village, Sardinia.*

BOHUS, B. (1974b) Behavioral and methodological factors influencing heart rate of freely moving rats. In *Biotelemetry. II. Proc. 2nd Int. Symp. on Biotelemetry*, P. A. NEUKOMM (Ed.), Karger, Basel, pp. 185–187.

BOHUS, B. (1974c) The influence of pituitary peptides on brain centers controlling autonomic responses. In *Integrative Hypothalamic Activity, Progress in Brain Research, Vol. 41*, D. F. SWAAB AND J. P. SCHADÉ (Eds.), Elsevier, Amsterdam, pp. 175–183.

Bohus, B., Ader, R. and de Wied, D. (1972) Effects of vasopressin on active and passive avoidance behavior. *Horm. Behav.*, **3**, 191–197.

Bohus, B., Gispen, W. H. and de Wied, D. (1973) Effect of lysine vasopressin and ACTH$_{4-10}$ on conditioned avoidance behavior of hypophysectomized rats. *Neuroendocrinology*, **11**, 137–143.

Brain, P. F. (1972) Mammalian behavior and the adrenal cortex — a review. *Behav. Biol.*, **7**, 453–477.

Caul, W. F. and Miller, R. E. (1968) Effects of shock probability on heart rate of rats during classical conditioning. *Physiol. Behav.*, **3**, 865–869.

Fitzgerald, R. D., Vardaris, R. M. and Brown, J. S. (1966) Classical conditioning of heart rate deceleration in the rat with continuous and partial reinforcement. *Psychon. Sci.*, **6**, 437–438.

Garrud, P., Gray, J. A. and de Wied, D. (1974) Pituitary–adrenal hormones and extinction of rewarded behavior in the rat. *Physiol. Behav.*, **12**, 109–119.

Greven, H. M. and de Wied, D. (1973) The influence of peptides derived from corticotrophin (ACTH) on performance. Structure activity studies. In *Drug Effects on Neuroendocrine Regulation, Progress in Brain Research, Vol. 39*, E. Zimmermann, W. H. Gispen, B. H. Marks and D. de Wied (Eds.), Elsevier, Amsterdam, pp. 429–442.

Harris, A. H. and Brady, J. V. (1974) Animal learning-visceral and autonomic conditioning. *Ann. Rev. Psychol.*, **25**, 107–133.

Kastin, A. J., Miller, L. M., Nockton, R., Sandman, C. A., Schally, A. V. and Stratton, L. O. (1973) Behavioral aspects of melanocyte-stimulating hormone (MSH). In *Drug Effects on Neuroendocrine Regulation, Progress in Brain Research, Vol. 39*, E. Zimmermann, W. H. Gispen, B. H. Marks and D. de Wied (Eds.), Elsevier, Amsterdam, pp. 461–470.

King, A. R. and de Wied, D. (1974) Localized behavioral effects of vasopressin on maintenance of an active avoidance response in rats. *J. comp. physiol. Psychol.*, **86**, 1008–1018.

Lande, S., Witter, A. and de Wied, D. (1973) Pituitary peptides. An octapeptide that stimulates conditioned avoidance acquisition in hypophysectomized rats. *J. biol. Chem.*, **246**, 2058–2062.

Levine, S., Goldman, L. and Coover, G. D. (1972) Expectancy and the pituitary–adrenal system. In *Physiology, Emotion and Psychosomatic Illness, Ciba Foundation Symposium 8*, Elsevier/Excerpta Medica/North Holland, Amsterdam, pp. 281–296.

Mason, J. W. (1968) A review of psychoendocrine research on the pituitary–adrenal cortical system. *Psychosom. Med.*, **30**, 576–607.

McDonald, D. G., Stern, J. A. and Hahn, W. W. (1963) Classical heart rate conditioning in the rat. *J. psychosom. Res.*, **7**, 97–106.

Mowrer, O. H. (1947) On the dual nature of learning. A reinterpretation of conditioning and problem solving. *Harvard Educ. Rev.*, **17**, 102–148.

Rescorla, R. A. and Solomon, R. L. (1967) Two-process learning theory: relationships between Pavlovian conditioning and instrumental learning. *Psychol. Rev.*, **74**, 151–182.

Sandman, C. A., Kastin, A. J., Schally, A. V., Kendall, J. W. and Miller, L. H. (1973) Neuroendocrine responses to physical and psychological stress. *J. comp. physiol. Psychol.*, **84**, 386–390.

Smith, O. A. (1974) Reflex and central mechanisms involved in the control of the heart and circulation. *Ann. Rev. Physiol.*, **36**, 93–123.

Spevack, A. A. and Subovski, M. D. (1969) Retrograde effects of electroconvulsive shock on learned responses. *Psychol. Bull.*, **72**, 66–76.

Thompson, E. A. and de Wied, D. (1973) The relationship between the antidiuretic activity of rat eye plexus blood and passive avoidance behavior. *Physiol. Behav.*, **11**, 377–380.

de Wied, D. (1969) Effects of peptide hormones on behavior. In *Frontiers in Neuroendocrinology*, W. F. Ganong and L. Martini (Eds.), Oxford University Press, London, pp. 97–140.

de Wied, D. (1971) Long term effect of vasopressin on the maintenance of a conditioned avoidance response in rats. *Nature (Lond.)*, **232**, 58–60.

de Wied, D., van Delft, A. M. L., Gispen, W. H., Weijnen, J. A. W. M. and van Wimersma Greidanus, Tj. B. (1972a) The role of pituitary–adrenal system hormones in active avoidance conditioning. In *Hormones and Behavior*, S. Levine (Ed.), Academic Press, New York, N.Y., pp. 135–171.

de Wied, D., Greven, H. M., Lande, S. and Witter, A. (1972b) Dissociation of the behavioural and endocrine effects of lysine vasopressin by tryptic digestion. *Brit. J. Pharmacol.*, **45**, 118–122.

de Wied, D., Bohus, B. and van Wimersma Greidanus, Tj. B. (1974) The hypothalamo-neurohypophyseal system and the preservation of conditioned avoidance behavior in rats. In *Integrative Hypothalamic Activity, Progress in Brain Research, Vol. 41*, D. F. Swaab and J. P. Schadé (Eds.), Elsevier, Amsterdam, pp. 417–428.

Central Inhibitory Noradrenergic Cardiovascular Control*

WYBREN DE JONG, PIETER ZANDBERG AND BÉLA BOHUS

Rudolf Magnus Institute for Pharmacology, University of Utrecht, Medical Faculty, Vondellaan 6, Utrecht (The Netherlands)

The concept of physiological regulation of systemic arterial blood pressure already exists for a long time (Adolph, 1961; Cournand, 1964). Although some earlier experimental data indicating the importance of the brain in the control of blood pressure had been reported, it was the work of Bernard, Brown-Sequard and Schiff in the middle of the 19th century that laid the basis for further studies of central control mechanisms of blood pressure (see Heymans and Folkow, 1964). Over the past hundred years the study of cardiovascular function and its control received a great many contributions of a large number of brilliant students (for review: Alexander, 1946; Bard, 1960; Oberholzer, 1960; Uvnäs, 1960; Leake, 1962; Peiss, 1965; Wang and Chai, 1967; Korner, 1971; Koizumi and Brooks, 1972; Smith, 1974). The role of the brain in arterial hypertension, on the contrary, for many years received rather limited attention (Oberholzer, 1960; Tyler and Dawson, 1961; Page and McCubbin, 1962; Pickering, 1964; Katsuki, 1966). However, the recent rapid development of the knowledge of brain neurotransmission and the fact that some of the newer hypotensive drugs may act via a central mechanism (van Zwieten, 1973) greatly stimulated interest in this field. High density of the neurotransmitters noradrenaline and serotonin (Dahlström and Fuxe, 1964; Fuxe, 1965; Andén *et al.*, 1969) and probably adrenaline (Hökfelt *et al.*, 1973; Saavedra *et al.*, 1974) was observed in some areas crucial for central cardiovascular control. The involvement of brain monoamines in hypertension has been suggested. Based mainly on findings in a strain of genetic hypertensive rats, Sjoerdsma and his coworkers postulated that a deficiency of noradrenaline in certain parts of the brain may lead to hypertension (Yamori *et al.*, 1970). In addition, a number of observations suggests that α-methyldopa (α-methyl 3,4,dihydroxyphenylalanine) (Henning and van Zwieten, 1968; Henning, 1969; Henning and Rubenson, 1971; Heise and Kroneberg, 1972; Yamori *et al.*, 1972a; Day *et al.*, 1973), clonidine (Kobinger, 1967; Schmitt *et al.*, 1967; Sattler and van Zwieten, 1967; Constantine and McShane, 1968; Sherman *et al.*, 1968; Andén *et al.*, 1970; Sinha *et al.*, 1973; Schmitt *et al.*, 1973a) and related compounds (Hoyer and van Zwieten, 1972; van Zwieten, 1973; Schmitt *et al.*, 1973a) exert their hypotensive action via a

---

* Part of this work was done by the first author in collaboration with Drs. A. Sjoerdsma, W. Lovenberg and H. Yamabe in the Experimental Therapeutics Branch, National Heart and Lung Institute, National Institute of Health, Bethesda, Md., U.S.A.

References p. 295–298

central effect. Because the central hypotensive effects could be blocked by α-adrenoreceptor blocking agents (Schmitt and Schmitt, 1970; Bolme and Fuxe, 1971; Schmitt
et al., 1971; Heise and Kroneberg, 1972; Finch and Haeusler, 1973) it was suggested
that stimulation of central α-receptors is the mechanism of action of these hypotensive drugs (Henning and Rubenson, 1971; Schmitt *et al.*, 1971; Haeusler, 1973;
Sinha *et al.*, 1973; van Zwieten, 1973; Schmitt *et al.*, 1973a). These data in addition
to the central hypotensive action observed in patients receiving L-DOPA treatment
(Calne *et al.*, 1970; Watanabe *et al.*, 1970) favor the existence of a central inhibitory
noradrenergic control of blood pressure.

The hypotensive effect of L-DOPA has also been shown in rats, dogs and cats
(Henning and Rubenson, 1970a, b; Watanabe *et al.*, 1971; Yamori *et al.*, 1972a;
Schmitt *et al.*, 1972, 1973b). Inhibition of extracerebral decarboxylase activity to
prevent the peripheral effects of dopamine and noradrenaline, which generate from
L-DOPA, is required for the expression of the hypotensive effect of L-DOPA in the
rat. Chronic treatment with L-DOPA and a peripheral decarboxylase inhibitor decreased systolic blood pressure of genetic hypertensive rats while it increased brain
stem noradrenaline level (Yamori *et al.*, 1972a). Similar results were obtained after
acute oral administration of L-DOPA and the peripheral decarboxylase inhibitor
L-α-methyldopa hydrazine (MK-486) in genetic hypertensive rats. Systolic blood
pressure of unanesthetized rats was measured with a tail plethysmographic method.
Noradrenaline was assayed according to de Champlain *et al.* (1967). The decrease
in blood pressure was again associated with an increase in brain stem noradrenaline
(Fig. 1). Regimens of L-DOPA and MK-486 that did not increase brain stem noradrenaline level failed to change blood pressure significantly. A relationship between

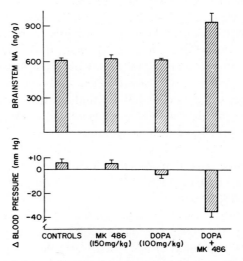

Fig. 1. Effect of single oral doses of L-DOPA and MK-486, alone and in combination, on systolic
blood pressure and brain stem noradrenaline (NA) levels of spontaneously hypertensive rats. Eight-
week-old male rats with systolic blood pressures averaging about 180 mm Hg were divided into
groups of 7. L-DOPA and MK-486 were administered by stomach tube in 5 ml water. Values shown
represent means ± S.E.M. of measurements made 4 hr after treatment.

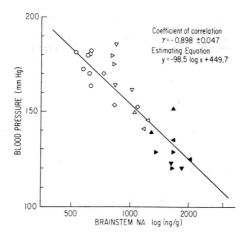

Fig. 2. Correlation between systolic blood pressure and brain stem noradrenaline (NA) level in adult male spontaneously hypertensive rats treated with L-DOPA, MK-485 and a monoamine oxidase inhibitor. The circles represent data of untreated controls (from Yamori *et al.*, 1972a).

brain stem noradrenaline level and blood pressure was also found after chronic administration of L-DOPA, MK-485 (D,L-α-methyldopa hydrazine) and a mono-amine oxidase inhibitor (Yamori *et al.*, 1972a). As shown in Fig. 2, blood pressure values over a considerable range were related to brain stem noradrenaline level. These data suggest that the increase in the noradrenaline level in the brain stem may be causally related to the decrease of blood pressure after L-DOPA administration.

A number of experiments was performed to investigate whether low levels of brain noradrenaline would lead to opposite effects. That is to say, whether a reduction of brain noradrenaline would be followed by an elevation of blood pressure. We failed to demonstrate the development of hypertension under these conditions (Table I).

TABLE I

EFFECT OF INTRAVENTRICULAR ADMINISTRATION OF 200 μg 6-HYDROXYDOPAMINE (6-OHDA) ON SYSTOLIC BLOOD PRESSURE AND BRAIN STEM NORADRENALINE (NA)

Figures in parentheses indicate number of animals. Data in part from Yamori *et al.*, 1972b.

		Blood pressure (mm Hg)	Brain stem NA (ng/g)	
Neonate Wistar rats	Vehicle	131 ± 3*	669 ± 24	(9)
	6-OHDA	125 ± 3	354 ± 64	(7)
Adult Wistar rats	Vehicle	125 ± 3	837 ± 14	(6)
	6-OHDA	129 ± 2	352 ± 75	(5)
Adult spontaneously	Vehicle	183 ± 7	595 ± 24	(4)
hypertensive rats	6-OHDA	185 ± 2	222 ± 27	(4)

* Mean ± S.E.M.

Brain noradrenaline depletion was induced by intraventricular administration of 6-hydroxydopamine. In the first group of animals this treatment was given on days 1 and 2 after birth. Data from these male rats were obtained at an age of 3 months. Despite considerable reduction in brain stem noradrenaline level blood pressure did not change. A similar conclusion was reached for the same treatment in adult female normotensive rats and genetic hypertensive rats. Blood pressure of these groups of rats was followed for 20 days after the treatment. These results do not support the hypothesis that low levels of noradrenaline in the brain are associated with an increase of blood pressure. However, noradrenaline depletion was not complete and super-sensitivity to noradrenaline may have developed (Palmer, 1972; Schoenfeld and Uretsky, 1973; Schoenfeld and Zigmond, 1973). One should also realize, that the intraventricular administration of 6-hydroxydopamine is not specific for brain stem noradrenaline depletion, but depletes noradrenaline in other brain areas and in the spinal cord as well.

It is possible, therefore, that the presence of noradrenaline at other sites in the central nervous system is essential in this respect. For example, administration of 6-hydroxydopamine (600 μg/kg) intracisternally was found to decrease blood pressure of neurogenic hypertensive rabbits (Chalmers and Reid, 1972). Haeusler *et al.* (1972) reported that intraventricular 6-hydroxydopamine (3 $\times$ 250 μg) in rats prevented the development of desoxycorticosterone–NaCl hypertension and of renal hyper-tension. Interestingly, the hypotensive action of noradrenaline following intra-ventricular administration is reversed into a hypertensive response when administered to reserpinized cats (Gagnon and Melville, 1968). Intraventricular clonidine in dogs decreased blood pressure and this effect was also reversed into a large hypertensive response when passage through the cerebral aqueduct was blocked so that the clonidine could not reach the medullary structures (Bousquet and Guertzenstein, 1973). Data from the literature on the influence of noradrenaline and other putative transmitters on central blood pressure regulation are summarized in Table II (Toivola and Gale, 1970; Struyker Boudier and Van Rossum, 1972; Philippu *et al.* 1973; Neumayr *et al.*, 1974). Inhibitory effects of serotonin in the medulla oblongata (Ito and Schanberg, 1972; Yamori *et al.*, 1972a) and the spinal cord have been implicated (Hare *et al.*, 1972; Neumayr *et al.*, 1974). Cholinergic mechanisms in the whole brain stem may contribute to blood pressure elevation (Varagić, 1955), although inhibitory

TABLE II

PUTATIVE ROLES OF NORADRENALINE (NA), 5-HYDROXYTRYPTAMINE (5-HT) AND ACETYLCHOLINE IN BLOOD PRESSURE CONTROL AT DIFFERENT CENTRAL SITES

↑, increase of blood pressure. ↓, decrease of blood pressure. — —, no data available.

	NA	5-HT	Acetylcholine
Hypothalamus	↑↓	— —	↑↓
Brain stem	↓↓	↓	↑
Spinal cord	↑	↓	— —

effects of hypothalamic application of carbachol have also been found (Brezenoff, 1972).

At present we do not know precisely which brain structures are involved in the mediation of the hypotensive effects of noradrenaline. However, on the basis of elegant animal studies it was suggested (Sattler and van Zwieten, 1967; Henning and van Zwieten, 1968; Schmitt and Schmitt, 1969; Henning *et al.*, 1972; Schmitt *et al.*, 1973a; van Zwieten, 1973), that in particular the lower brain stem is involved. The important role of the medulla oblongata in cardiovascular control is well known from early studies employing brain stem transections or electrical stimulation (Dittmar, 1870, 1873; Owsjannikow, 1871; Alexander, 1946; Bard, 1960; Oberholzer, 1960; Fallert and Bucher, 1966; Schmitt *et al.*, 1973a). It was shown that in a large region in the medulla electrical stimulation resulted in a pressor response and in a smaller region in a depressor response. In the cat the larger pressor region occupies mainly

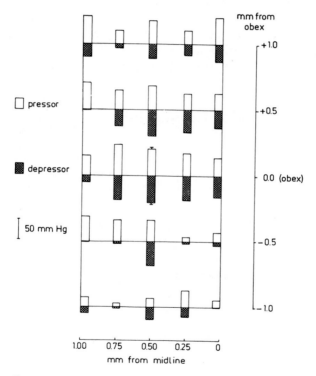

Fig. 3. Magnitude of pressor and depressor responses evoked by unilateral electrical stimulation of 25 different locations in the medulla oblongata of urethanized rats. Data shown are means of the maximal responses of mean blood pressure observed in each location. A bipolar stainless steel electrode with a diameter of 0.2 mm, insulated except at the tip, was used. The distance between the two electrode tips was maximally 0.1 mm. A current intensity of 130–200 μA (4–6 V) was employed. Stimulation was delivered during 5 sec with a pulse duration of 1 msec. In each location the electrode was lowered to a depth of 2.0–2.5 mm below the dorsal surface and responses were subsequently evoked in localizations at 0.3 mm distance in depth. Bars depict results from 3–6 rats, except for the localization 0.5 mm lateral of the obex where means ± S.E.M. of 18 animals are shown. Adult male rats were used. The location of the electrode tracks was verified histologically.

lateral and rostral parts of the reticular formation of the medulla. The smaller depressor area occupies more mediocaudal structures in the medulla oblongata (Alexander, 1946). The same kind of results was obtained in several other mammalian species (Bard, 1960; Oberholzer, 1960; Calaresu and Pearce, 1965).

In the rat a similar localization of the depressor area has been reported (Scherrer, 1967a) although this author could differentiate between two well defined depressor regions. The largest area corresponds to the location of the nucleus tractus solitarii. We confirmed this in intact rats anesthetized with urethane. The same distribution of the depressor area was found which had its largest extension at the obex. A bipolar electrode was introduced stereotaxically and blood pressure and heart rate were monitored from an iliac cannula using a Statham transducer (P23 AC) and a Grass polygraph. The cannula had been implanted 20–24 hr before the experiment. The cardiovascular responses to stimulation in 25 different unilateral locations were determined at the obex and 0.5 mm and 1.0 mm rostral and caudal from the obex. Locations in each of these fronto-caudal levels were: in the midline, and 0.25 mm, 0.50 mm, 0.75 mm and 1.00 mm lateral from the midline (Fig. 3). A stimulation frequency of 50 Hz was generally used because both 10 Hz as well as 50 Hz evoke depressor responses but significant pressor responses were usually not obtained with

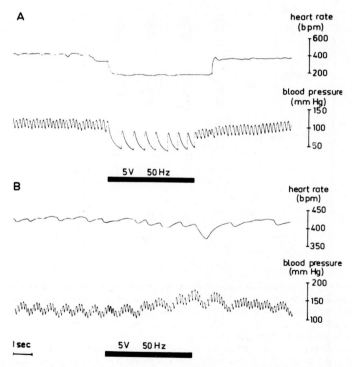

Fig. 4. Examples of a depressor response (A) and a pressor response (B). The electrode localization was 0.5 mm lateral of the obex at a depth of 0.5 mm (A) and 1.1 mm (B). For details see legend of Fig. 3.

a frequency of 10 Hz. An example of a depressor response is shown in Fig. 4A. Usually the depressor response was associated with a marked bradycardia. Depressor responses without heart rate changes were occasionally observed. Up to 1 mm rostral and caudal of the obex the depressor and bradycardia response could still be evoked but from a more restricted area (Fig. 3). The depressor responses with a few exceptions were found only in the most dorsal part, *i.e.* the upper 0.7 mm. Thus, it appears that in the rat in contrast to other species, the depressor area is restricted to a more superficial layer of the dorsal medulla. All areas immediately adjacent to the depressor area gave distinct pressor responses upon stimulation (Fig. 4B). The pressor responses varied between 20 and 90 mm Hg and occurred with a latency of approximately 0.8–1.4 sec. The depressor responses, which varied between 30 and 90 mm Hg had a shorter latency of 0.3–0.7 sec. Pressor responses generally occurred without major changes of heart rate. Bradycardia was often associated with the larger pressor responses while a moderate tachycardia (20–70 bpm) was observed frequently upon stimulation of the lower parts of the area explored.

The depressor area may exert an inhibition of sympathetic tone and of reflex activity and thereby decrease blood pressure. Transection experiments are in favor of such a possibility (Alexander, 1946). Later on, Fallert and Bucher (1966) reported a clear elevation of blood pressure in rabbits following a bilateral lesion in the depressor area. These lesions were located in the nucleus tractus solitarii. Doba and Reis (1973) showed that a similar lesion in the rat at the level of the obex resulted in a fulminating hypertension. These authors suggested that structures above the midbrain were essential for the development of this hypertension since it could be blocked by general anesthesia and by mid-collicular transection of the brain stem.

We also studied the cardiovascular effect of bilateral electrolytic brain stem lesions at the level of the obex in rats anesthetized with ether. The size of the lesions was approximately 1 mm. They destroyed the most dorsal region of the medulla including the nucleus and tractus solitarii. Immediately after completion of the operation the ether anesthesia was ended. Blood pressure in the conscious rats was recorded from a permanent indwelling iliac cannula. Lesioning this area was followed by an acute and severe hypertension. The heart rate showed only minor changes (Fig. 5). Data from 3 groups of 6 rats are summarized in Fig. 6. Mean blood pressure did not change in the sham-operated animals. In lesioned rats mean blood pressure rose from 115 to

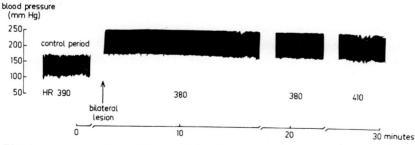

Fig. 5. Blood pressure recording and heart rate showing the effect of bilateral electrolytic lesion in the area of the nucleus tractus solitarii. For details see legend of Fig. 6.

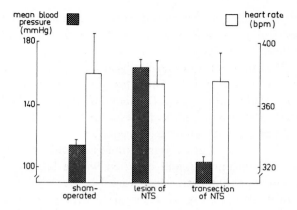

Fig. 6. Effect of bilateral electrolytic lesion and of bilateral transection of the area of the nucleus tractus solitarii (NTS) on mean blood pressure and heart rate. Data shown are means $\pm$ S.E.M. of 6 adult male rats. A stainless steel electrode (outer diameter 0.3 mm) with a bare tip of 0.2 mm was placed stereotaxically 0.5 mm lateral at a depth of 0.5 mm below the obex. Current was applied through a radionics lesion generator (13 V during 1 min). Location and size of the lesions was verified histologically.

164 mm Hg. Larger lesions were less effective or did not increase blood pressure. Lesions located more rostrally or more laterally also failed to elicit hypertension. In the third group of rats the nucleus and tractus solitarii were transected at the level of the obex. The transection failed to raise blood pressure or to change heart rate. Thus, a mere interruption of the tractus at this level is not sufficient to cause hypertension. Probably not enough fibers were transected and experiments in which the cut is placed more rostrally and/or laterally should be performed.

Taken together these data indicate that the area of the nucleus tractus solitarii at the obex is an important site for the central control of arterial blood pressure. It appears to exert a tonic inhibitory effect on sympathetic outflow. It is conceivable that damage to this area may result in hypertension. This region is also known to contain the first synapse of the afferent pathways from the carotid sinus baroreceptors (Oberholzer, 1955; Miura and Reis, 1969; Seller and Illert, 1969) and an increase or a decrease of the discharge rate of some neurons in this location were found to be related to cardiovascular changes (Salmoiraghi, 1962; Preobrazhenskii, 1966; Scherrer, 1967b; Koepchen *et al.*, 1967; Seller and Illert, 1969). Furthermore, a high noradrenaline content of this region has been reported (Vogt, 1954) while histochemical studies revealed that it contains dense noradrenergic terminals (Dahlström, 1964; Dahlström and Fuxe, 1964; Fuxe, 1965). Thus, one may infer from these data that the area of the nucleus tractus solitarii is an important site for the noradrenergic inhibitory control mechanism of blood pressure.

To substantiate this hypothesis we studied the effect of direct noradrenaline application in the area of the nucleus tractus solitarii. Bilateral microinjections of 1 μl of noradrenaline were given through a stereotaxically inserted cannula at 0.5 mm lateral to the obex. The rats were anesthetized with ether. The effect of a dose of 5 nmoles of noradrenaline is shown in Fig. 7. In this animal a rapid decrease in heart rate occurred

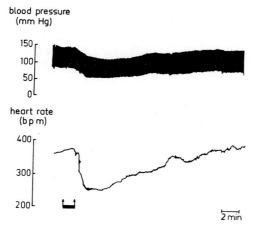

Fig. 7. Blood pressure and heart rate recording showing the effect of bilateral microinjection of 5.0 nmoles noradrenaline (at arrows) into the area of the nucleus tractus solitarii.

with a more gradual decline in blood pressure. In general, the maximal effect on both parameters was reached in 5 min. Both slowly returned to the initial control level within 30 min. No significant effect was observed after bilateral microinjections given 0.5 mm more lateral or 1.0 mm more rostral or caudal. The inhibitory cardiovascular action of noradrenaline microinjection at 0.5 mm lateral of the obex is dose related.

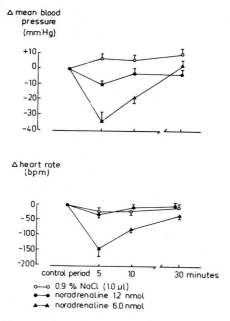

Fig. 8. Effect of bilateral microinjection of noradrenaline (1.2 or 6.0 nmoles) into the area of the nucleus tractus solitarii on mean blood pressure and heart rate. Data shown are means ± S.E.M. of 6 adult male rats. Cannula locations were verified histologically.

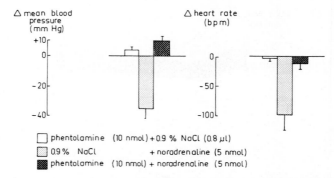

Fig. 9. Effect of bilateral microinjection of noradrenaline into the area of the nucleus tractus solitarii on mean blood pressure and heart rate after prior administration of phentolamine at the same site Data shown are means ± S.E.M. of 5–6 adult male rats.

The lowest dose of 1.2 nmoles caused a significant decrease of blood pressure without a clear bradycardia. The higher dose decreased both blood pressure and heart rate and the effect of this dose lasted longer (Fig. 8).

In order to determine whether α-receptor blockade could prevent the inhibitory effect of noradrenaline the α-blocking agent phentolamine was injected into the nucleus tractus solitarii followed 10 min later by a dose of 5.0 nmoles (0.8 μl) of noradrenaline at the same site. The dose of phentolamine was 10.0 nmoles. Phentolamine followed by 0.9% NaCl had no significant effect (Fig. 9). Saline followed by 5.0 nmoles noradrenaline resulted in a decrease of blood pressure and heart rate. In the last group the preceding injection of phentolamine completely blocked the effect of noradrenaline. The effect on blood pressure was reversed into an increase, amounting to 11 mm Hg (Fig. 9).

CONCLUSION

Our results lend further support to the existence of a central noradrenergic inhibitory control of blood pressure. They also point to a possible role of the area of the nucleus tractus solitarii at the obex in the control mechanism. The pronounced effect of minor quantities of noradrenaline and the blockade by phentolamine suggest a role of an α-adrenoreceptor. Tonic inhibition of the spinal cord sympathetic vasomotor outflow as well as interference with baroreceptor reflex control are likely to be involved.

SUMMARY

Experiments are presented which indicate that the central hypotensive effect of L-DOPA may be related to an increase of brain stem noradrenaline level. Depletion of brain noradrenaline in neonate or adult rats by intraventricular administration of 6-hydroxydopamine did not affect blood pressure. The region of the depressor area in the medulla oblongata in rats was explored for pressor and depressor responses using electrical stimulation. The largest extension of the depressor area was found to be in the region of the nucleus tractus solitarii at the obex. The important role of this region in blood pressure control was also indicated by ablation of this area by electrolytic lesions causing a severe hypertension without a significant change of heart rate. Microinjection of noradrenaline into this area caused a dose-related decrease of blood pressure and heart rate. The inhibitory cardiovascular action of centrally administered noradrenaline was blocked by prior administration of the α-adrenoreceptor blocking agent, phentolamine.

REFERENCES

ADOLPH, E. F. (1961) Early concepts of physiological regulations. *Physiol. Rev.*, **41**, 737–770.

ALEXANDER, R. S. (1946) Tonic and reflex functions of medullary sympathetic cardiovascular centers. *J. Neurophysiol.*, **9**, 205–217.

ANDÉN, N.-E., CARLSSON, A. AND HÄGGENDAL, J. (1969) Adrenergic mechanisms. *Ann. Rev. Pharmacol.*, **9**, 119–134.

ANDÉN, N.-E., CORRODI, H., FUXE, K., HÖKFELT, B., HÖKFELT, T., RYDIN, C. AND SVENSSON, T. (1970) Evidence for a central noradrenaline receptor stimulation by clonidine. *Life Sci.*, **9**, 513–523.

BARD, P. (1960) Anatomical organization of the central nervous system in relation to control of the heart and blood vessels. *Physiol. Rev.*, **40**, **Suppl. 4**, 3–26.

BOLME, P. AND FUXE, K. (1971) Pharmacological studies on the hypotensive effects of clonidine. *Europ. J. Pharmacol.*, **13**, 168–174.

BOUSQUET, P. AND GUERTZENSTEIN, P. G. (1973) Localization of the central cardiovascular action of clonidine. *Brit. J. Pharmacol.*, **49**, 573–579.

BREZENOFF, H. E. (1972) Cardiovascular responses to intrahypothalamic injections of carbachol and certain cholinesterase inhibitors. *Neuropharmacology*, **11**, 637–644.

CALARESU, F. R. AND PEARCE, J. W. (1965) Effects on heart rate of electrical stimulation of medullary vagal structures in the cat. *J. Physiol. (Lond.)*, **176**, 241–251.

CALNE, D. B., BRENNAN, J., SPIERS, A. S. D. AND STERN, G. M. (1970) Hypotension caused by L-DOPA. *Brit. med. J.*, **1**, 474–475.

CHALMERS, J. P. AND REID, J. L. (1972) Participation of central noradrenergic neurons in arterial baroreceptor reflexes in the rabbit. *Circulat. Res.*, **31**, 789–804.

CHAMPLAIN DE, J., KRAKOFF, L. R. AND AXELROD, J. (1967) Catecholamine metabolism in experimental hypertension in the rat. *Circulat. Res.*, **20**, 136–145.

CONSTANTINE, J. W. AND MCSHANE, W. K. (1968) Analysis of the cardiovascular effects of 2-(2,6-dichlorophenylamino)-2-imidazoline hydrochloride (Catapres®). *Europ. J. Pharmacol.*, **4**, 109–123.

COURNAND, E. (1964) Air and blood. In *Circulation of the Blood*, A. P. FISHMAN AND D. W. RICHARDS (Eds.), Oxford University Press, London, pp. 3–70.

DAHLSTRÖM, A. (1964) Evidence for the existence of monoamine-containing neurons in the central nervous system — I. Demonstration of monoamines in the cell bodies of brain stem neurons. *Acta physiol. scand.*, **62**, **Suppl. 232**, 1–55.

DAHLSTRÖM, A. AND FUXE, K. (1964) Evidence for the existence of monoamine neurons in the central nervous system. II. Experimentally induced changes in the intraneuronal amine levels of bulbo-spinal neuron systems. *Acta physiol. scand.*, **64**, **Suppl. 247**, 1–36.

DAY, M. D., ROACH, A. G. AND WHITING, R. L. (1973) The mechanism of the antihypertensive action of α-methyldopa in hypertensive rats. *Europ. J. Pharmacol.*, **21**, 271–280.

DITTMAR, C. (1870) Ein neuer Beweis für die Reizbarkeit der centripetalen Fasern des Rückenmarks. *Ber. Sächs. Ges. Wiss. Mat. Phys. Kl.*, **22**, 18–48.

DITTMAR, C. (1873) Ueber die Lage des sogenannten Gefässcentrums in der Medulla oblongata. *Ber. Sächs. Ges. Wiss. Mat. Phys. Kl.*, **25**, 449–469.

DOBA, N. AND REIS, D. J. (1973) Acute fulminating neurogenic hypertension produced by brainstem lesions in the rat. *Circulat. Res.*, **32**, 584–593.

FALLERT, M. UND BUCHER, V. M. (1966) Lokalisation eines blutdruckaktiven Substrats in der Medulla oblongata des Kaninchens. *Helv. physiol. Acta*, **24**, 139–163.

FINCH, L. AND HAEUSLER, G. (1973) Further evidence for a central hypotensive action of α-methyldopa in both the rat and cat. *Brit. J. Pharmacol.*, **47**, 217–228.

FUXE, K. (1965) Evidence for the existence of monoamine neurons in the central nervous system. IV. The distribution of monoamine terminals in the centra lnervous system. *Acta physiol. scand.*, **64, Suppl. 247**, 38–85.

GAGNON, D. J. AND MELVILLE, K. I. (1968) A possible dual role of noradrenaline in cardiovascular responses mediated by the central nervous system. *Canad. J. physiol. Pharmacol.*, **46**, 595–599.

HAEUSLER, G., FINCH, L. AND THOENEN, H. (1972) Central adrenergic neurones and the initiation and development of experimental hypertension. *Experientia (Basel)*, **28**, 1200–1203.

HAEUSLER, G. (1973) Activation of the central pathway of the baroreceptor reflex, a possible mechanism of the hypotensive action of clonidine. *Naunyn-Schmiedeberg's Arch. exp. Path. Pharmak.*, **278**, 231–246.

HARE, B. D., NEUMAYR, R. J. AND FRANZ, D. N. (1972) Opposite effects of L-DOPA and 5-HTP on spinal sympathetic reflexes. *Nature (Lond.)*, **239**, 336–337.

HEISE, A. AND KRONEBERG, G. (1972) α-Sympathetic receptor stimulation in the brain and hypotensive activity of α-methyldopa. *Europ. J. Pharmacol.*, **17**, 315–317.

HENNING, M. AND VAN ZWIETEN, P. A. (1968) Central hypotensive effect of α-methyldopa. *J. Pharm. Pharmacol.*, **20**, 409–417.

HENNING, M. (1969) Interaction of DOPA decarboxylase inhibitors with the effect of α-methyldopa on blood pressure and tissue monoamines in rats. *Acta pharmacol. (Kbh.)*, **27**, 135–148.

HENNING, M. AND RUBENSON, A. (1970a) Evidence for a centrally mediated hypotensive effect of L-DOPA in the rat. *J. Pharm. Pharmacol.*, **22**, 241–243.

HENNING, M. AND RUBENSON, A. (1970b) Central hypotensive effect of L-3,4-dihydroxyphenylalanine in the rat. *J. Pharm. Pharmacol.*, **22**, 553–560.

HENNING, M. AND RUBENSON, A. (1971) Evidence that the hypotensive action of methyldopa is mediated by central actions of methylnoradrenaline. *J. Pharm. Pharmacol.*, **23**, 407–411.

HENNING, M., RUBENSON, A. AND TROLIN, G. (1972) On the localization of the hypotensive effect of L-DOPA. *J. Pharm. Pharmacol.*, **24**, 447–451.

HEYMANS, C. J. F. AND FOLKOW, B. (1964) Vasomotor control and the regulation of blood pressure. In *Circulation of the Blood*, A. P. FISHMAN AND D. W. RICHARDS (Eds.), Oxford University Press, London, pp. 407–486.

HÖKFELT, T., FUXE, K., GOLDSTEIN, M. AND JOHANSSON, O. (1973) Evidence for adrenaline neurons in the rat brain. *Acta physiol. scand.*, **89**, 286–288.

HOYER, I. AND VAN ZWIETEN, P. A. (1972) The central hypotensive action of amphetamine, ephedrine, phentermine, chlorphentermine and fenfluramine. *J. Pharm. Pharmacol.*, **24**, 452–458.

ITO, A. AND SCHANBERG, S. M. (1972) Central nervous system mechanisms responsible for blood pressure elevation induced by p-chlorophenylalanine. *J. Pharmacol. exp. Ther.*, **181**, 65–74.

KATSUKI, S. (1966) Role of the brain stem in pathogenesis of hypertension. *Jap. Circulat. J. (Ni)*, **30**, 175–178.

KOBINGER, W. (1967) Über den Wirkungsmechanismus einer neuen antihypertensiven Substanz mit Imidazolinstruktur. *Naunyn Schmiedeberg's Arch. exp. Path. Pharmak.*, **258**, 48–58.

KOEPCHEN, H. P., LANGHORST, P., SELLER, H., POLSTER, J. UND WAGNER, P. H. (1967) Neuronale Aktivität im unteren Hirnstamm mit Beziehung zum Kreislauf. *Pflügers Arch. ges. Physiol.*, **294**, 40–64.

KOIZUMI, K. AND BROOKS, C. M. (1972) The integration of autonomic system reactions: A discussion of autonomic reflexes, their control and their association with somatic reactions. *Ergebn. Physiol.*, **67**, 1–68.

KORNER, P. I. (1971) Integrative neural cardiovascular control. *Physiol. Rev.*, **51**, 312–367.

LEAKE, C. D. (1962) The historical development of cardiovascular physiology. In *Handbook of Physiology, Section 2: Circulation, Vol. I*, W. F. HAMILTON AND P. DOW (Eds.), American Physiological Society, Washington, D.C., pp. 11–22.

MIURA, M. AND REIS, D. J. (1969) Termination and secondary projections of carotid sinus nerve in the cat brain stem. *Amer. J. Physiol.*, **217**, 142–153.

NEUMAYR, R. J., HARE, B. D. AND FRANZ, D. N. (1974) Evidence for bulbospinal control of sympathetic preganglionic neurons by monoaminergic pathways. *Life Sci.*, **14**, 793–806.

OBERHOLZER, R. J. H. (1955) Lokalisation einer Schaltstelle für den Depressor-reflex in der Medulla oblongata des Kaninchens. *Helv. physiol. pharmacol. Acta*, **13**, 331–353.

OBERHOLZER, R. J. H. (1960) Circulatory centers in medulla and midbrain. *Physiol. Rev.*, **40, Suppl. 4,** 179–195.

OWSJANNIKOW, P. (1871) Die tonischen und reflectorischen Centren der Gefässnerven. *Ber. Sächs. Ges. Wiss. Mat. Phys. Kl.*, **23**, 135–147.

PAGE, I. H. AND MCCUBBIN, J. W. (1962) The physiology of arterial hypertension. In *Handbook of Physiology, Section 2: Circulation, Vol. III*, W. F. HAMILTON AND P. DOW (Eds.), American Physiological Society, Washington, D.C., pp. 2163–2208.

PALMER, G. C. (1972) Increased cyclic AMP response to norepinephrine in the rat brain following 6-hydroxydopamine. *Neuropharmacology*, **11**, 145–149.

PEISS, C. N. (1965) Concept of cardiovascular regulation: past, present and future. In *Nervous Control of the Heart*, W. C. RANDALL (Ed.), Williams and Wilkins, Baltimore, Md., pp. 154–197.

PHILIPPU, A., ROENSBERG, W. AND PRZUNTEK, H. (1973) Effects of adrenergic drugs on pressor responses to hypothalamic stimulation. *Naunyn Schmiedeberg's Arch. exp. Path. Pharmak.*, **278**, 373–386.

PICKERING, G. (1964) Systemic arterial hypertension. In *Circulation of the Blood*, A. P. FISHMAN AND D. W. RICHARDS (Eds.), Oxford University Press, London, pp. 487–541.

PREOBRAZHENSKII, N. N. (1966) Microelectrode recording of activity from neurons in vasomotor center. *Fed. Proc.*, **25**, T18–T22.

SAAVEDRA, J. M., PALKOVITS, M., BROWNSTEIN, M. J. AND AXELROD, J. (1974) Localisation of phenylethanolamine N-methyl transferase in the rat brain nuclei. *Nature (Lond.)*, **248**, 695–696.

SALMOIRAGHI, G. C. (1962) "Cardiovascular" neurones in brain stem of cat. *J. Neurophysiol.*, **25**, 182–197.

SATTLER, R. W. AND VAN ZWIETEN, P. A. (1967) Acute hypotensive action of 2-(2,6-dichlorophenyl-amino)-2-imidazoline hydrochloride (St. 155) after infusion into the cat's vertebral artery. *Europ. J. Pharmacol.*, **2**, 9–13.

SCHERRER, H. (1967a) Inhibition of sympathetic discharge by stimulation of the medulla oblongata in the rat. *Acta neuroveg. (Wien)*, **29**, 56–74.

SCHERRER, H. (1967b) Responses of bulbar reticular units to hypothalamic stimulation in the rat. *Acta neuroveg. (Wien)*, **29**, 45–55.

SCHMITT, H., SCHMITT, H., BOISSIER, J. R. AND GIUDICELLI, J. F. (1967) Centrally mediated decrease in sympathetic tone induced by 2(2,6-dichlorophenylamino)-2-imidazoline (St. 155, Catapresan®). *Europ. J. Pharmacol.*, **2**, 147–148.

SCHMITT, H. AND SCHMITT, H. (1969) Localization of the hypotensive effect of 2-(2,6-dichlorophenyl-amino)-2-imidazoline hydrochloride (St. 155, Catapresan®). *Europ. J. Pharmacol.*, **6**, 8–12.

SCHMITT, H. AND SCHMITT, H. (1970) Interactions between 2-(2,6-dichlorophenylamino)-2-imidazoline hydrochloride (St. 155, Catapresan®) and α-adrenergic blocking drugs. *Europ. J. Pharmacol.*, **9**, 7–13.

SCHMITT, H., SCHMITT, H. AND FENARD, S. (1971) Evidence for an α-sympathomimetic component in the effects of catapresan on vasomotor centres: antagonism by piperoxane. *Europ. J. Pharmacol.*, **14**, 98–100.

SCHMITT, H., SCHMITT, H. AND FENARD, S. (1972) New evidence for an α-adrenergic component in the sympathetic centres. Centrally mediated decrease in sympathetic tone by L-DOPA and its antagonism by piperoxane and yohimbine. *Europ. J. Pharmacol.*, **17**, 293–296.

SCHMITT, H., SCHMITT, H., FENARD, S. AND LAUBIE, M. (1973a) Evidence for a sympathomimetic component inhibiting the sympathetic centres: Nature of the receptor. In *Symposium on Pharmacological Agents and Biogenic Amines in the Central Nervous System*, J. KNOLL AND K. MAGYAR (Eds.), Akadémiai Kiadó, Budapest, pp. 177–194.

SCHMITT, H., SCHMITT, H. AND FENARD, S. (1973b) Localization of the site of the central sympatho-inhibitory action of L-DOPA in dogs and cats. *Europ. J. Pharmacol.*, **22**, 212–216.

SCHOENFELD, R. I. AND URETSKY, N. J. (1973) Enhancement by 6-hydroxydopamine of the effects of DOPA upon the motor activity of rats. *J. Pharmacol. exp. Ther.*, **186**, 616–624.

SCHOENFELD, R. I. AND ZIGMOND, M. J. (1973) Behavioral pharmacology of 6-hydroxydopamine. In *Frontiers in Catecholamine Research*, E. USDIN AND S. SNYDER (Eds.), Pergamon Press, New York, N.Y., pp. 695–700.

SELLER, H. AND ILLERT, M. (1969) The localization of the first synapse in the carotid sinus baroreceptor reflex pathway and its alteration of the afferent input. *Pflügers Arch. ges. Physiol.*, **306**, 1–19.

SHERMAN, G. P., GREGA, G. J., WOODS, R. J. AND BUCKLEY, J. P. (1968) Evidence for a central hypotensive mechanism of 2-(2,6-dichlorophenylamino)-2-imidazoline (Catapresan, St. 155). *Europ. J. Pharmacol.*, **2**, 326–328.

SINHA, J. N., ATKINSON, J. M. AND SCHMITT, H. (1973) Effects of clonidine and L-DOPA on spontaneous and evoked splanchnic nerve discharges. *Europ. J. Pharmacol.*, **24**, 113–119.

SMITH, O. A. (1974) Reflex and central mechanisms involved in the control of the heart and circulation. *Ann. Rev. Physiol.*, **36**, 93–123.

STRUYKER BOUDIER, H. A. J. AND VAN ROSSUM, J. M. (1972) Clonidine-induced cardiovascular effects after stereotaxic application in the hypothalamus of rats. *J. Pharm. Pharmacol.*, **24**, 410–411.

TOIVOLA, P. AND GALE, C. C. (1970) Effect on temperature of biogenic amine infusion into hypothalamus of baboon. *Neuroendocrinology*, **6**, 210–219.

TYLER, H. R. AND DAWSON, D. (1961) Hypertension and its relation to the nervous system. *Ann. intern. Med.*, **55**, 681–694.

UVNÄS, B. (1960) Central cardiovascular control. In *Handbook of Physiology, Section 1: Neurophysiology, Vol. II*, J. FIELD, H. W. MAGOUN AND V. E. HALL (Eds.), American Physiological Society, Washington, D.C., pp. 1131–1162.

VARAGIĆ, V. (1955) The action of eserine on the blood pressure of the rat. *Brit. J. Pharmacol.*, **10**, 349–353.

VOGT, M. (1954) The concentration of sympathin in different parts of the central nervous system under normal conditions and after the administration of drugs. *J. Physiol. (Lond.)*, **123**, 451–481.

WANG, S. C. AND CHAI, C. Y. (1967) Central control of baroreceptor reflex mechanism. In *Baroreceptors and Hypertension*, P. KEZDI (Ed.), Pergamon Press, Oxford, pp. 117–130.

WATANABE, A. M., CHASE, T. N. AND CARDON, P. V. (1970) Effects of L-DOPA alone and in combination with an extracerebral decarboxylase inhibitor on blood pressure and some cardiovascular reflexes. *Clin. Pharmacol. Ther.*, **11**, 740–746.

WATANABE, A. M., PARKS, L. C. AND KOPIN, I. J. (1971) Modification of the cardiovascular effects of L-DOPA by decarboxylase inhibitors. *J. clin. Invest.*, **50**, 1322–1328.

YAMORI, Y., LOVENBERG, W. AND SJOERDSMA, A. (1970) Norepinephrine metabolism in brainstem of spontaneously hypertensive rats. *Science*, **170**, 544–546.

YAMORI, Y., DE JONG, W., YAMABE, H., LOVENBERG, W. AND SJOERDSMA, A. (1972a) Effects of L-DOPA and inhibitors of decarboxylase and monoamine oxidase on brain noradrenaline levels and blood pressure in spontaneously hypertensive rats. *J. Pharm. Pharmacol.*, **24**, 690–695.

YAMORI, Y., YAMABE, H., DE JONG, W., LOVENBERG, W. AND SJOERDSMA, A. (1972b) Effect of tissue norepinephrine depletion by 6-hydroxydopamine on blood pressure in spontaneously hypertensive rats. *Europ. J. Pharmacol.*, **17**, 135–140.

ZWIETEN, P. A. VAN (1973) The central action of antihypertensive drugs, mediated via central α-receptors. *J. Pharm. Pharmacol.*, **25**, 89–95.

Relationships of Perception, Cognition, Suggestion and Operant Conditioning in Essential Hypertension

ALVIN P. SHAPIRO, DANIEL P. REDMOND,
ROBERT H. McDONALD, Jr. AND MICHAEL GAYLOR

Division of Hypertension and Clinical Pharmacology, Department of Medicine, University of Pittsburgh School of Medicine, Pittsburgh, Pa. 15261 (U.S.A.)

INTRODUCTION

That emotional factors influence blood pressure and may play a role in the pathogenesis and perpetuation of hypertension is well known. Clinicians and investigators have regularly contributed anecdotal and experimental data which emphasize these relationships, although they have been minimized in the face of the more dramatic physiological and therapeutic attainments of recent years. Yet these latter developments have served to elucidate the psychological linkages and place behavioral factors in an appropriate scientific perspective. As a result, the role of behavioral change has increasingly been defined in the spectrum of events which constitute hypertensive disease. For instance the data on placebo effects of drugs have permitted more meaningful assays of the clinical pharmacology of a variety of new agents employed in treatment (Moutsos *et al.*, 1967), while studies of the pressor effects of noxious stimuli of behavioral nature have permitted greater understanding of the mechanisms causing acceleration of hypertension (Shapiro, 1961). Furthermore, studies demonstrating the production of hypertension by avoidance conditioning in monkeys (Forsyth, 1969), and in mice by a sociologic stress, namely crowding of living space (Henry *et al.*, 1967), have outlined sequences pertinent to the etiology of hypertension.

Regardless of how behavioral events manifest themselves peripherally on the cardiovascular system and the mechanisms which control blood pressure — or in fact how environmental or interpersonal conflicts do indeed become noxious psychologic stimuli — they affect the organism through the central nervous system and the integrating functions of the hypothalamus. However, although this is a psychoneuroendocrinology conference, we do not intend to review these mechanisms in any detail since they have not been the area of our interest. Others have devoted major efforts to these areas, and I would refer you to work of Zanchetti (1970), of Reis (1972) and of Korner (1972) and their respective collaborators.

We would rather confine our discussion to two areas which have been subjects of our own studies in recent years; namely the phenomenon of perception of conflict in the hypertensive subject, and secondly the role of operant conditioning and biofeedback in the manipulation of blood pressure.

References p. 310–312

(1) Perception of conflict

The personality pattern of the hypertensive individual has been variously described by many authors, but a common theme runs through most of these descriptions. Thus the "hypertensive personality" is marked by a characteristic inability to express anger, or an ineffectual expression of anger, and indeed at times by an obsequious type of behavior as a retreat from potentially hostile expression (Shapiro, 1960). In the classical hypothesis, this anger is "turned inward" and in keeping with Cannon's hypothesis of the effect of rage on sympathetic activity, takes its expression on the cardiovascular system as an integrated pressor response. Both the ease of producing pressor responses by noxious stimuli and the many personality surveys of hypertensive patients which demonstrate the described "personality pattern", lend support to these linkages.

Some years ago Weiner *et al.* (1962) put these observations together in a somewhat different manner. They observed that hypertensive subjects, when asked to react to the Thematic Apperception Test (TAT), told relatively uninvolved stories and showed minimal blood pressure responses. In fact their pressor responses were somewhat less than those of normotensive individuals and of patients with peptic ulcer, in spite of the well-known observation that hypertensives generally have an increased cardiovascular reactivity. The stories which the patients told were rather flat and generally devoid of the obvious conflicts apparent in the TAT pictures. When interviewed by the investigators, who increasingly involved the patients, pressor responses often occurred. On the basis of these findings, the investigators suggested that the hypertensive patient, aware of his tendency to hyperreact, managed to "insulate himself" from conflict whenever it was possible.

In a study which we have reported previously (Sapira *et al.*, 1971), we investigated this interesting suggestion in the following manner. A pair of movies was developed in which contrasting doctor–patient attitudes were displayed. The movies demonstrated a simulated office visit of a hypertensive patient to a doctor. In one of the movies the doctor played the part of a rough, gruff, unsympathetic individual; in the contrasting movie he was a gentle, and obviously considerate person. The various aspects of the movie sequences developed to bring out these contrasts were exaggerated to the point of making them easily recognizable caricatures. When these movies were shown to hypertensive patients minimal pressor responsivity was noted which was no greater than that seen in a comparable group of normotensives. However, when the patient was interviewed it was discovered that the hypertensive denied the very obvious contrasts between the physician behaviors demonstrated in the two movies whereas the normotensive easily recognized the differences. In the course of the interviews pressor responses occurred in the hypertensives which were now significantly greater than those in the normotensives.

Subsequently, this observation of the apparent inability of the hypertensive to "perceive the conflict" was confirmed in a large group of hypertensive out-patients who were compared to patients with other diseases, as well as to healthy normotensive subjects. In a subsequent study, we developed a similar pair of movies concerned with a dermatologic problem. The hypertensive patients now recognized the contrasting roles of the physician as easily as did the normotensives suggesting that their "failure to perceive" was specific to their own disease, namely hypertension.

These data, it seems to us, lend strong confirmation to the hypothesis that Weiner *et al.* proposed, namely that the hypertensive insulates himself from situations of conflict. Carried further such insulation may represent the behavioral awareness of innate hyperreactivity, *i.e.* by "failing to perceive" a conflict, the subject will not react to it and therefore will not suffer the physiological consequences. Such an individual would present manifest behavior in which he seems somewhat withdrawn from conflict and unable to express anger and hostile expression in situations obviously calling for it. Thus this sequence takes into account the observations about the hypertensive personality described previously but turns the relationship around so that the behavior stems from the hyperreactivity rather than the hyperreactivity arising from the behavior. When one then examines the studies of John Lacey the hypothesis becomes increasingly attractive. Lacey has argued that the state of autonomic reactivity of the individual influences behavior through hypothalamic cortical pathways and has suggested "that cardiovascular depressor responses go along with responsiveness to external environment, whereas cardiovascular pressor responses go along with rejection or non-responsiveness to the external environment" (Lacey, 1964).

Obviously, additional data are needed to further support this hypothesis. However, the concept is testable in many ramifications. Techniques such as that described can be used to study behavioral and pressor responses in appropriate situations. They may serve to pick out cardiovascular hyperreactors even before the subjects necessarily show the clinical evidence, and to assess their potential for the targeting of the cardiovascular system to stress.

(II) Operant conditioning and biofeedback in blood pressure control

Recent interest in this area appears to stem from the studies of Neal Miller and his colleagues on control of autonomic function in rats through visceral conditioning (Miller, 1969). This was followed by the work of the Boston group consisting of David Shapiro, Tursky, Schwartz, Benson and others (Benson *et al.*, 1971; Schwartz, 1973; Schwartz and D. Shapiro, 1973; Schwartz *et al.*, 1971; D. Shapiro *et al.*, 1969; 1970a, b; 1972) who reported blood pressure reduction and elevation in man by biofeedback techniques. However, there is a considerable prior literature on the effect of behavioral stimuli on blood pressure both in individual patients and in experimental studies as well as data related to psychotherapeutic attempts to lower blood pressure and to the placebo effects associated with pharmacological studies (Reiser *et al.*, 1951; Shapiro, 1960; 1961; Moutsos *et al.*, 1967; Pilewski *et al.*, 1971). Much of the latter experience, and the well known marked lability of blood pressure in hypertensives, both of which have considerable pertinence to biofeedback studies, seem to have been ignored by the new groups of investigators. Our own studies therefore approached this problem with the intent of relating these recent experiments in biofeedback to previous clinical and experimental data, particularly after our own initial studies, in

References p. 310–312

avoidance conditioning in animals (Shapiro and Melhado, 1958) and man (Moustos *et al.*, 1964) and more recently with operant conditioning (Shapiro, 1970) had not been particularly rewarding.

In the recent literature, the effects reported on heart rate and blood pressure utilize an "external biofeedback" system which detects change and immediately informs or rewards the subject. Although the data suggest that learned directional control of these cardiovascular measures may be achievable, critical reviews by Blanchard and Young (1973) and Katkin and Murray (1968) raise several theoretical and practical issues with the methods used and results obtained to date. Taken together with the aforementioned well-known variability of blood pressure in the course of the hypertensive patient, the data in human subjects may be criticized along several lines: (1) the magnitude of changes, although statistically significant, are as a rule clinically insignificant; (2) statistical significance is often obtained by comparison of oppositely directed groups, rather than by analysis against a stable baseline or a nonfeedback control group; (3) in multi-session studies the nonspecific effects of repeated visits and treatments are not controlled; (4) reward or reinforcement systems are variable, of uncertain value, and perhaps arbitrary; (5) the influence of task awareness or instructional set if not always clearly defined or controlled; (6) maintenance of changes has not been demonstrated.

Thus in a series of reports by David Shapiro and his colleagues small differences (4–8 mm Hg) occurred between upward and downward directed groups in systolic (D. Shapiro *et al.*, 1969; 1970a, b; Schwartz *et al.*, 1971) and diastolic (D. Shapiro *et al.*, 1972) blood pressure. Nonfeedback control was omitted from these studies. In one of the reports (D. Shapiro *et al.*, 1970a), a comparison of performance under a randomized feedback condition showed that neither directional condition differed significantly from this control. Randomized feedback also was applied to subjects in another study (D. Shapiro *et al.*, 1972), but the statistical comparison is not reported. In another report by this group (Benson *et al.*, 1971), 7 hypertensive patients underwent from 8 to 34 consecutive sessions in which a decrease in systolic pressure was rewarded. Although the pressure fell by a mean of 16.5 mm Hg (range $+0.9$ to -33.8) from an average of 5 antecedent nonfeedback sessions, two factors impair a valid conclusion from this study. First, although the use of several preconditioning sessions seemed to indicate a stability of the baseline, control data are lacking in which subjects are exposed to a comparable number of sessions with meaningful events (*e.g.*, flashing lights and tones) and encouragement. Second, the subjects were expressly aware that downward changes were desired.

The problem of instructional effects pertains to the paper by Brener and Kleinman (1970) in which normotensive students achieved a 15 mm Hg drop in systolic pressure against both baseline and a control group. Indeed, while both the experimental and control groups received valid feedback to their pressure changes, the difference between the groups appears to be the results of the instructions on how to use that information. Interestingly, in D. Shapiro *et al.* (1972), the blood pressure difference was increased during extinction among those subjects who were instructed to "continue to make correct responses". Such data indicate that instruction and directional task awareness may play a major confounding role in the assessment of the efficacy of external feedback. Bergman and Johnson (1971, 1972) have explored this question in relation to heart-rate control. Significant changes occurred appropriate to directional instructions in the absence of feedback, while the addition of feedback did not seem to augment the response to instruction.

In order to resolve some of these objections, and particularly to look at the potential "placebo effect" in biofeedback, we studied a small group of hypertensives in a series of weekly sessions. Several of these sessions dealt with the ability to recognize and report spontaneous changes in blood pressure and will be discussed later. Five sessions involved the response of these subjects to verbal instruction in the absence of biofeedback, which resulted in sustained directional changes in blood pressure. Progressive muscular relaxation (PMR) was induced in one of these sessions and the separate effects of this technique were noted.

The methodology employed in these sessions has been described in a detailed publication (Redmond et al., 1974). Briefly, the patients — 3 men and 3 women with mild to moderate essential hypertension — were selected for their willingness to participate, without compensation, in a study of "some of the psychological aspects of high blood pressure". After reporting to the laboratory, the patients assumed a semi-recumbent position in a quiet, dimly lit room and the instrumentation was attached. Indirect blood pressure was recorded automatically every 30 sec by the Doppler-ultrasonic transducer system (Arteriosonde) and heart rate by ECG (electrocardiogram) chest leads; the rate was averaged for the period between systolic and diastolic blood pressure measurements.

In session I, after a 15-min rest period (R-1), the investigator entered the room and engaged in non-specific conversation for 5 min (E-1). He then instructed the patient to "change his blood pressure", by delivering a repetitive monologue in which a monotonous emphasis was directed to having the patient change the "rate and force of heart beat and resistance of vessels to flow.

It is well known that people can control their blood pressure by concentrating on the parameters in their body which control their pressure, namely, the speed of the heart, the force with which the heart beats, and the degree to which the vessels resist the flow of blood. Now, I want you to raise (lower) your blood pressure by concentrating hard on making your heart beat faster (slower) and more (less) forcefully, and your blood vessels more (less) resistant to the flow of blood. Make your heart beat faster (slower) and more (less) forcefully, and your vessels resist (lessen resistance to) the flow of blood . . ."

This initial instruction period was aimed at raising blood pressure (U-1) and then direction was reversed in the instructions (D-1). After a rest period (R-2), the sequence was repeated but with the down instructions first (E-2, D-2, U-2). After a third rest period (R-3), the patient was disconnected from the apparatus and briefly interviewed. In the subsequent session (II) training in PMR was introduced; this was followed by two sessions (III and IV) in one of which PMR was induced by the experimenter, and in the next was "self-induced" by the patient. In a final session (V), directional instruction according to the protocol in session I was given following induction of PMR.

(1) Cardiovascular results

The cardiovascular data obtained in the two directional sessions (I and V) are illustrated in Figs. 1 and 2. These data were handled by an analysis of variance.

In session I, direction of change for UP periods was positive in 9 of 12 instances for systolic pressure and 9 of 11 for diastolic, while for DOWN periods, it was negative in 11 of 12 instances for systolic and 10 of 12 for diastolic.

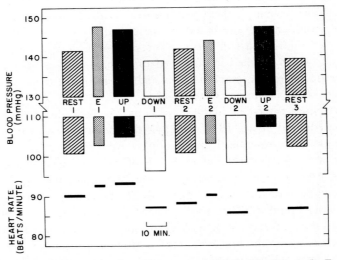

Fig. 1. Session I: first instruction session. Group mean period data (N = 6); E = ENTRY of experimenter. Least significant period differences (*P* = 0.05) are 8.5 mm Hg systolic BP, 5.5 mm Hg diastolic BP, and 6.1 bpm heart rate.

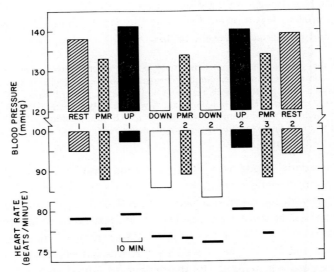

Fig. 2. Session V: second instruction session with PMR. Group mean period data (N = 5). Least significant period differences (*P* = 0.05) are 6.2 mm Hg systolic BP, 7.1 mm Hg diastolic BP and 7.2 bpm heart rate.

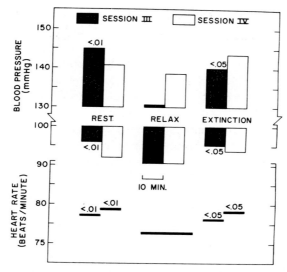

Fig. 3. Sessions III and IV: response to relaxation. Induction, with (session III) and without (session IV) active monologue by the experimenter. Significant differences shown are with respect to the RELAX period.

The average magnitudes of these changes in the 6 subjects were 9/9 mm Hg for UP_1 *vs.* $DOWN_1$ differences ($P = 0.05$), and 14/9 mm Hg for UP_2 *vs.* $DOWN_2$ differences ($P = 0.01$). UP periods generally were not significantly higher than ENTRY periods. DOWN periods however were significantly lower than ENTRY and REST periods with average magnitudes up to 14/7 mm Hg ($P = 0.01$) and 8/6 mm Hg ($P = 0.05$) respectively.

Pulse rate changes were directionally similar to those of blood pressure but magnitude of the changes only occasionally reached statistically significant levels.

In session V, in which directional instruction was administered following induction of PMR, results were similar except that a depressor response to PMR replaced the "pressor response" to ENTRY. The direction of change was positive for UP periods in 10 out of 10 instances for both systolic and diastolic, and negative for DOWN periods in 9 of 10 and 10 of 10 for systolic and diastolic, respectively. The magnitude of the changes between the various periods was not significantly greater in this session than in session I, except for a slightly greater diastolic fall. (All UP × DOWN differences in session I averaged 12/9 mm Hg and in Session II, 10/12 mm Hg and for heart rate 5 and 6 bpm, respectively.)

The effects of relaxation (PMR) alone are demonstrated in Fig. 3. Blood pressure fell 14/6 mm Hg in session III when PMR was induced by the experimenter, but did not decline significantly when PMR was self-induced.

(2) Interview data

In response to instructions to raise or lower blood pressure, subjects associated mental imagery with directional shifts in blood pressure. When asked how they tried to raise

References p. 310–312

their pressures, subjects reported that although they concentrated on their heart beat and blood flow, they visualized themselves in certain psychologically or physically stimulating activities, *e.g.* climbing a hill, seeing one's mother die, singing before an audience, taking an examination, falling off a cliff, being hit by a truck, lying in a coffin. Similarly, during DOWN periods, subjects stated that they pictured their heart and blood flow, but while lying on a beach, or on soft, blue blankets, in a warm bath, descending in a slow elevator, or floating in space. In session V, when subjects were told to maintain relaxation, similar imagery was reported, especially for UP periods. For DOWN periods, they reported more concentration on lowering muscular tension than on other images. Subjects stated that it was difficult or impossible to maintain muscular relaxation during UP periods, but that during DOWN periods, the opposite was true.

After "self-induced" relaxation in session IV, all subjects believed they had relaxed as well as they ever had by themselves (by an estimate of "depth" on a scale of 1–10), but not as well as they had previously in the presence of the investigator. All subjects stated that in the absence of the relaxation monologue, they were more easily distracted by various noises, thoughts of current problems, or the inflation of the BP cuff.

(3) Recognition of blood pressure level

It would seem to us that one of the basic questions involved in biofeedback study is whether the subject can indeed recognize changes in his level of blood pressure. Although in clinical practice, many patients report that they can tell when their blood pressure is "up (or down)", most of my own clinical experience at least had lead me to believe that any coincidence occurs by chance. Accordingly, we have studied the phenomenon in this group of 6 hypertensive subjects in 3 additional sessions. These sessions consisted of an initial session (I) which was primarily a rest period although a few stimuli were introduced (*i.e.* a venipuncture and the aforementioned set of doctor–patient movies); a PMR session (II) in which PMR was induced; and a suggestion session (III) in which PMR was maintained but it was suggested to the patient that he could "recognize better" if he attended to his perception of "heart rate, force of contraction and tightness of his vessels".

Instrumentation used was identical to that described previously and recordings were made every 30 sec. In addition, the patient was supplied with a set of buttons to push 10 sec after each blood pressure cycle was recorded indicating whether he "recognized" that his blood pressure was up, down or unchanged. Each session lasted approximately 30 min.

The results provide some evidence that recognition during session III was slightly better than in I and II, but the differences were small and of doubtful significance so that for the purpose of this presentation of the data all sessions and periods have been pooled.

For all responses in which the subjects reported UP, the rise in mean blood pressure (MBP) was 2.2 mm Hg. For all DOWN responses, the fall in MBP was −1.7 mm Hg and for all zero responses, the delta was −0.3 mm Hg. The differences between these values were highly significant ($P = 0.001$). When the subjects were "Correct" in their responses, MBP change was $\pm$ 5.1 mm Hg; when they were "Wrong", change was $\pm$ 3.4 mm Hg. Again this was a significant difference.

Still using all the pooled data, 651 of 1418 trials were "Correct" or 46.0%. Expected percent correct was estimated at 36.3 and the difference is significant with a P value of 0.01. When zero responses were eliminated, the percent correct was 70% (expected 50%). If only the responses greater than 2 mm Hg are considered, 53% were correct and if zero responses are eliminated in this calculation, the score becomes 67%.

These data would suggest that subjects were able to recognize blood pressure change at a level somewhat better than chance. Looking at individual subjects, several were quite striking, one subject achieving levels of 53.4–58.5% "Correct" responses in the 3 sessions and 72.5–82.5% when zero responses were eliminated. However, the true meaning of these observations remains for further study. Questions which are obvious include the degree of individual variation, the recognition ability of non-hypertensives and the potential for this "talent" to be improved by training. The attractive hypothesis to us is that recognition is a behavioral manifestation of a physiological set, which moves through hypothalamic–cortical pathways. On the other hand, the ability to recognize may arise, if indeed it does exist, from cues having to do with awareness of muscle tension, of increased heart rate, or other peripheral sensations which have been learned or taught as indicating elevated blood pressure.

DISCUSSION

The studies reported herein speak to several different areas of the relationship between blood pressure and behavior. Two of the studies — that concerned with perception of conflict and that concerned with recognition of the physiological setting of the blood pressure — are related in that they bear on the hypothesis that central nervous system "awareness" of blood pressure may in turn have an effect on behavior of the organism. Obviously any inferences drawn from these observations must remain tentative until more data have been procured and to make further claims from them at this time is rather premature.

The recognition data further relate to our study on suggestion and relaxation as factors involved in the reported results of biofeedback and operant conditioning. Because of these reports, considerable excitement has been engendered, as pointed out earlier, about the potential of conditioning as a treatment modality. The fact that some degree of recognition of blood pressure may occur, offers some evidence of an "internal feedback" loop.

However, since blood pressure is a function of a complex array of variable humoral, neurological and psychological factors (Shapiro, 1973), measurement of its changes in man is subject to numerous additional problems of experimental control. The well-documented lability of blood pressure, which is even more evident in hypertensive patients, complicates the evaluation of any drug, agent or device which is purported to alter the blood pressure (Shapiro, 1960). Furthermore, an extensive literature demonstrates the variety of psychological manipulations which can result in systematic directional shifts in blood pressure, both acutely and chronically. Such influences may be termed "placebo effects" in their relation to the evaluation of any single psychologic manipulation, *e.g.*, "biofeedback". Among several relevant studies are the observations of Reiser *et al.* (1951) regarding the correlation of the course of hypertensive disease with emotional factors including doctor–patient interactions. The enthusiasm of both parties in a treatment situation are closely related to the effects of antihypertensive drugs (Shapiro *et al.*, 1954), and the setting of treatment, *e.g.* hospitalization, itself will lower the blood pressure (Moutsos *et al.*, 1967). In a study in 1956 by Goldring *et al.* (1956), the hypotensive effect of reassurance coupled with a dramatic but innocuous electronic device was demonstrated; this clever experiment bears a special relation to the report by Benson *et al.* (1971) of blood pressure conditioning in hypertensives. Regarding studies of the more acute effects of psychological variables, consistent directional changes occur with application and removal of noxious stimuli (Shapiro, 1961) and hypnotic suggestion of attitudes (Stern *et al.*, 1961). Lowering of blood pressure is associated with progressive muscular relaxation (Jacobson, 1939), autogenic training (Luth, 1960), "yogi" or transcendental meditation (Wallace, 1970), and hypnotically suggested relaxation (Paul, 1969).

The subjects in our study were highly selected: young, cooperative, mildly hypertensive and in a doctor–patient relationship. From the foregoing discussion, these factors probably played a role in the achievement of consistent results. However, similar factors (age, motivation, therapeutic expectation) operate in conditioning studies, in which students or hypertensives are subjects. The presence, degree and specificity of autonomic perception have a basic relation to the problem of voluntary control, which may well have operated in this study. However, in the literature of voluntary control, it is implicitly assumed, that such recognition either does not exist, or requires exteroceptive augmentation. Thus, to the extent that internal cardiovascular perception is a factor, as suggested in our "movie study" and in the recognition study, further issue with external feedback methods is raised.

Our data coincide with other studies indicating the quantitative significance of blood pressure responses to psychological variables. In this instance, consistent directional changes were associated with continuous verbal instructions to concentrate upon and alter the blood pressure and heart rate. Critics of biofeedback studies (Katkin and Murray, 1968; Blanchard and Young, 1973) suggest that the reported changes may be too small to have clinical value, especially if they are not sustained chronically. Perhaps a more serious difficulty is that changes achieved in such studies are of the same order as those associated with numerous other experimental manipulations, including direct, forceful instructions to perform the task. Hence, the specificity, as well as the utility, of feedback is subject to question.

In our study, instructions admittedly differed from those used in most studies of instructional set (Jacobson, 1938; Bergman and Johnson, 1972). Monotonous and repetitive, they may have been more forceful and suggestive, thus serving as a more potent and direct stimulus. The behavioral mechanisms by which the responses occurred are by no means clear, but are surely complex. A direct and specific response to the literal meaning of the instructions is not likely, while the intervention of associative imagery is suggested by interview data. Whatever the mechanism, the influence of instructional set on cardiovascular performance in the feedback paradigm has been demonstrated by other data (Lang *et al.*, 1967; Brener and Kleinman, 1970; Bergman and Johnson, 1971, 1972). Whether mere awareness of the physiological task at hand influences success has not been studied systematically, to our knowledge. However, since the verbal instructions in our study were restricted to the physiological factors involved, the results suggest that in these selected hypertensives at least, task awareness (*e.g.*, "to change the blood pressure") can alter the results. If this is generally true, it is an effect difficult to avoid since a degree of common knowledge, added to the application of a blood pressure cuff and EKG electrodes will lead usually to the subject's own conclusion that cardiovascular parameters are involved and thus narrow down his uncertainty to the direction of change desired. Given only two choices, a subject might learn the correct direction by trial and error from the feedback display and then proceed independently of feedback, as did the patients in our study. In such a case, the feedback merely completes the instructional set, and the continuation of the display thereafter may be superfluous.

Our data related to PMR should be viewed in reference only to the technique employed and not to the physiological effects reported by Jacobson (1939). Of interest was the fact that lowering of blood pressure seemed to require the presence of one of the investigators, a result which concurred with that of Paul and Trimble (1970). PMR did not remarkably influence the performance during instructional sessions of our patients as measured by UP–DOWN differences. On the other hand, performance against baseline was altered in that lower pressures during DOWN periods were obtained with PMR and greater pressures in UP periods occurred without it. Furthermore, DOWN responses did not exceed the depressor effect of PMR, while UP responses did not exceed those to ENTRY. Such parallelism underscores the broad, and perhaps non-specific stimulus basis for pressure changes as recorded in a given experiment.

In summary, in the instruction and relaxation studies predictable directional changes in blood pressure and heart rate were shown to occur in response to forceful verbal instruction to alter cardiovascular functions. These data indicate that potent directional effects, apart from feedback, operate in studies of operant conditioning of blood pressure and heart rate in man. It is frequently assumed in such studies that feedback serves as the effector agent but efficacy tested against "placebo" effects must surely be studied further before projections of clinical utility are seriously entertained. The present study is consistent with the speculation that external feedback procedures are, to borrow a remark of Blanchard and Young (1973), merely less efficient methods for telling the subject what to do.

Taken together, the work which we have reported has importance in indicating areas of research into which studies of relationships of blood pressure and behavior can proceed. As indicated earlier, such relationships have long been known and discussed, but data have largely been anecdotal, descriptive and not lending themselves either to fresh hypotheses or therapeutic consequences. Moreover, the relationships have been studied often separately from their bearing on the overall problem

References p. 310–312

of hypertensive disease. Indeed some investigators have argued that psychological stress can be a unitary cause of hypertension, or of a particular type of hypertension, much as others have sought the "holy grail" of single causation in the kidney, the adrenal, or the autonomic nervous system. However, present theories of the etiology of essential hypertension indicate with increasing clarity that it is a disease which develops from a failure of integration of a variety of known homeostatic mechanisms (Shapiro, 1973). Psychological and behavioral factors in the disease need to be studied in relationship to these other mechanisms and hopefully we have outlined several directions towards this goal.

SUMMARY

A series of studies pertaining to several different aspects of the relationship of behavior and hypertension are reported. Exposure of hypertensive subjects to a contrived conflictual situation demonstrated a failure of the subject to fully perceive the conflict; it is suggested that this phenomenon represents a behavioral "awareness" of the hypertensive's physiological hyperreactivity. A study of recognition of blood pressure level suggested that some hypertensives at least can recognize up and down change at a somewhat better than chance percentage. In a third study, results mimicking those achieved in hypertensive subjects with operant conditioning and biofeedback were produced simply by relaxation and by instruction and suggestion. Taken as a whole, the work indicates new avenues for investigation of physiological and psychological mechanisms in hypertensive disease which interrelate to each other in a reversible fashion.

ACKNOWLEDGEMENTS

Studies supported by research and training grants from the USPHS (HL-13604, HL-05711, HL-05467).

REFERENCES

BENSON, H., SHAPIRO, D., TURSKY, B. AND SCHWARTZ, G. E. (1971) Decreased systolic blood pressure through operant conditioning techniques in patients with essential hypertension. *Science*, **173**, 740.
BERGMAN, J. S. AND JOHNSON, H. J. (1971) The effects of instructional set and autonomic perception on cardiac control. *Psychophysiology*, **8**, 180.
BERGMAN, J. S. AND JOHNSON, H. J. (1972) Sources of information which affect training and raising of heart rate. *Psychophysiology*, **9**, 30.
BLANCHARD, E. B. AND YOUNG, L. D. (1973) Self-control of cardiac functioning: a promise as yet unfulfilled. *Psychol. Bull.*, **79**, 145.
BRENER, J. AND KLEINMAN, R. A. (1970) Learned control of decreases in systolic blood pressure. *Nature (Lond.)*, **226**, 1063.
FORSYTH, R. (1969) Blood pressure responses to long term avoidance schedules in the restrained Rhesus monkey. *Psychosom. Med.*, **31**, 300.

GOLDRING, W., CHASIS, H., SCHREINER, G. E. AND SMITH, H. W. (1956) Reassurance in the management of benign hypertensive disease. *Circulation*, **14**, 260.

HENRY, J. P., MEEHAN, J. P. AND STEPHENS, P. (1967) The use of psychosocial stimuli to induce prolonged systolic hypertension in mice. *Psychosom. Med.*, **29**, 408.

JACOBSON, E. (1938) *Progressive Relaxation*, University of Chicago Press, Chicago, Ill.

JACOBSON, E. (1939) Variation of blood pressure with skeletal muscle tension and relaxation. *Ann. intern. Med.*, **12**, 1194.

KATKIN, E. S. AND MURRAY, E. N. (1968) Instrumental conditioning of autonomically mediated behavior; theoretical and methodological issues. *Psychol. Bull.*, **70**, 52.

KORNER, P. I. (1972) The central nervous system and physiological mechanisms of optimal cardiovascular central. In *Neural and Psychological Mechanisms in Cardiovascular Disease*, A. ZANCHETTI (Ed.), Il Ponto, Milan, p. 321.

LACEY, J. (1964) Methodological approaches to the role of the central nervous system in cardiovascular disease. *Proceedings of the Timberline Conference, 1963, Psychosom. Med.*, **26**, 445.

LANG, P. J., SROUFE, A. AND HASTINGS, J. E. (1967) Effects of feedback and instructional set of the control of cardiac rate variability. *J. exp. Psychol.*, **75**, 425.

LUTH, E. W. (1960) Physiological and psychodynamic effects of autogenic training. In *Topical Problems of Psychotherapy, Vol. 3*, B. STOKZIS (Ed.), Karger, Basel, p. 174.

MILLER, N. E. (1969) Learning of visceral and glandular responses. *Science*, **163**, 434.

MOUTSOS, S. E., KRIFCHER, E., MILLER, R. E. AND SHAPIRO, A. P. (1964) An experimental study of conditioning and reactivity as determinants of pressor responses to noxious stimuli. *Psychosom. Med.*, **26**, 274.

MOUTSOS, S. E., SAPIRA, J. D., SCHEIB, E. T. AND SHAPIRO, A. P. (1967) An analysis of the placebo effect in hospitalized hypertensive patients. *Clin. Pharmacol. Ther.*, **8**, 676.

PAUL, G. L. (1969) Physiologic effects of relaxation training and hypnotic suggestion. *J. abnorm. soc. Psychol.*, **74**, 425.

PAUL, G. L. AND TRIMBLE, R. W. (1970) "Recorded" *vs.* "live" relaxation training and hypnotic suggestion: comparative effectiveness for reducing physiological arousal and inhibiting stress response. *Behav. Ther.*, **1**, 285.

PILEWSKI, R. M., SCHEIB, E. T., MISAGE, J. R., KESSLER, E., KRIFCHER, E. AND SHAPIRO, A. P. (1971) Technique of controlled drug assay in hypertension. V. Comparison of hydrochlorothiazide with a new quinethazone diuretic, metolazone. *Clin. Pharmacol. Ther.*, **12**, 843 (and references in this paper to earlier studies in this series).

REDMOND, D., GAYLOR, M., MCDONALD, R. H. AND SHAPIRO, A. P. (1974) Blood pressure and heart rate response to verbal instruction and relaxation in hypertension. *Psychosom. Med.*, **36**, 285.

REIS, D. (1972) Central neural mechanisms governing the circulation with particular reference to the lower brain stem and cerebellum. In *Neural and Psychological Mechanisms in Cardiovascular Disease*, A. ZANCHETTI (Ed.), Il Ponto, Milan, p. 255.

REISER, M. F., BRUST, A. A., SHAPIRO, A. P., BAKER, H. M., RANSOHOFF, W. AND FERRIS, E. B. (1951) Life situations, emotions and the course of patients with arterial hypertension. *Psychosom. Med.*, **13**, 133.

SAPIRA, J. D., SCHEIB, E. T., MORIARTY, R. AND SHAPIRO, A. P. (1971) Differences in perception between hypertensive and normotensive populations. *Psychosom. Med.*, **33**, 239.

SCHWARTZ, G. E. (1972) Voluntary control of human cardiovascular integration and differentiation through feedback and rewards. *Science*, **175**, 90.

SCHWARTZ, G. E. AND SHAPIRO, D. (1973) Biofeedback and essential hypertension: current findings and theoretical concerns. *Semin. Psychiat.*, **5**, 493.

SCHWARTZ, G. E., SHAPIRO, D. AND TURSKY, B. (1971) Learned control of cardiovascular integration in man through operant conditioning. *Psychosom. Med.*, **33**, 57.

SHAPIRO, A. P. (1960) Psychophysiologic mechanisms in hypertensive vascular disease. *Ann. intern. Med.*, **53**, 65.

SHAPIRO, A. P. (1961) An experimental study of comparative responses of blood pressure to different noxious stimuli. *J. chron. Dis.*, **13**, 293.

SHAPIRO, A. P. (1970) Psychologic aspects of hypertension (Discussion). *Circulat. Res.*, **27**, **Suppl. I**, 1–36.

SHAPIRO, A. P. (1973) Essential hypertension — Why idiopathic? *Amer. J. Med.*, **54**, 1.

SHAPIRO, A. P. AND MELHADO, J. (1958) Observations on blood pressure and other physiological and biochemical mechanisms in rats with behavioral disturbances. *Psychosom. Med.*, **20**, 303.

SHAPIRO, A. P., MYERS, T., REISER, M. F. AND FERRIS, E. B. (1954) Comparison of blood pressure to Veriloid and to the doctor. *Psychosom. Med.*, **16**, 478.

SHAPIRO, D., SCHWARTZ, G. E. AND TURSKY, B. (1972) Control of diastolic blood pressure in man by feedback and reinforcement. *Psychophysiology*, **9**, 296.

SHAPIRO, D., TURSKY, B. AND SCHWARTZ, G. E. (1970a) Control of blood pressure in man by operant conditioning. *Circulat. Res.*, **27, Suppl. I**, 1–27.

SHAPIRO, D., TURSKY, B. AND SCHWARTZ, G. E. (1970b) Differentiation of heart rate and systolic blood pressure in man by operant conditioning. *Psychosom. Med.*, **32**, 417.

SHAPIRO, D., TURSKY, B., GERSHON, E. AND STERN, M. (1969) Effects of feedback and reinforcement on the control of human systolic blood pressure. *Science*, **163**, 588.

STERN, J. A., WINOKUR, G., GRAHAM, D. T. AND GRAHAM, F. K. (1961) Alterations in physiological measures during experimentally induced attitudes. *J. Psychosom. Res.*, **5**, 73.

WALLACE, R. K. (1970) Physiologic effects of transcendental meditation. *Science*, **167**, 1751.

WEINER, H., SINGER, M. T. AND REISER, M. F. (1962) Cardiovascular responses and their psychophysiologic correlates. A study in healthy young adults and patients with peptic ulcer and hypertension. *Psychosom. Med.*, **24**, 477.

ZANCHETTI, A. (1970) Control of the cardiovascular system. In *The Hypothalamus*, L. MARTINI, M. MOTTA AND F. FRASCHINI (Eds.), Academic Press, New York, N.Y., p. 233.

Changes in Myocardial Function as a Consequence of Prolonged Emotional Stress

K. D. CAIRNCROSS AND J. R. BASSETT

School of Biological Sciences, Macquarie University, North Ryde, N.S.W. 2113 (Australia)

Activation of the pituitary–adrenal cortical system and a resulting elevation of plasma glucocorticoids has been established as a sequel typical to stress situations. Recent work from this laboratory has demonstrated that such elevation can be quantitated, the degree of plasma steroid elevation relating to the type of stress to which the animal is exposed. Thus, regular signalled footshock induces an intermediate elevation (50–60 μg/100 ml blood plasma), whereas irregular signalled footshock with the possibility of escape induces extreme steroid elevation (85–95 μg/100 ml plasma) (Bassett *et al.*, 1973). It should be noted that the degree of steroid elevation in the intermediate range is independent of the intensity of the physical stressor, and that extreme steroid elevation occurs only with irregular signalled footshock with the possibility of escape. The contention is made, therefore, that extreme steroid elevation is dependent on a psychological component, and that an increment in the psychological stressor can induce a further increase in corticosterone output. The emotional response, however, is not concerned solely with the hypothalamic–hypophyseal–adrenal axis but also with the sympathetic adreno-medullary system, with an associated increase in catecholamine secretion and release. In this regard, several workers have demonstrated a corticosterone–catecholamine interaction *in situ* using exogenous steroid administration (Nicol and Rae, 1972; Iwasawa and Gillis, 1973). One site of such interaction is the heart, and it was decided to examine myocardial sensitivity to noradrenaline (NA) and adrenaline in the presence of extreme corticosterone elevation. Accordingly male rats (Carworth CSF strain) 90 days old at the start of the experiment were placed on a reverse 12-hr night–day schedule, and housed in conditions of constant temperature and humidity. Following 14 days equilibration the stress group of rats was placed in an automated one-way avoidance box (Lafayette Model 85200) described in detail by Potts and McKown (1969). The animals were stressed on 4 consecutive days in a treatment session of 35 min, in which they received 7 CS–UCS exposures randomly placed. Animals were sacrificed immediately following the stress session, or after 3 and 48 hr. Myocardial sensitivity was measured using a driven atrial strip as described by Blinks (1966). The results are presented in Table I in which it can be seen that the mean ED_{50} for adrenaline and noradrenaline is significantly reduced following irregular signalled stress. The enhanced myocardial sensitivity to both catecholamines was observed in naive animals, and persisted un-

TABLE I

MYOCARDIAL SENSITIVITY TO CATECHOLAMINES IN RATS SUBJECTED TO 4 DAYS OF IRREGULAR-SIGNALLED ESCAPE STRESS

Number of animals/group = 6.

Time (hr)		Mean ED_{50} ($\times 10^{-8}$ M) $\pm$ S.E.M.		P (by t-test)
		Control	Stressed	
0	Adrenaline	13.5 ± 2.0	5.5 ± 0.6	< 0.01
	NA	21.0 ± 2.6	6.2 ± 0.8	< 0.005
	11-OHCS*	7.9 ± 1.8	83.0 ± 6.3	
3	Adrenaline	19.6 ± 2.4	10.1 ± 1.6	< 0.005
	NA	24.1 ± 3.1	13.1 ± 1.6	< 0.005
	11-OHCS*	6.3 ± 1.3	3.0 ± 0.5	
48	Adrenaline	12.6 ± 1.1	12.1 ± 2.5	> 0.8
	NA	17.4 ± 3.3	14.5 ± 2.6	> 0.3
	11-OHCS*	11.5 ± 4.4	6.4 ± 1.1	

* Concentration in μg/100 ml plasma.

changed in animals stressed daily over a 25-day period. No enhanced myocardial sensitivity was observed in rats subjected to regular stress (*i.e.* intermediate corticosterone elevation).

This experiment demonstrated that it was possible to induce an increased sensitivity of the heart to catecholamines in an experimental model utilizing endogenously released corticosterone. Two questions which could be asked of such a model presented themselves. Firstly, how does corticosterone induce increased myocardial sensitivity, and secondly what physiological changes would be observed following long term stress associated with increased emotionality?

In answer to the first question two experiments were undertaken. One experiment related to the endogenous levels of adrenaline and NA in the rat myocardium following exposure to irregular-signalled escape stress. In this experiment the stress procedure previously described was repeated daily for periods of 1, 4 and 10 days and the animals were sacrificed immediately following the last stress period. The atria and ventricles were removed and snap frozen in liquid nitrogen. Catecholamines were separated using a modified aluminum oxide chromatographic method after Anton and Sayre (1962) and assayed fluorimetrically after the method of Häggendal (1963).

The results of this experiment are illustrated in Fig. 1 which demonstrates a significant atrial NA reduction on the first day of stress ($P < 0.01$, $df = 18$), which was maintained for at least 4 days ($P < 0.005$, $df = 18$) and thereafter a degree of recovery occurred. Ventricular NA showed a similar trend. Adrenaline values were too low for analysis.

The possibility that neuronal uptake of NA into stores can be inhibited by corticosterone has not been reported in the literature, although other workers have suggested that corticosterone can inhibit uptake into extraneuronal NA stores (Iversen and Salt,

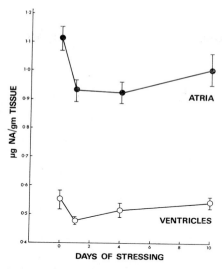

Fig. 1. Endogenous levels of noradrenaline in rat atria and ventricles of control animals (0 days), and animals exposed to 1, 4 and 10 days of irregular-signalled escape stress. Each point represents the mean value, horizontal bars designate ± S.E.

Number of analyses/group.

	Control	1 day	4 days	10 days
Atria	11	9	9	8
Ventricles	10	8	9	8

1970). The results reported here indicate that the depletion of NA is more pronounced in the atria, and such a conclusion implicates neuronal rather than extraneuronal uptake mechanisms.

In order to examine this question more closely, a second experiment was undertaken in which the effect of the stress procedure on the uptake of [³H]NA into the rat myocardium was examined. Such an experiment was feasible because the uptake characteristics of tritiated NA into neuronal and extraneuronal stores have been well documented (Iversen 1963, 1965a, b; Burgen and Iversen, 1965). Both processes saturate with increasing external concentrations of NA, and can be described with Michaelis–Menten kinetics. Accordingly, isolated atria were prepared from rats exposed to 4 consecutive days of irregular-signalled stress, the animals being sacrificed immediately following the last stress session.

Such atria were compared with atria obtained from control rats, in that accumulation of radioactivity was measured as a function of time following incubation with varying concentrations of L-[7-³H]NA. Standard liquid scintillation techniques were followed. Results obtained in this experiment establish that a significant reduction in the accumulation of NA occurs in the stressed atria. These results when plotted in the form of the Michaelis–Menten equation as S/v against S (Fig. 2) show on linear

References p. 318

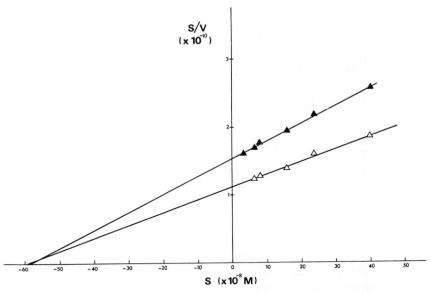

Fig. 2. Michaelis–Menten analysis of uptake results. S = incubation concentration of noradrenaline (molar bath conc.); v = initial rate of noradrenaline uptake by atria (disint./min/mg/min). Intercept on baseline = $-K_m$. Slope = $1/V_{max}$. ▲ = stressed animals (plasma corticosterone = 90.3 ± 4.8 μg/ 100 ml plasma); △ = control animals (plasma corticosterone = 20.8 ± 1.4 μg/100 ml plasma).

regression analysis straight lines with the following correlation coefficients: $r = 0.996$ (control) and $r = 0.987$ (stressed). The values of K_m calculated using the regression equations (± 95 % confidence limits) were 59.2 (± 13.7) × 10^{-8} M for control atria, and 58.7 (± 6.1) × 10^{-8} M for stressed atria. A test for parallelism on the two regression equations indicated the two lines were not parallel, the two gradients (V_{max} stressed and control) being significantly different.

The results described confirm the postulate suggested by the previous experiment, that the neuronal uptake of NA is inhibited in animals with extreme corticosterone elevation following irregular-signalled stress. The inhibition, however, appears to reflect an interference with the rate of neuronal uptake, rather than a change in storage capacity. While the accumulation of radioactivity is initially less in stressed atria, prolongation of the incubation time shows no difference between stress and control atria. This conclusion is confirmed by the kinetic studies. Atria from stressed animals show a significant lowering of the maximum rate of NA uptake (V_{max}) but no change in the affinity of NA for the uptake mechanism. These results may be interpreted on the basis that in both control and stressed preparations NA is competing for the same uptake sites, but that in stress situations there may be fewer sites available. This reduction in uptake sites may reflect the binding to such sites of 11-hydroxycortico-sterone (11-OHCS), ACTH (corticotropin), or some other metabolite liberated in response to stress.

Thus it is apparent that a glucocorticoid–catecholamine interaction can occur in the myocardium, and as suggested by Raab (1966) such an interaction could be implicated in the stress-induced pathogenesis of the cardiovascular disease process. As intimated earlier in this paper, an experiment was initiated to examine this possibility. Rats were placed on an irregular-signalled footshock regimen, as previously described. The treatment was continued 7 days per week for a total period of 70 days. In addition, the opportunity arose to compare a saturated fat diet with a polyunsaturated fat diet in the stress situation. Both diets had a fat content of 22.5–23.2%, but one diet (P) had an unsaturated fat content (linoleic acid) of 21.6%, whereas the second diet (S) had an unsaturated fat content of 2.9%. Rats (20 per group) were randomly assigned to each diet which was available *ad lib.*

Histological examination of the hearts of the P group after 70 days showed marked changes in the micro-circulation of the coronary vasculature. These changes included congestion and dilatation of the large venules, collecting venules and veins, accumulation of PAS-positive material, consistent with platelet aggregation, margined in the venous endothelium, mild edema of the intima and media of some arterioles with the presence of vacuoles, and evidence of mast cell infiltration of the myocardium. No infarct-like lesions were observed.

Similar examination of the S group revealed all the changes described for the P group and in addition a number of infarct-like lesions were observed. These changes included a loss of myocardial definition, fibrosis, leucocyte infiltration and an excess of PAS-positive material in the perivascular areas adjacent to the lesion. Also observed in the S group was fatty infiltration into the myocardium, such infiltration being both extracellular and intracellular.

Thus it may be concluded that prolonged unpredictable stress can induce pathological changes in the myocardium, and this may be associated with extreme glucocorticoid elevation. It has been demonstrated that extreme glucocorticoid elevation retards the uptake of NA into its stores, thus increasing the availability of NA in the extracellular space. This, in turn, could account for many of the pathological changes described in the prolonged stress situation.

SUMMARY

Exposure of male CSF rats to an irregular-signalled footshock regimen induced extreme plasma corticosterone elevation. It was demonstrated that cardiac muscle sensitivity to noradrenaline is enhanced in this situation, and studies using tritiated noradrenaline suggest that corticosterone can retard the uptake of this amine into its neuronal stores (uptake$_1$). Long term studies (70 days) to examine myocardial pathogenesis development were undertaken using a saturated and a polyunsaturated fat diet. Both diet groups demonstrated changes in the coronary micro-circulation, but only the saturated fat group developed infarct-like lesions.

ACKNOWLEDGEMENTS

The skilled technical assistance of Mrs. Carol Martin is gratefully acknowledged.

References p. 318

This research was supported by the Australian Research Grants Committee, Grant No. D173/15017, to the authors.

REFERENCES

ANTON, A. H. AND SAYRE, D. F. (1962) A study of the factors affecting the aluminium oxide–trihydroxy indol procedure for the analysis of catecholamines. *J. Pharmacol. exp. Ther.*, **138**, 360–375.

BASSETT, J. R., CAIRNCROSS, K. D. AND KING, M. G. (1973) Parameters of novelty, shock predictability and response contingency in corticosterone release in the rat. *Physiol. Behav.*, **10**, 901–907.

BLINKS, J. R. (1966) Field stimulation as a means of affecting the graded release of autonomic transmitters in isolated heart muscle. *J. Pharmacol. exp. Ther.*, **151**, 221–235.

BURGEN, A. S. V. AND IVERSEN, L. L. (1965) The inhibition of noradrenaline uptake by sympathomimetic amines in rat isolated heart. *Brit. J. Pharmacol.*, **25**, 34–39.

HÄGGENDAL, J. (1963) An improved method for fluorimetric determination of small amounts of adrenaline and noradrenaline in plasma and tissues. *Acta physiol. scand.*, **59**, 242–254.

IVERSEN, L. L. (1963) The uptake of noradrenaline by the isolated perfused heart. *Brit. J. Pharmacol.*, **21**, 523–537.

IVERSEN, L. L. (1965a) The uptake of adrenaline by the rat isolated heart. *Brit. J. Pharmacol.*, **24**, 387–394.

IVERSEN, L. L. (1965b) The uptake of catecholamines at high perfusion concentrations in the rat isolated heart; a novel catecholamine uptake process. *Brit. J. Pharmacol.*, **25**, 18–33.

IVERSEN, L. L. AND SALT, P. J. (1970) Inhibition of catecholamine uptake by steroids in the isolated rat heart. *Brit. J. Pharmacol.*, **40**, 528–530.

IWASAWA, Y. AND GILLIS, C. N. (1973) Effects of steroid and other hormones on lung removal of noradrenaline. *Europ. J. Pharmacol.*, **22**, 367–370.

NICOL, C. J. M. AND RAE, R. M. (1972) Inhibition of accumulation of adrenaline and noradrenaline in arterial smooth muscle by steroids. *Brit. J. Pharmacol.*, **44**, 361–362P.

POTTS, W. J. AND McKOWN, J. (1969) Effect of platform exposure duration on acquisition performance in an automated one-way avoidance procedure. *Psychol. Rep.*, **24**, 959–964.

RAAB, W. (1966) Emotional and sensory stress factors in myocardial pathology. Neurogenic and hormonal mechanisms in pathogenesis, therapy and prevention. *Amer. Heart J.*, **72**, 538–564.

Free Communications

Effect of the renin–angiotensin system on sodium appetite

EMMA CHIARAVIGLIO — *Instituto de Investigación Médica M. y M. Ferreyra, Córdoba (Argentina)*

Saline consumption by rats depleted of sodium by intraperitoneal dialysis, given a two-bottle choice test of water and 1% NaCl solution, was reduced during the 3 h following bilateral nephrectomy compared with unoperated controls. The water intake of thirsty rats was not affected by nephrectomy. Unilateral nephrectomy as well as ureteric ligature did not affect sodium intake. The intraperitoneal injection of 3 U. of renin re-established the sodium appetite abolished by nephrectomy. Angiotensin I (3 ng) or angiotensin II (5–40 ng), injected into the 3rd brain ventricle, also restored the sodium appetite. The effect was dose-dependent. The subcutaneous injection of 1 mg/kg of the angiotensin converting-enzyme inhibitor, SQ 20,881, before the intracranial administration of angiotensin, inhibited the response to angiotensin I, but not that to angiotensin II. The kidneys might, therefore, play a role in the regulation of sodium intake via the renin–angiotensin system.

Physiological mechanisms involved in psychological stress

I. T. KURTSIN — *I. P. Pavlov Institute of Physiology, Academy of Sciences U.S.S.R., Leningrad (U.S.S.R.)*

Psychological stress arises in man due to the effect of various factors on the neocortex. Physiological mechanisms underlying stress are identical in man and animals. Experiments in animals have shown that deep and prolonged psychosomatic disturbances arise from psychological stress[1]. The metabolism of acetylcholine (ACh) and other biologically active substances, activity of ACh-esterase, brain nuclease and other enzymes are altered under psychological stress. The ultrastructure of cells (membranes, cytoplasm) as well as blood flow and gaseous exchanges are disturbed under stress in limbic, premotor, and orbital zones of the cortex. These changes give rise to functional depletion of nerve cells, abnormalities in the gross activity of the CNS and corticovisceral pathology. The intensity and duration of the psychological stress may be accounted for by disturbances in (1) hormonal regulatory mechanisms, (2) vascular homeostasis, (3) permeability of histohematic barriers of the internal organs, (4) blood–brain barrier, (5) tropic processes in the cells, (6) efferent and afferent neural transmission, (7) inter-relationships between neocortex and subcortex centers[2].

1 BYKOV, K. M. AND KURTSIN, I. T., *Patologica Cortico-Visceral*, Editorial Atlante, Madrid, 1968.
2 KURTSIN, I. T., *Theoretical Bases of the Psychosomatic Medicine*, Science, Leningrad, 1973.

Inhibition of adrenocortical responses following sciatic nerve stimulation in rats with complete and partial hypothalamic deafferentation

S. FELDMAN — *Department of Neurology, Hadassah University Hospital, Jerusalem (Israel)*

Previous studies from this laboratory have demonstrated that in rats with hypothalamic islands the adrenocortical response to photic and acoustic stimulation was partially inhibited indicating that they were at least to a certain degree neurally mediated. In the same preparation anoxia, immobilization and ether-stress produced normal adrenocortical responses. With the purpose of determining to what extent afferent somatosensory connections to the hypothalamus participate in the activation of adrenocortical responses following sciatic nerve stimulation, the effects of this stimulus applied through chronically implanted electrodes were studied on plasma corticosterone levels in pentobarbital anesthetized intact animals and in rats with hypothalamic islands. A 2-min ether-stress or sciatic nerve stimulation in intact rats produced a rise of plasma corticosterone to 32.1 ± 1.2 and 32.1 ± 1.8 $\mu g/100$ ml, respectively. However, in animals with hypothalamic islands the corresponding values were 29.2 ± 1.8 and 12.4 ± 0.8 $\mu g/100$ ml, respectively. The latter value was not significantly different from the basal corticosterone levels (13.0 ± 1.2 $\mu g/100$ ml) found in rats 15 min after pentobarbital anesthesia, the time when the sciatic stimulus was applied. Partial hypothalamic deafferentation has demonstrated that the adrenocortical responses were inhibited following sciatic stimulation in rats with anterolateral and anterior cuts, however no such effects were obtained with posterior and posterolateral deafferentations.

The present data would indicate that the adrenocortical discharge following sciatic nerve stimulation is totally inhibited by complete hypothalamic deafferentation and that the afferent input is mediated by anterior neural pathways entering the hypothalamus.

Aggression and psychoneuroendocrine factors

E. TOMORUG — *Hospital "Gh. Marinescu", Bucharest (Rumania)*

Cases of aggressive acts have lately become extremely numerous. This increase in aggression is most marked among younger age groups.

In young people, aggressive incidents are more superficial in nature, whereas adults generally commit more violent actions such as attempted murder or murder.

Four hundred such cases have been analyzed from a forensic-psychiatric standpoint. It appears that states of aggressiveness both in young people and adults occur especially during periods involving a biological crisis. In most cases of aggressiveness it is possible to identify an endocrine factor. Even if this psychoneuroendocrine factor does not always play the main part, it nevertheless contributes to aggressiveness as suggested by present data.

All cases studied clearly indicated a psychoneuroendocrine disturbance. The case studies of 200 women included 43% superficial aggressive acts connected with jealousy, 37% brutal and violent actions (attempted murder and murder), 17% acts of larceny and 3% various other misdemeanors.

It is emphasized that psychoneuroendocrine disturbances are of major importance for understanding the causes of aggressiveness.

Disturbances of homeostasis by heat stress or aging and its treatment with minidoses of MAO blockers

F. G. SULMAN, Y. PFEIFER AND E. SUPERSTINE — *Bioclimatology Unit, Department of Applied Pharmacology, School of Pharmacy, Hebrew University, Jerusalem (Israel)*

We have observed that elderly patients or young people when exposed to extreme climatic heat stress can suffer from lack of adrenaline and noradrenaline. This was shown by daily urinalysis[1]. Having ascertained that the people were suffering from lack of monoamines, we found all the symptoms of catecholamine deficiency, *i.e.*, hypotension, fatigue, exhaustion, apathy, depression, lack of concentration, confusion, hypoglycemic spells, and ataxia.

We have been treating 300 patients for 5 years with minidoses of MAO blockers (1–10 mg/day). A low dosage of ¼–1 tbl/day completely cures the patients of their disability and adynamia, without any danger of a cheese tyramine reaction[2]. We have singled out the following preparations which produce relief within 30 min without producing any signs of tolerance or addiction: isocarboxazid (Marplan, Roche), mebanazine (Actomol, ICI) or tranylcypromine (Parnate, SKF).

1 SULMAN, F. G., DANON, A., PFEIFER, Y., TAL, E. AND WELLER, C. P., *Int. J. Biometeorol.*, 14 (1970) 45–53.
2 SULMAN, F. G., *Aerztl. Praxis*, 23 (1971) 998–999.

Interactions of self-stimulation behavior and some humoral factors

G. HARTMANN, M. FEKETE AND K. LISSÁK — *Institute of Physiology, University Medical School, Pécs (Hungary)*

Changes in plasma corticosterone levels, hypothalamic and mesencephalic serotonin contents, and self-stimulation (SS) behavior have been investigated in rats after electrical stimulation (ES) or SS of the medial forebrain bundle (MFB) region, and following injection of cholinergic drugs into the nucleus raphe dorsalis or the lateral ventricle.

(1) SS behavior appears first in 14–15-day-old rats.

(2) The plasma corticosterone level increased in 13–14-day-old rats following ES of MFB, and in 14–17-day-old animals following ES and SS.

(3) In 13-day-old rats the serotonin contents of the hypothalamus and mesencephalon showed no change following ES of the MFB.

(4) In 17-day-old rats the hypothalamic serotonin content increased following ES, but did not change after SS. The serotonin content of the mesencephalon in both cases increased.

(5) Cholinergic stimulation of the nucleus raphe dorsalis increased the plasma corticosterone level and the mesencephalic serotonin content in adult rats, but caused no change in the hypothalamic serotonin content. The rate of SS decreased.

(6) Cholinergic drugs injected into the lateral ventricle increased the plasma corticosterone level and decreased the hypothalamic and the mesencephalic serotonin contents, and the rate of SS.

The results indicate that both serotoninergic and cholinergic systems are important in the organization of SS behavior.

Changes in the EEG during menstrual cycle of women with and without oral contraceptives

W. WUTTKE, P. M. ARNOLD, D. BECKER, O. D. CREUTZFELDT, S. LANGENSTEIN, S. PÖPPL AND W. TIRSCH — *Max-Planck-Institute for Biophysical Chemistry, and Institute of Psychology, Göttingen (G.F.R.)*

Bipolar temporo-central EEG records were made from 32 young and healthy women at 2-day intervals. One-half of the women had spontaneous menstrual cycles, the others were under combined oral contraceptives (o. C's). A period of 2 min at the beginning and at the end of each 10 min record was analyzed and the power spectra of each period were plotted. For proper timing of the follicular and luteal phases the serum levels of LH, FSH, prolactin, progesterone and estradiol were measured by radioimmunoassays. Power-spectral analysis of the α-rhythm of the EEG revealed the following results: in spontaneously cycling women, the absolute power of the α-rhythm in the 10.5–13 Hz range (fast α-component) was about twice as high as in the 8–10.5 Hz range (slow α-component), whereas in women under o. C's the power of the fast and slow α-component was evenly distributed. Correspondingly, the α-peak-frequency was higher in women with spontaneous menstrual cycles (11.5 Hz) when compared to those under o. C's (10.9 Hz). Further analysis during the spontaneous cycles revealed increasing fast α-components during the luteal phase, *i.e.* the quotient "power of fast α-component/power of slow α-component" was smaller during the follicular phase than during the luteal phase, which correlates with the circulating serum progesterone levels. The fast α-component dropped suddenly 1–2 days before menstruation. A minor but steady acceleration of the α-peak-frequency during the luteal phase was also noted. The only cyclical changes of the α-rhythm in women under o. C's were a slight acceleration 1–2 days prior to menstruation; this is the period following discontinuation of the oral contraceptive.

Variations of performance in psychological tests during the menstrual cycle in women with and without oral contraceptives

D. BECKER, P. M. ARNOLD, O. D. CREUTZFELDT, S. LANGENSTEIN AND W. WUTTKE — *Institute of Psychology and Max-Planck-Institute for Biophysical Chemistry, Göttingen (G.F.R.)*

The same 32 young women as in the EEG study were tested for variations in automatized psychological performance tests (EPS 73). These tests covered different performances such as reaction time, concentration, integration and learning abilities. The group with spontaneous menstrual cycles performed significantly better in both speed and accuracy of all tests compared to the group under combined oral contraceptives (o. C's). During spontaneous menstrual cycles, significantly better performances were achieved during the luteal phase compared to the follicular phase. Best scores in both speed and accuracy of reaction were obtained 1–2 days prior to menstruation; thus, the ability to react fast and accurately correlated with serum progesterone levels and was also linked to the acceleration of the α-rhythm in the EEG. More complex performances such as integrating and learning ability also showed cyclical changes, whereas none of the parameters tested in women under o. C's showed any such fluctuations.

Neural and humoral interactions between basal prechiasmatic area and median eminence

Y. SAKUMA AND M. KAWAKAMI — *Department of Physiology, Yokohama City University School of Medicine, Yokohama (Japan)*

In the Wistar female rat during proestrus, two types of neuronal responses were recorded in the basal prechiasmatic area (PVA), a part of organum vasculosum laminae terminalis, following electrical stimulation of the arcuate nucleus (ARC)–median eminence (ME) region, namely, antidromic and orthodromic responses. In the antidromically activated units, high frequency stimuli inhibited somadendritic spikes and subsequent spontaneous activity. Orthodromically activated units were facilitated by the stimulation.

Microiontophoresis of LH-RH, LH, FSH, TRH and prolactin was performed on both units. LH-RH and FSH elicited inhibition in about 15% of antidromically activated units respectively, whereas LH excited about 20%. TRH and prolactin caused excitation or inhibition in 20%. None of the orthodromically activated units responded to the hormones.

These results, when taken in conjunction with our earlier observation[1] that LH-RH affected the ARC–ME activity, suggest that the responsiveness to LH-RH might characterize these structures. It also appears likely that the inhibitory effect of the ARC–ME on the PVA is mediated by an inhibitory interneuron.

1 KAWAKAMI, M. AND SAKUMA, Y., In *Proc. Workshop Conference of ISPNE, September 1973,* Karger, Basel, in press.

Session V

AMINES, STEROIDS AND THE BRAIN

ABSTRACTS OF FREE COMMUNICATIONS

Free Communications

Effect of pineal principles on avoidance and exploratory activity in the rat

G. L. Kovács, G. Telegdy and K. Lissák — *Department of Physiology, University Medical School, Pécs (Hungary)*

Melatonin (5-methoxy-N-acetyltryptamine) facilitates the extinction of conditioned active avoidance reflex and decreases the intertrial activity during extinction. However, it has no effect on learning and intertrial activity during acquisition. Pinealectomy has no effect on acquisition, extinction or intertrial activity.

Melatonin facilitates the passive avoidance behavior (thirst drive *versus* fear) in two different experimental situations. Surgical removal of the pineal gland is without effect on passive avoidance behavior.

Neither melatonin treatment nor pinealectomy has any influence on water intake or on exploratory (open-field) activity.

The action of melatonin seems to be a pharmacological rather than a physiological one. DL-*p*-chlorophenylalanine treatment, which inhibits serotonin synthesis, in the passive avoidance situation has an effect opposite to that of melatonin, suggesting that the action of melatonin might be mediated via serotonin.

Effect of midbrain raphe lesion on diurnal and stress-induced changes in serotonin content of discrete regions of the limbic system and adrenal function in the rat

K. Lissák, I. Vermes and G. Telegdy — *Department of Physiology, University Medical School, Pécs (Hungary)*

In the normal animal, the serotonin levels in the mesencephalon, hippocampus, septum, amygdala and hypothalamus showed a diurnal rhythm having the highest level between 8 h and 16 h in the mesencephalon, septum and amygdala, and between 8 h and 12 h in the hippocampus and hypothalamus. The lowest values were observed at 20 h in each brain area investigated. Plasma corticosterone showed an opposite trend having the minimum level at 8 h and maximum at 20 h.

The diurnal variation of brain serotonin and plasma corticosterone disappeared after lesion of the midbrain raphe nuclei. The serotonin level in the different brain areas investigated decreased by 50–75 % and the plasma corticosterone level increased to about three times the morning level.

The stress response was facilitated in the raphe-lesioned animal and return to the resting value was delayed. The hypothalamic serotonin level did not change during stress.

The results suggest that the mesencephalic raphe nuclei play an important role in the maintenance of the serotonin rhythm in the brain, which is in negative correlation with the diurnal adrenal rhythm.

Mechanism of reserpine-induced changes in the pituitary–gonadal axis in rats

Cs. Nyakas, Zs. Kovács and F. Tallián — *Central Research Division, Postgraduate Medical School, Budapest (Hungary)*

Reserpine treatment produced a significant reduction of the estradiol-induced increase in uterus weight in both infantile and adult ovariectomized rats. In contrast to these observations, it was found that reserpine administration resulted in an increase in pituitary hypertrophy as a result of estradiol treatment or of the introduction of estradiol into the median eminence region.

Reserpine administration to ovariectomized rats led to a significant decrease of the accumulation of labeled estradiol by the uterine slices. Similarly, the reserpine treatment produced an inhibition of the estradiol uptake by the nuclear fraction of the uterus.

Pituitary uptake of labeled estradiol was significantly higher following reserpine administration than in untreated ovariectomized rats. Moreover, it was found that reserpine administration resulted in an increased accumulation of estradiol by the nuclear fraction of the pituitary under *in vitro* conditions.

It is assumed that reserpine exerts its influence on the transfer of cytosol receptor–steroid complex into the nuclear compartment. This influence seems to be opposite in the pituitary and the uterus under both *in vivo* and *in vitro* conditions.

Comparison of binding of [³H]corticosterone and [³H]dexamethasone by rat brain cytosol

B. I. Grosser, D. J. Reed and W. Stevens — *Departments of Psychiatry, Pharmacology, and Anatomy, University of Utah College of Medicine, Salt Lake City, Utah (U.S.A.)*

A protein "receptor" for corticosterone (B_k) has been demonstrated in cytoplasm and nuclei of rat brain. Since dexamethasone (D_x) has important central nervous system effects, it is important to determine whether there are specific receptor molecules for D_x and whether these are the same as the receptors for B_k. Adult male adrenalectomized (adrex) or non-adrenalectomized (intact) rats were perfused ventriculocisternally with $[1,2,4-^3H]D_x$ (0.1 μg/ml, spec. act., 30 Ci/mmole). After a 1 h perfusion, the animals were sacrificed and brain cytosols were prepared. Binding was determined by chromatography on Sephadex G-25. In the adrex rats, 11,069 disint./min/mg protein were bound whereas the comparable figure for intact rats was only 404 disint./min/mg protein indicating that the available binding sites were filled by endogenous B_k. Data obtained from competitive binding experiments *in vitro* appear to indicate a difference in the binding characteristics of "receptor sites" for $[^3H]D_x$ and $[^3H]B_k$. From Scatchard plots, the K_{dissoc} of $[^3H]D_x$ was 4.2×10^{-10} M and 0.24 pmoles were bound/mg protein. The comparable figures for $[^3H]B_k$ were 2.7×10^{-10} M and 0.47 pmoles/mg protein. The cytosol from hippocampus bound more $[^3H]D_x$ and $[^3H]B_k$ than comparable fractions from other brain regions.

Supported by 5-K02 MH 18270, NS 07761, 5-K3-NB7779, NB-04554, and U.S.A.E. C. Contract AT(11-1)-119.

Influence of hypothalamic extract on the uptake of steroid hormones by the anterior pituitary gland in rats

I. HEGEDÜS AND E. ENDRÖCZI — *Central Research Division, Postgraduate Medical School, Budapest (Hungary)*

Incubation of the acid extract of median eminence tissue with anterior pituitary gland produced a marked increase in the accumulation of labeled estradiol and corticosterone by the pituitary. It was found that the binding capacity of the nuclear fraction increased to a greater extent than that of the cytosol fraction. Using the same quantity of median eminence extract, a greater increase in estradiol uptake resulted than could be observed in the case of corticosterone uptake.

Lysine-8-vasopressin did not induce changes in the accumulation of labeled steroids by the anterior pituitary gland under *in vitro* conditions. Larger doses of vasopressin produced a slight suppression of estradiol uptake.

On studying the mechanism of the effect of the median eminence extract, it was concluded that the active principle(s) exert their influence on the transfer of the cytosol receptor–steroid complex into the nuclear compartment. Further investigations are required to decide whether the effect is closely related to the action of hypothalamic factors or whether it may be attributed to a non-specific stimulatory effect of the hypothalamic extract on the steroid uptake of the anterior pituitary gland.

Regulation of estradiol-binding receptor synthesis at the hypothalamic–pituitary–gonad level in rats

I. MARTON, G. SZABÓ, Á. HRASCHEK AND E. ENDRÖCZI — *Central Research Division, Postgraduate Medical School, Budapest (Hungary)*

Estradiol uptake by the uterus showed a significant increase during the first postnatal week, followed by a decline in the consecutive period. This increase could be attributed to an increase in the cytosol receptor sites, and it could be observed after ovariectomy. It was found that the administration of estradiol to ovariectomized rats produced an increase in the binding capacity of the cytosol fraction for estradiol when the uptake was tested 16–24 h after the last injection. These findings indicated that estradiol has a facilitatory influence on the synthesis of estradiol-binding receptor in the uterus, anterior pituitary and the hypothalamus. After a transient increase in estradiol-binding capacity of the cytosol fraction, there is a significant decline in estradiol uptake by the target tissues.

It was found that the pituitary gonadotropins play a role in controlling estradiol receptor synthesis. Administration of pituitary FSH or HCG to ovariectomized rats resulted in a marked influence on the estradiol-binding capacity of the cytosol fraction at the hypothalamic–pituitary–uterus level. A complex feedback regulation of the synthesis of estradiol receptors by estrogens and gonadotropins is assumed at the cellular level of the target organs.

Metabolism of androstenedione and testosterone in human fetal brain

ADOLF E. SCHINDLER* — *Universitäts-Frauenklinik, 74 Tübingen (G.F.R.)*

Since extraglandular steroid metabolism may play an important role in target organ functions, the metabolism of androstenedione (A) and testosterone (T) was measured in cerebral and hypothalamic tissue from 38 human male and female fetuses between the 9th and 40th week of gestation.

The conversions of A to estrone (E_1) and T to 5α-dihydrotestosterone (DHT) were measured by double isotope methods previously described (Schindler and Friedrich[1]). Isolation, identification and quantitation of E_1 and DHT were carried out by celite column chromatography, thin-layer chromatography, acetylation and repeated crystallization to constant isotope ratio.

The conversion of A to E_1 was significantly lower in cerebral tissue (0.016%) than in hypothalamic tissue (0.479%). For the conversion of T to DHT the evaluation of the data according to the sex of the fetus did reveal a higher conversion of male hypothalamic tissue (4.6%) *versus* female hypothalamic tissue (3.4%). In the cerebrum, no difference was found.

Comparing male cerebrum and hypothalamus the 5α-reductase activity was found to be higher in hypothalamic tissue (4.46% *versus* 1.63%). Such a difference was not seen in female fetuses (3.70% *versus* 2.13%).

The data indicate a distinct difference between cerebrum and hypothalamus for essential steps in extraglandular steroid metabolism. Together with the peculiarities of HCG (human chorecnic gonadotropin) production during human pregnancy these metabolic events may play an important role in the intrauterine development of these endocrine and paraendocrine tissues.

1 SCHINDLER, A. E. AND FRIEDRICH, *Acta endocr. (Kbh.)*, Suppl. 177 (1973) 177.

* Supported by DFG (Schi 129/1).

EARLY HORMONAL INFLUENCES ON ONTOGENESIS OF BEHAVIOR AND BRAIN DEVELOPMENT

Chairmen: R. ADER (Rochester, N.Y., U.S.A.)
A. SOULAIRAC (Paris, France)

Neonatal Stimulation and Maturation of the 24-Hour Adrenocortical Rhythm

ROBERT ADER

Department of Psychiatry, University of Rochester School of Medicine and Dentistry, Rochester, N.Y. 14642 (U.S.A.)

Experimentally imposed stimulation of the infant rat during the first 3 weeks of life is capable of modifying a variety of developmental processes, subsequent behaviors and physiological function, and ultimate susceptibility to experimentally induced organic disease (Ader, 1970; Denenberg, 1972). Based on the consistent finding that infant rats subjected to handling or electric shock stimulation show a reduced adreno-cortical response to "stress" experienced later in life, several attempts have been made to relate adult adrenocortical and emotional reactivity to the release of steroids by the neonate in response to the stimulation or "stress" experienced during development (Levine and Mullins, 1966; Denenberg and Zarrow, 1971). A critical review of this literature has been presented in a previous volume in this series (Ader and Grota, 1973).

Thus far the effects of early life experiences on subsequent adrenal function have been primarily concerned with adrenocortical *reactivity*. "Reactivity", however, is a difficult dimension of adrenal function to define. Several studies (*e.g.*, Zarrow *et al.*, 1966, 1967; Ader *et al.*, 1967; Friedman and Ader, 1967; Ader and Friedman, 1968) have shown that the adrenocortical response to environmental stimulation is determined by a complex interaction among several factors. These include the nature of the stimulus used to elicit an adrenal response, the duration or intensity of that stimulation, the time following stimulation when steroid samples are obtained, and the point in the 24-hr adrenocortical rhythm upon which the stimulation is superimposed. One might also question the criteria defining "reactivity". Is "reactivity" reflected by the magnitude of the adrenocortical response, the latency of the responses and/or the duration of the elevation in steroid level? All of the above factors are relevant in defining and evaluating adrenocortical reactivity, particularly if one is interested in comparing differentially treated groups of animals. In view of these practical issues, studies of the neuroendocrine mediation of the behavioral and physiological effects of early life experiences become difficult to execute and to interpret. Many of these difficulties may be circumvented by studying the development of normal endocrine function. That is, by analyzing the effects of early experiences on the maturation of normal biologic processes one can obviate the need to make a series of essentially arbitrary decisions. More positively, the study of neuroendocrine development might also be expected to generate additional hypotheses regarding the means by which early life experiences influence subsequent psychophysiological processes. Instead of measuring the adrenocortical response to some environmental stimulus or stressor, we were, therefore, led to a study of the effects of early life experiences on the development of the 24-hr rhythm in adrenocortical activity.

An outstanding characteristic of normal endocrine function is its daily rhythm. Such circadian rhythms are thought to be endogenous and merely synchronized by environmental cues, the most prepotent of which is the daily light–dark cycle. Nevertheless, these rhythms are not necessarily present at birth. Presumably, the development and maintenance of normal rhythmicity depend upon the functional maturation and integrity of central nervous system areas which are presently unknown or incompletely defined.

In the nocturnal rat, maintained under a 12-hr light–dark cycle, there is a precise 24-hr rhythm in adrenocortical activity. Plasma corticosterone levels are at their maximum approximately 2 hr before the 12-hr period of darkness begins and at their nadir approximately 2 hr before the onset of the 12-hr period of light (*e.g.*, Guillemin *et al.*, 1959; Critchlow *et al.*, 1963; Saba *et al.*, 1963; Ader *et al.*, 1967). Infant rats were sampled at these times in the light–dark cycle to determine when, during the course of development, the adrenocortical rhythm could first be observed (Ader, 1969). Experimentally naive animals were reared in modified office cabinets which provided for independent control of light–dark cycles. Under these conditions rhythmicity was first evident at 21 days of age. The difference between values sampled 2 hr before darkness and 2 hr before light gradually increased to the magnitude seen in adult animals. The characteristic sex difference in steroid levels developed sometime after 21 days and was evident in samples obtained when the animals were 30 days old. Although the development of rhythmicity at approximately 3 weeks of age is considerably earlier than had previously been observed (Allen and Kendall, 1967), these observations have been confirmed by Hiroshige and Sato (1970a) and by Krieger (1973).

In a second study (Ader, 1969), litters of rats born within a 24-hr period were split, randomly reassigned to mothers in litters of 10 animals, and randomly divided into handled, shocked, and control groups. This entire population was housed in an open colony room. Handled animals were removed individually from the nest and simply held in the experimenter's hand for a period of 3 min daily up to but not including the day of sacrifice. Shocked animals were subjected to 3 min of daily electric shock stimulation (0.1 mA increasing with age to a maximum of 1.0 mA) through the grid floor of a separate chamber. Control animals remained undisturbed. Randomly selected litters of handled, shocked, and control animals were sacrificed at 16, 18, 20, 22, and 25 days of age. Trunk blood was collected and plasma levels of corticosterone were assayed according to the method of Glick *et al.* (1964) as modified in our laboratory (Friedman *et al.*, 1967).

The results of this study are shown in Fig. 1. The unmanipulated control animals did not show any evidence of rhythmicity until 25 days of age. The difference between these data and those of the preceding experiment might be a reflection of the greater

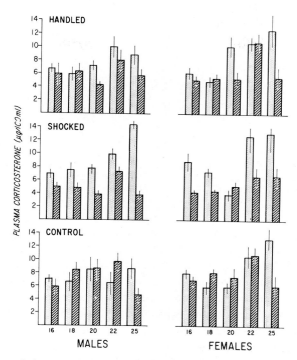

Fig. 1. Development of the 24-hr rhythm in adrenocortical activity in handled, shocked, and undisturbed control rats reared under a 12-hr light–dark cycle (from Ader, 1969). Light bars = crest values obtained 2 hr before dark; hatched bars = trough values obtained 2 hr before light; vertical lines = standard error of the mean. Mean values are based on groups of 8–17 animals. (Reprinted by permission of the American Association for the Advancement of Science.)

degree of environmental control afforded by the separate office cabinets used to house the animals in contrast to the housing of these litters in the usual open colony room.

In contrast to the control group, handled animals showed a significant difference between the steroid values obtained 2 hr before the onset of darkness and 2 hr before the onset of light at 20 days of age, but there was no significant difference at 22 days of age. At 25 days the rhythm was again evident. The failure to uncover a difference at 22 days appears to be due to the relatively high steroid level observed during the period of darkness. Since relatively innocuous stimulation superimposed upon the trough in the 24-hr adrenal cycle is sufficient to cause a significant elevation in corticosterone level (Ader *et al.*, 1967; Ader and Friedman, 1968), this inconsistency in the data may have been the result of extraneous stimulation.

With the single exception of the group of females sampled at 20 days of age, animals that had been subjected to daily electric shock stimulation showed a consistent rhythm in corticosterone concentrations beginning at 16 days of age. Electric shock stimulation experienced during the first 2 weeks of life had, then, accelerated the development of the 24-hr light-synchronized rhythm in adrenocortical activity.

The animals that experienced handling or electric shock were stimulated at approximately the same time each day. It was possible, therefore, that such repetitive stimula-

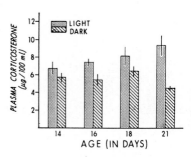

Fig. 2. Development of the 24-hr rhythm in adrenocortical activity in animals reared under a 12-hr light–dark cycle and subjected to electric shock stimulation at random times on each of the first 14 days of life.

tion could have served as a cue to 24 hr and facilitated the development of rhythmicity by virtue of its significance as a "time giver" rather than as neurogenic stimulation, *per se*. To eliminate this possibility an additional population of animals was subjected to electric shock stimulation at a different time each day. As can be seen in Fig. 2, a consistent rhythm in steroid levels was again observed beginning at 16 days of age. These data indicated that early life experiences, particularly electric shock stimulation, could influence the development of the 24-hr adrenocortical rhythm, a basic biologic process and a hormonal system with wide ranging influence on behavioral as well as physiologic processes. In order to further define the parameters of stimulation that might be optimal in accelerating this maturational process, the next experiment investigated the effects of different frequencies of stimulation experienced during the first 2 weeks of life on development of the 24-hr light-synchronized rhythm in adrenocortical activity.

In order to maintain a constant time for sampling, half the population of pregnant rats were housed under a 12-hr light–dark schedule that was 180° out of phase with the remaining animals. At parturition the litters within a single light–dark schedule were randomly redistributed to the lactating females in litters of 8–10 pups. Four litters each were randomly assigned to groups in which the pups were subjected to a 3-min period of electric shock stimulation every other day, once daily, twice daily, or to a control group which remained unmanipulated. Stimulation was imposed during the first 2 weeks of life. On days 14, 16, 18, 21 and 25 two complete litters were decapitated either 2 hr before the lights went off or 2 hr before the lights went on, *i.e.*, at the crest and trough, respectively, of the adult rat's 24-hr adrenocortical cycle.

As before, control animals did not display adrenocortical rhythmicity until 25 days of age. For the animals that were stimulated every other day, the crest values were higher than the trough values at the 0.10 level on days 18 and 21, but did not reach a statistically significant level until 25 days. Animals subjected to a single daily period of stimulation displayed an accelerated development of adrenocortical rhythmicity; there was a consistent difference between crest and trough values beginning at 16 days of age. In animals stimulated twice daily, crest values were significantly higher than trough values beginning at 18 days of age.

The development of adrenocortical rhythmicity at 25 days in unmanipulated control animals and an accelerated maturation in animals subjected to a single daily period of stimulation replicates our previous data. Beyond this, the findings of this experiment suggest that less frequent stimulation during infancy is less effective in accelerating this developmental process, but such infrequent stimulation does have some facilitating effect. Stimulation twice each day, however, did not further influence the rate of development of the adrenocortical rhythm. The observation that animals stimulated twice daily did not evidence rhythmicity until 18 days (*i.e.*, after the animals stimulated once each day) could suggest that there is a curvilinear function relating amount of stimulation during infancy to developmental processes. This would be consistent with observations of a curvilinear function relating the intensity or frequency of early stimulation to adult emotional reactivity (Ader, 1966; Goldman, 1969). Such a common relationship should not, however, be taken to imply that there is any necessary relationship between adrenocortical rhythmicity and emotional reactivity in the rat.

In a further effort to define the conditions under which early life experiences would accelerate maturation of the light-synchronized adrenocortical rhythm, a study was designed to determine if there was a "critical" or sensitive period during which stimulation would be maximally effective in accelerating development. Randomly selected split litters of rats were subjected to 3 min of electric shock stimulation each day during the first week of life, during the second week of life, or during the first and second weeks of life. Control litters remained totally undisturbed. At 16, 18, 20, and 22 days of age randomly selected litters from each group were sacrificed either 2 hr

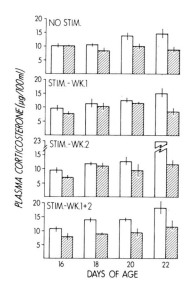

Fig. 3. Development of the 24-hr rhythm in adrenocortical activity in rats subjected to electric shock stimulation during different periods of early life. Light bars = crest values; hatched bars = trough values. Mean values are based on groups of 4–10 litters.

before the lights went on or 2 hr before the lights went off in the 12-hr light–dark schedule. The results are shown in Fig. 3.

Unmanipulated control animals evidenced adrenocortical rhythmicity at 20 days of age which is somewhat earlier than usual for our animals that are maintained in an open colony room. In the animals that experienced electric shock stimulation during the first 2 weeks of life the difference between crest and trough values reached statistically significant levels beginning at 18 days of age, which is somewhat later than had been observed previously. Nonetheless, as before, the animals that had been stimulated showed the expected accelerated maturation of adrenocortical rhythmicity relative to unmanipulated controls. Electric shock stimulation experienced only during the first week of life or only during the second week of life was not sufficient to accelerate the development of rhythmicity; neither of these groups showed evidence of a daily rhythm until 22 days of age.

It would appear, then, that stimulation throughout the first 2 weeks of life is necessary for the accelerated development of the 24-hr adrenocortical rhythm and that there is no evidence for a single period within the first 2 weeks of life when environmental stimulation is especially effective in accelerating rhythmicity. The previous experiment indicated that increasing the amount (*i.e.*, the number of periods of daily stimulation) experienced by the animals did not further accelerate rhythmicity or provide for a more delineated rhythm than was obtained from a single period of daily stimulation. In this instance, however, what now appears to have been a relatively moderate amount of stimulation was distributed over the first 2 weeks of life. The possibility remains, therefore, that a major increase in the amount or intensity of stimulation experienced during a shorter period of time could reveal a "critical" period for the effects of stimulation on the maturation of adrenal rhythmicity. It is likely, however, that normal anatomic or functional development within the central nervous system may place a limit on maturation rate.

Although the present data provide no evidence for a critical period for the effects of early experience on maturation of the 24-hr adrenocortical rhythm, they have consistently shown that stimulation of the infant rat during the first 2 weeks of life can accelerate the development of this rhythm and, presumably, other rhythmic phenomena. While these studies derived from observations of reduced adrenocortical reactivity in animals stimulated during early life, the present data on accelerated maturation of adrenal function may have no bearing on the mechanisms underlying attenuated adrenocortical reactivity. Several studies have directly or indirectly indicated that different mechanisms appear to be responsible for the ontogenesis of periodicity and the ontogenesis of adrenal responsiveness to environmental or "stressful" stimulation.

The means by which early life experiences might hasten the display of rhythmicity remain unknown. There are, however, some parallel data which are of interest and, perhaps, of some import. For example, Hiroshige and Sato (1970a, b) have shown that, like corticosterone, the circadian rhythm in hypothalamic corticotropin-releasing factor (CRF) also develops during the third week of life in the rat. While plasma corticosterone levels typically follow changes in CRF activity in the hypothalamus, the circadian rhythm in CRF is not controlled by a feedback mechanism. It is evidently under direct control of the central nervous system since the rhythm in CRF activity is present in hypophysectomized as well as in adrenalectomized animals (Hiroshige and Sakakura, 1971; Seiden and Brodish, 1972). Such data suggest that stimulation of the infant rat could be influencing maturation within the central nervous system.

Krieger (1973) has shown that a light–dark cycle is necessary for the development and maintenance of normal periodicity in adrenal activity and that the eyes are necessary for the expression of such rhythmicity. Light must, then, be processed by the central nervous system. In this connection, it is of interest to note that Fiske and Leeman (1964) found that neurosecretory material in the supraoptic and paraventricular nuclei of the hypothalamus begins to appear between 14 and 18 days of age which is about the time that the eyes open in the infant rat. By 22 days of age the entire neurosecretory system was functioning actively. As these authors pointed out, "a marked development of the neurosecretory system occurred just as the diurnal corticosteroid rhythm was initiated." (p. 237). More recently, Campbell and Ramaley (1974) were able to demonstrate a relationship between the development of the 24-hr light-synchronized adrenocortical rhythm and changes in visual input to the hypothalamus. Direct retinohypothalamic projections to the suprachiasmatic nuclei were first observed when the rat was about 17 days of age.

Given the temporal relationship between anatomical and functional maturation within the central nervous system and the ontogeny of adrenocortical rhythmicity, it seems possible that the environmental stimulation experienced by the infant rat may be accelerating maturation by accelerating the development of sensory capacity and/or by accelerating anatomical and/or functional development within the central nervous system. There are some data which indicate that early life experiences can influence development of the central nervous system. Using the amount of cholesterol present in whole brain as a reflection of the process of myelination, Levine and Alpert (1959) observed a more rapid development in rats subjected to a handling procedure than in undisturbed controls. Schapiro and Vukovich (1970) studied the development of dendritic spines of cortical pyramidal cells. In the rats subjected to a variety of sensory stimuli several times each day, there was an accelerated development reflected in an increase in the number of dendritic spines observable at 8 days of age and an increase in the number of neurons staining at 8–16 days. It was suggested that the accelerated development of dendritic spines could represent a neuroanatomical basis for the effects of early stimulation upon subsequent behavioral processes.

The present data indicate that early life experiences are capable of accelerating the development of adrenocortical rhythmicity. There is no evidence, however, for a critical period for this effect of early stimulation — at least in terms of the brief daily stimulation that has been used thus far. Still, there is accelerated rhythmicity. To the extent that the development and maintenance of the adrenocortical rhythm are a reflection of integrated neuroendocrine function, stimulation during early life would appear to be facilitating the maturation of neuroendocrine mechanisms which, if not directly controlling periodicity, are necessary for the expression of rhythmic processes.

References p. 340–341

SUMMARY

The 24-hr light-synchronized rhythm in plasma levels of corticosterone is first observed in experimentally naive rats between 22 and 25 days of age. Environmental stimulation of the infant rat by handling or, particularly, electric shock stimulation accelerates development of the adrenocortical rhythm. In animals subjected to daily electric shock stimulation rhythmicity is apparent by 16 days of age. Stimulation experienced every other day during the first 2 weeks of life is not quite as effective as daily stimulation, nor does an increase in the frequency of stimulation further accelerate development. Stimulation during the first, second, or first and second weeks of life uncovered no evidence for a "critical" period for the effects of early experiences on the accelerated maturation of adrenocortical rhythmicity.

Normal development of the adrenal rhythm is associated with maturational processes within the central nervous system. Although the mechanism remains unknown, it is suggested that early life experiences influence the development of these processes which are necessary for the expression of rhythmic phenomena.

ACKNOWLEDGEMENTS

Preparation of this manuscript and research conducted by the author were supported by U.S.P.H.S. Grant MH-16,741 and a Research Scientist Award (MH-6318) from the National Institute of Mental Health, and a research grant from the Grant Foundation, Inc.

REFERENCES

ADER, R. (1966) Frequency of stimulation during early life and subsequent emotionality in the rat. *Psychol. Rep.*, **18**, 695–701.

ADER, R. (1969) Early experiences accelerate maturation of the 24-hour adrenocortical rhythm. *Science*, **163**, 1225–1226.

ADER, R. (1970) The effects of early life experiences on developmental processes and susceptibility to disease in animals. In *Minnesota Symposium on Child Psychology*, J. P. HILL (Ed.), Univ. of Minnesota Press, Minneapolis, Minn., pp. 3–35.

ADER, R. AND FRIEDMAN, S. B. (1968) Plasma corticosterone response to environmental stimulation: effects of duration of stimulation and the 24-hour adrenocortical rhythm. *Neuroendocrinology*, **3**, 378–386.

ADER, R., FRIEDMAN, S. B. AND GROTA, L. J. (1967) "Emotionality" and adrenal cortical function: effects of strain, test, and the 24-hour corticosterone rhythm. *Anim. Behav.*, **15**, 37–44.

ADER, R. AND GROTA, L. J. (1973) Adrenocortical mediation of the effects of early life experiences. In *Drug Effects on Neuroendocrine Regulation, Progress in Brain Research*, Vol. 39, E. ZIMMERMANN, W. H. GISPEN, B. H. MARKS AND D. DE WIED (Eds.), Elsevier, Amsterdam, pp. 395–405.

ALLEN, C. AND KENDALL, J. W. (1967) Maturation of the circadian rhythm of plasma corticosterone in the rat. *Endocrinology*, **80**, 926–930.

CAMPBELL, C. B. G. AND RAMALEY, J. A. (1974) Retinohypothalamic projections: correlations with onset of the adrenal rhythm in infant rats. *Endocrinology*, **94**, 1201–1204.

CRITCHLOW, V., LIEBELT, R. A., BAR-SELA, M., MOUNTCASTLE, W. AND LIPSCOMB, H. D. (1963) Sex differences in resting pituitary-adrenal function in the rat. *Amer. J. Physiol.*, **205**, 807–815.

DENENBERG, V. H. (Ed.) (1972) *The Development of Behavior*, Sinauer, Stanford, Conn.

DENENBERG, V. H. AND ZARROW, M. X. (1971) Effects of handling in infancy upon adult behavior and adrenocortical activity: suggestions for a neuroendocrine mechanism. In *Early Childhood: the Development of Self-Regulatory Mechanisms*, D. H. WALCHER AND D. L. PETERS (Eds.), Academic Press, New York, pp. 39–64.

FISKE, V. M. AND LEEMAN, S. (1964) Observations on adrenal rhythmicity and associated phenomena in the rat: effect of light on adrenocortical functions; maturation of the hypothalamic neurosecretory system in relation to adrenal secretion. *Ann. N.Y. Acad. Sci.*, **117**, 231–240.

FRIEDMAN, S. B. AND ADER, R. (1967) Adrenocortical response to novelty and noxious stimulation. *Neuroendocrinology*, **2**, 209–212.

FRIEDMAN, S. B., ADER, R., GROTA, L. J. AND LARSON, T. (1967) Plasma corticosterone response to parameters of electric shock stimulation in the rat. *Psychosom. Med.*, **29**, 323–328.

GLICK, D., VON REDLICH, D. AND LEVINE, S. (1964) Fluorometric determination of corticosterone and cortisol in 0.02–0.05 milliliters of plasma or submilligram samples of adrenal tissue. *Endocrinology*, **74**, 653–655.

GOLDMAN, P. S. (1969) The relationship between amount of stimulation in infancy and subsequent emotionality. *Ann. N.Y. Acad. Sci.*, **159**, 640–650.

GUILLEMIN, R., DEAR, W. E. AND LIEBELT, R. (1959) Nychthermal variations in plasma free corticosteroid levels of the rat. *Proc. Soc. exp. Biol. (N.Y.)*, **101**, 394–395.

HIROSHIGE, T. AND SAKAKURA, M. (1971) Circadian rhythm of corticotropin-releasing activity in the hypothalamus of normal and adrenalectomized rats. *Neuroendocrinology*, **7**, 25–36.

HIROSHIGE, T. AND SATO, T. (1970a) Circadian rhythm and stress-induced changes in hypothalamic content of corticotropin-releasing activity during postnatal development in the rat. *Endocrinology*, **86**, 1184–1186.

HIROSHIGE, T. AND SATO, T. (1970b) Postnatal development of circadian rhythm of corticotropin-releasing activity in the rat hypothalamus. *Endocr. jap.*, **17**, 1–6.

KRIEGER, D. T. (1973) Effect of ocular enucleation and altered lighting regimens at various ages on the circadian periodicity of plasma corticosteroid levels in the rat. *Endocrinology*, **93**, 1077–1091.

LEVINE, S. AND ALPERT, M. (1959) Differential maturation of the central nervous system as a function of early experience. *Arch. gen. Psychiat.*, **1**, 403–405.

LEVINE, S. AND MULLINS, JR., R. J. (1966) Hormonal influence on brain organization in infant rats. *Science*, **152**, 1585–1592.

SABA, G. S., SABA, P., CARNICELLI, A. AND MARESCOTTI, V. (1963) Diurnal rhythm in the adrenal cortical secretion and in the rate of metabolism of corticosterone in the rat. I. In normal animals. *Acta endocr. (Kbh.)*, **44**, 409–412.

SCHAPIRO, S. AND VUKOVICH, K. R. (1970) Early experience effects upon cortical dendrites: a proposed model for development. *Science*, **167**, 292–294.

SEIDEN, G. AND BRODISH, A. (1972) Persistence of a diurnal rhythm in hypothalamic corticotropin-releasing factor (CRF) in the absence of hormone feedback. *Endocrinology*, **90**, 1401–1403.

ZARROW, M. X., DENENBERG, V. H., HALTMEYER, G. C. AND BRUMAGHIN, J. T. (1967) Plasma and adrenal corticosterone levels following exposure of the two-day-old rat to various stressors. *Proc. Soc. exp. Biol. (N.Y.)*, **125**, 113–116.

ZARROW, M. X., HALTMEYER, G. C., DENENBERG, V. H. AND THATCHER, J. (1966) Response of the infantile rat to stress. *Endocrinology*, **79**, 631–634.

Neuroendocrine Effects of Perinatal Androgenization in the Male Ferret

M. J. BAUM AND P. SCHRETLEN

Department of Endocrinology, Growth and Reproduction, Medical Faculty, Erasmus University, Rotterdam (The Netherlands)

INTRODUCTION

It is widely believed that the tonic pattern of gonadotropin secretion and testicular function characteristic of adult males of such species as the mouse, rat and guinea pig develops only if the brain is exposed to androgen during a critical perinatal period (reviewed by Barraclough, 1967; Johnson, 1972). In contrast to these rodent species, the male ferret, like its female counterpart, displays an annual cycle of reproductive activity (Allanson, 1932; Bissonnette, 1935; Rust and Shackelford, 1969). The present experiment was conducted to see whether (a) related annual fluctuations in testosterone secretion and the display of sexual behavior occur in male ferrets, and whether (b) the administration of androgen during perinatal life would in any way disrupt the male ferret's normal capacity to display annual reproductive cycles in adulthood.

MATERIALS AND METHODS

Animals

Male albino ferrets were born in the laboratory during the summer of 1971 and were reared under "short-day" photoperiod (lights on between 08.30 and 16.30 hr) in groups of 2–3 males as described previously (Baum and Goldfoot, 1974). Three groups of males were used: for one group 7 pregnant females were injected s.c. with 5 mg testosterone propionate (TP) on days 16–21 and with 1 mg TP on days 22–34 of the 42-day gestation period. Five of these females delivered live litters; however, postnatal mortality was high in these as well as in litters from other, untreated mothers used to form the other groups. All surviving offspring of TP-treated mothers received a single injection of 1 mg TP 3 days after birth. Four males so treated (from 3 litters) were successfully weaned and used in the experiment. A second group of 4 males born of untreated mothers received 1 mg TP s.c. 3 days after birth and a third group of 9 control males from 3 litters received no perinatal TP injections. Five of these control ferrets (nos. 10, 11, 12, 14 and 31) received a sham-lesion of the hypothalamus at

References p. 354–355

16 weeks of age in conjunction with another experiment (Baum and Goldfoot, 1974), and 4 control males, one of which died at age 33 weeks, underwent no brain operation.

Blood collection and testosterone estimation

Males were anesthetized with sodium pentobarbitone, and 1–4 ml blood was withdrawn from the right ophthalmic venous plexus into a heparinized glass tube. Samples were stored at $-15\,°C$ prior to being assayed for testosterone content using the radio-immunoassay described by Verjans *et al.* (1973). Briefly, the procedure was as follows: each sample was assayed in duplicate using 10–1000 μl blood. Following addition of internal standard [1,2-^{3}H]testosterone, the samples were extracted with 1 ml *n*-hexane–ether (4:1, v/v) for 1 min with a Vortex mixer, centrifuged, and the super-natants collected. Samples for the standard curve were prepared in duplicate by dissolving [1,2-^{3}H]testosterone together with known amounts of unlabeled testosterone (0, 20, 50, 100, 150, 250, 500 and 750 pg) in 1 ml *n*-hexane–ether, and these were treated the same way as the unknown samples. Extracts of all samples were chromato-graphed on alumina microcolumns in order to eliminate steroids such as 5α-dihydro-testosterone which otherwise would have cross-reacted with testosterone in the assay. Recovery of [1,2-^{3}H]testosterone after extraction and chromatography was $72.8 \pm 0.3\%$ (mean $\pm$ S.E.M.). Incubation of the samples with antiserum and separation of bound and free testosterone using dextran-coated charcoal were performed as described by Verjans *et al.* (1973). The concentration of testosterone in unknown blood samples was read directly off the standard curve and corrected for recovery and sample volume. The concentrations of testosterone measured in samples of male ferret blood using this radioimmunoassay correlated highly with values for the same samples obtained with a gas chromatographic method using electron capture detection of testosterone heptafluorobutyrate (Baum and Goldfoot, 1974) (for 28 blood samples $r = 0.89$, $P < 0.01$).

Procedure

Ferrets were inspected and weighed weekly beginning at 6 weeks of age. As soon as it could be found, each testis was rated for size by palpating it and comparing this impression with a set of 8 clay models. Each animal received a single weekly testicular rating ranging from 1 (smallest) to 8 (largest). In males with completely descended testes the rating assigned was the mean of the two testes' ratings. In other ferrets descent of the testes was incomplete, and the rating assigned was the larger of the individual's two ratings. The occurrence of both growth and color changes of the pelage was also noted weekly. As will be seen in Fig. 1, all ferrets were hemicastrated in May 1973 toward the end of the second season of maximal testicular ratings in order to obtain material for histological examination. In September 1973 the photo-period was switched from "short" to "long days" (lights on between 20.00 and 12.00 hr) in an attempt to hasten a final period of testicular recrudescence. The remaining testis was removed at the end of February 1974, after recrudescence and subsequent regression had occurred. Testes were fixed in Susa solution, sectioned at 5 μm, mounted and stained using the periodic acid–fuchsin sulfurous acid technique.

Each ferret received tests of sexual behavior beginning at 4 months of age and continuing at monthly intervals until intromission first occurred or until a regression in testicular size to a minimal rating had occurred. Males were tested with a female in natural estrus in a large box with a Plexiglass front and a mirror positioned beneath it to enable viewing of the animals' ventral surface. Several parameters of the male's mating behavior (listed under Results) were scored using an event recorder. Tests were scheduled to the last 15 min; however, if a male displayed pelvic thrusting the test was extended to 30 min or until intromission was achieved, whereupon the test was terminated. Males which displayed an initial intromission were retested in subsequent weeks with an estrous female in an *ad libitum* test which was terminated 15 min after the male spontaneously stopped intromitting with the female. In addition each male received 3 mating tests spaced over 1 week: (a) during the first period of testicular regression when testicular size was rated at 4 or less, and (b) after full recrudescence of the testes when testicular ratings had reattained the maximum achieved previously during the first period of reproductive activity. Ferrets which failed to intromit in any of these tests were given daily s.c. injections of TP (5 mg/kg in 0.1 ml oil) for 17 days after they had been hemicastrated and had shown maximal testicular ratings in response to "long-day" photoperiod (Fig. 1). Each of these males received a 1-hr test of sexual behavior on each of the last 2 days of TP treatment.

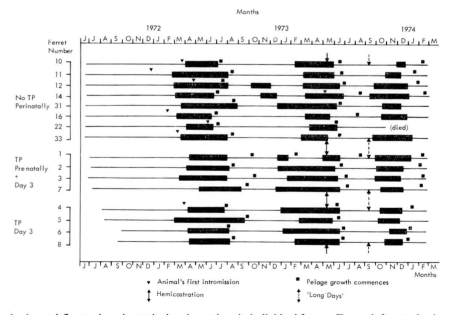

Fig. 1. Annual fluctuations in testicular size ratings in individual ferrets. For each ferret a horizontal line begins at the date of birth and indicates periods when the testicular size ratings were less than that animal's maximal value. A horizontal bar indicates periods when the testicular size ratings were maximal. "Short-day" photoperiod prevailed prior to the switch to "long days" in September 1973.

Blood samples were collected 24 hr after each of the initial monthly tests of sexual behavior. If an animal failed to achieve intromission during these 5 months, behavioral tests were continued and an additional blood collection was performed 24 hr after any initial intromission which occurred. In addition, a blood sample was collected from each animal 24 hr after the last of the 3 behavioral tests given both at the time of initial regression and following initial recrudescence of the testes.

RESULTS

Annual changes in testicular size and pelage growth

The testes of all ferrets were first palpable at an age of 8–9 weeks. In males which received TP on day 3 it was found that at least one testis (in two ferrets both testes) failed to descend completely into the scrotum. These incompletely descended testes were all palpable in the subcutaneous fat of the groin, and they showed annual changes in rated size while in this position. Fig. 1 shows that annual changes in testicular size ratings occurred in all animals, regardless of whether or not TP had been administered perinatally. Maximal testicular ratings in the ferrets of all 3 groups ranged from 6 to 8, and minimal ratings ranged from 3 to 4. For some unknown reason, a very brief period of recrudescence occurred in two control males and in one prenatally + day 3 TP-treated male shortly after the initial regression of the testes. Growth of new pelage accompanied by whitening of the fur occurred in all animals in conjunction with the first period of testicular regression (1972) as well as at the time of the second regression which followed hemicastration (1973). However, in some animals these pelage changes failed to occur during the third and final regression. Removal of one testis during the second season of maximal testicular size ratings did not appreciably affect the duration of that period of maximal testicular activity, as compared with the previous year. However, in hemicastrates the period of maximal ratings induced by "long days" was somewhat shorter in all animals.

TABLE I

TESTICULAR WEIGHTS AND PENILE DIMENSIONS IN THREE GROUPS OF MALE FERRETS

Group	N	% with incompletely descended testes	Left testis (when testicular ratings were maximal)	Right testis (when testicular ratings were minimal)	Os length	Glans diameter
			Median weight (g)		*Median penile dimensions (mm)**	
No TP perinatally	8	0	1.546	0.552	42.5	7
TP prenatally + day 3	4	0	1.317	0.605	42.5	6
TP day 3	4	100	Scrotal 1.418 (n = 2) Non-scrotal 0.394 (n = 2)	— 0.270 (n = 4)	42.5	6

* Penile measurements were made when the left testis was removed.

The weights of testes removed either during a period of maximal testicular ratings or at the end of the experiment when testicular ratings were low are given in Table I. The scrotal testes removed during the regressed period weighed on the average less than half as much as those removed during a period of maximal ratings. Similar results were obtained by Rust and Shackelford (1969) who studied the annual testicular cycle of ferrets housed out-of-doors. In the present experiment incompletely descended testes also tended to weigh less during a period of minimal testicular ratings than during a period of maximal ratings. There were no significant differences in the weights of scrotal testes among the 3 groups, nor were there significant differences in the dimensions of either the os or the glans penis. Also, there were no significant differences in body weight among the 3 groups; however, in all animals body weight was higher during periods of testicular regression than when testicular ratings were maximal. Examination of the histology of scrotal testes showed that spermatogenesis was complete in all ferrets at the time of maximal testicular ratings, whereas primary spermatocytes were the most advanced type of germ cell present in the seminiferous epithelium of testes when size ratings were minimal. Spermatogenesis was severely disrupted in testes which failed to descend completely, regardless of whether rated size was maximal or minimal.

Annual changes in blood testosterone concentration

Fig. 2 shows that an annual fluctuation in the blood concentration of testosterone was present in all 3 groups, although to different degrees. Testosterone concentrations in the prenatally + day 3 TP-treated males were extremely variable during the initial 5 collections. The comparatively low concentrations measured in the males treated with TP on day 3 may have been due to reduced testosterone secretion by incompletely descended testes, at least one of which was present in all 4 ferrets of this group. Even so, within each group the median concentration of testosterone in blood fell to a lower value at the time of testicular regression than at either the eighth month of life or following testicular recrudescence.

Sexual behavior

Description of normal mating responses
A brief description of the mating behavior of the ferret has previously appeared (Poole, 1967); however, no quantitative data were reported. Upon introduction of an estrous female, the male engages in a chain of responses which lead to intromission and the emission of sperm. Table II shows the timing of these behaviors during *ad libitum* tests in which intromission occurred. Usually the male begins by sniffing the female's vulval region. He then proceeds to nuzzle the female's neck whereupon he takes a grip on the dorsal surface of the female's neck and may drag her around the test chamber before finally mounting her. The estrous female's response to being gripped by the neck is one of postural passivity together with deviation of the tail. While maintaining a neck grip and mount, the male displays periods of rapid thrusting

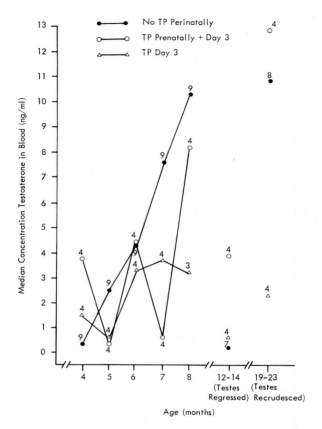

Fig. 2. Longitudinal data on the concentration of testosterone in the blood of 3 groups of male ferrets. The number above each point indicates the number of values included in the calculation of that particular median.

TABLE II

TIMING OF SEXUAL BEHAVIOR IN MALE FERRETS DURING UNINTERRUPTED TESTS WITH INTROMISSION

Time parameter (min)	No TP perinatally (N = 7)		Ferret no. 4 (TP day 3)
	Median	Range	
Vulval investigation latency	0.1*	0.1 — 1.0	—*
Neck grip latency	0.6	0.2 — 1.8	0.3
Mount latency	0.7	0.1 — 2.0	1.6
Pelvic thrusting latency	4.6	2.8 — 8.0	5.6
Intromission latency	16.5	11.0 — 29.6	12.5
Intromission duration	83.5	2.5 — 151.3	4.0
Inter-intromission interval	13.0**	—	—
Duration second intromission	62.8**	—	—

* Occurred neither in control ferret no. 10 nor in ferret no. 4.
** Value for one ferret (no. 10) in which a second intromission occurred within 15 min after termination of the first intromission.

of the pelvic region. This thrusting is frequently accompanied by extrusion of the glans penis from its sheath as it seeks out the female's swollen vulva. Once vulval penetration is achieved, pelvic thrusting ceases and intromission continues uninterrupted for many minutes. Although occasional postural adjustments are made by the intromitted male which appear to facilitate maximal penetration, no obvious behavioral pattern has been identified which signals the ejaculation of sperm. In tests in which intromission was interrupted by the experimenter within 1–2 min after it had begun, sperm was found in the vaginal smear. Copulating ferrets were always readily separated, suggesting that a penile lock does not occur in this species.

Initial development and annual changes in sexual behavior

Males in all 3 groups displayed neck grip and mount responses when first tested at 4 months of age. In subsequent months all ferrets began to display pelvic thrusting together with penile erection, although the development of these responses was delayed in males treated with TP prenatally + on day 3 (Fig. 3). The ability of perinatally androgenized males to intromit was severely deficient (Figs. 1 and 3). Whereas during the experiment 7/8 control males achieved intromission, 0/4 ferrets treated with TP prenatally + on day 3 and 1/4 males treated with TP on day 3

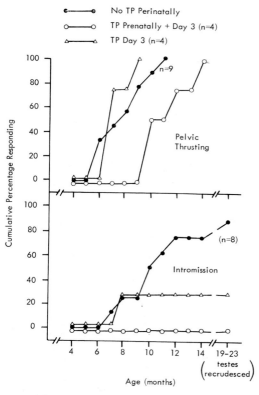

Fig. 3. The development of pelvic thrusting and intromission in 3 groups of male ferrets.

References p. 354–355

TABLE III

BLOOD TESTOSTERONE LEVELS IN INTROMITTING AND NON-INTROMITTING FERRETS

	Intromitting ferrets			Non-intromitting ferrets	
Treatment	Ferret's no.	Blood testosterone concentration 24 hr after first introm. (ng/ml)	Treatment	Ferret's no.	Highest concentration of testosterone measured in blood (ng/ml)
No TP perinatally	11	2.3	TP day 3	8	3.3
No TP perinatally	16	7.5	TP day 3	5	4.0
No TP perinatally	12	7.9	TP day 3	6	6.5
TP day 3	4	8.9	TP prenatally + day 3	3	8.4
No TP perinatally	14	9.5	No TP perinatally	31	10.3
No TP perinatally	22	18.2	TP prenatally + day 3	7	10.4
No TP perinatally	33	21.3	TP prenatally + day 3	1	17.6
No TP perinatally	10	29.5	TP prenatally + day 3	2	21.6
		Median = 9.2			Median = 9.3

successfully intromitted (P = 0.02, 2-tailed Fisher Exact Probability Test). The timing of the mating pattern in this single androgenized male during an *ad libitum* test fell within the range of the control males (Table II). It will be seen in Table III that the concentration of testosterone in the blood of non-intromitting ferrets was at some time, either during pubertal life or during the second season of maximal testicular ratings, well within the range of testosterone concentrations measured in responding males within 24 hr after initial intromission. Furthermore, daily injections of TP failed to induce intromission in non-responding animals (including one control male), although in the ferrets treated with TP on day 3 the duration of neck grip, mount and pelvic thrusting behavior during the first 15 min of these 60-min tests tended to be higher than during tests given when both testes were present and re-crudesced (Fig. 4). The administration of TP in adulthood together with the final behavioral tests was carried out only after the ferrets had been exposed to "long days" and the rated size of the remaining testis had become maximal, thus increasing the likelihood that the neural mechanisms controlling mating were maximally sensitive to the TP being injected.

Some males in all 3 groups occasionally displayed such seemingly aberrant behaviors as (a) mounts with pelvic thrusting oriented toward the female's side, (b) mounts with pelvic thrusting without maintaining a neck grip, and (c) gripping of the

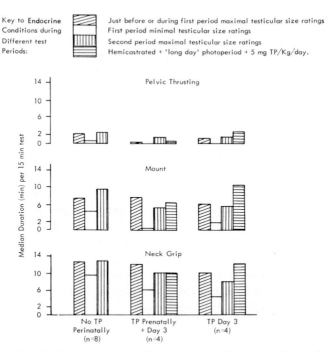

Fig. 4. Incidence of neck grip, mount and pelvic thrusting in 3 groups of male ferrets at different times during the annual reproductive cycle and following hemicastration + exposure to "long days" + administration of TP. Medians were calculated from data of the initial 15 min of mating tests, beginning for each ferret with that test in which pelvic thrusting was first displayed.

dorsal surface of the female's head instead of her neck. However, in individual males there was no reliable correlation between the incidence of such behavior and the ability of the male to achieve intromission.

In all 3 groups of males the incidence of several components of mating behavior fluctuated as a function of the annual changes in testicular size and function (Fig. 4). Although between groups comparisons were not significant for any of the 3 naturally occurring endocrine conditions listed, the within groups differences in the durations of neck grip and mount during tests given in different endocrine states were often significant when tested using the Friedman 2-way analysis of variance by ranks, with the shortest durations occurring when testicular ratings were minimal. Thus, the duration of neck grip fluctuated significantly both in control males and in ferrets treated with TP prenatally + on day 3 ($P < 0.01$). Also, the duration of mounting fluctuated significantly as a function of endocrine state in control ferrets ($P < 0.03$) and in males treated with TP on day 3 ($P < 0.05$). Although the duration of pelvic thrusting also tended to be lowest in tests given when testicular ratings were minimal, in no group was this difference statistically significant. Finally, except for two control males, each of which achieved intromission once when their testicular ratings were minimal, intromission was displayed exclusively during periods when ratings of testicular size were either increasing or maximal.

DISCUSSION

Annual fluctuations in testicular function and mating behavior occurred in male ferrets regardless of whether or not they had received TP perinatally. This finding suggests that there is no need for the level of testicular secretion of androgen to be particularly low during some critical perinatal period in order for annual reproductive cycles to occur in adulthood. It seems unlikely that the presence of testicular cyclicity in TP-treated males can be attributed to a failure of the injected TP to reach the fetal or neonatal ferret brain: female littermates of the males treated with TP prenatally + on day 3 displayed significantly increased amounts of aggressive behavior when tested as adults, in addition to possessing external genital organs which were severely masculinized (Baum, 1974). Furthermore, in the present experiment sexual behavior was disrupted in both groups of androgenized males, and this deficiency was not easily explained by a non-neural factor such as inadequate penile size or insufficient amounts of testosterone in the circulation. Instead, the results suggest that some factor other than the absence or reduction of gonadal secretion of androgen during perinatal life is responsible for establishing a gonadotropin control mechanism which in the adult ferret functions with an annual cycle of activity.

In the present experiment the initial development of sexual behavior in male ferrets as well as the subsequent annual fluctuation in the occurrence of these responses was found to correlate with the concentration of testosterone in the blood. Although the incidence of mating responses declined during the period when the testes were regressed in size and blood testosterone concentrations were low, they did not dis-appear completely. In this respect the male ferret resembles the ram, in which annual fluctuations in mating behavior and plasma testosterone concentration occur and are correlated, but in which a degree of sexual responsiveness remains even during the spring months when testosterone levels are lowest (Pepelko and Clegg, 1965; Katongole et al., 1974). It is not known whether the annual changes in sexual behavior of the ram and ferret are directly regulated by the level of circulating testosterone, or whether, as in the red deer stag (Lincoln et al., 1972), some other factor such as an annual fluctuation in the sensitivity of the brain to testosterone may play a crucial role.

The present results confirm a previous suggestion (Baum and Goldfoot, 1974) that an endogenous reproductive rhythm exists in the male ferret which operates even in the absence of seasonal changes in the length of day. Ferrets in all 3 groups showed periods of maximal testicular size ratings at approximately the same time and of approximately the same duration in two consecutive years, even though the photoperiod was maintained on "short days" from the time of birth. Also, it is interesting to note that removal of one testis, while testicular size ratings were maximal, seemed to have no effect on the duration of that period of maximal ratings. If confirmed, this observation would suggest that an inhibitory feedback effect of testicular steroids on gonadotropin secretion does not determine the period of the annual reproductive cycle of the male ferret.

As suggested above, the inability of perinatally androgenized ferrets to intromit is not readily explained by some gonadal or penile defect present in these males. Furthermore, beginning when behavioral tests were first given at 4 months of age, there was no deficiency evident in either the quality or quantity of such responses as neck grip, mount or pelvic thrusting. What was lacking in androgenized males was the capacity of these preliminary copulatory behaviors to culminate in intromission. One possibility is that the capacity for intromission develops only if the male ferret experiences a particular kind of androgen-stimulated social interaction early during prepubertal life. Speculating further, perinatal androgenization may have caused a change in the circulating concentration of testosterone well before the fourth month of life when blood levels were first measured, which in turn disrupted the normal development of social behavior. A related deficiency in mounting, intromission and ejaculation behavior has also been found in male rats which received TP in high doses either pre- and postnatally (E. I. Pollak and B. D. Sachs, personal communication, 1974) or only after birth (Wilson and Wilson, 1943; Diamond et al., 1973; A. K. Slob, P. E. Schenck and M. J. Baum, unpublished findings). Although the mechanism whereby perinatal androgenization disrupts mating behavior has yet to be identified, the available evidence indicates that the ontogeny of sexual behavior in male rats and ferrets proceeds in a normal fashion only if the amount of androgenic stimulation sustained by the developing brain remains below some critical upper limit.

SUMMARY

Reproductive function was studied for more than 2 consecutive years in 3 groups of male ferrets. One group received testosterone propionate (TP) both prenatally and on postnatal day 3; a second group received TP on postnatal day 3 only; and a control group received no hormone perinatally. Annual fluctuations in testicular size together with correlated changes in spermatogenesis, the concentration of testosterone in the blood and the incidence of neck grip, mount and pelvic thrusting behaviors occurred in all 3 groups, suggesting that there is no need for the level of testicular secretion of androgen to be particularly low during a critical perinatal period in order for annual reproductive cycles to occur in adulthood. The ability to achieve intromission was permanently impaired in both groups of androgenized ferrets, even though in adulthood penile size and blood testosterone concentrations were well within the range of the control animals. This suggests that the ontogeny of mating behavior in the male ferret proceeds in a normal fashion only if the amount of androgenic stimulation sustained perinatally by the brain remains below some critical upper limit.

ACKNOWLEDGEMENTS

We are indebted to Dr. B. A. Cooke for help in setting up the radioimmunoassay for testosterone and to Drs. J. J. van der Werff ten Bosch and D. A. Goldfoot for useful discussions during the course of this experiment. Also, the technical assistance of H. Nieuwenhuijsen, P. van der Vaart, M. Ooms and M. Huibrechtse-Zuidema is gratefully acknowledged.

This research was supported by the Dutch Foundation for Medical Research (FUNGO).

REFERENCES

ALLANSON, M. (1932) The reproductive processes of certain mammals. III. The reproductive cycle of the male ferret. *Proc. roy. Soc. B*, **110**, 295–312.

BARRACLOUGH, C. A. (1967) Modifications of reproductive function after exposure to hormones during the prenatal and early postnatal period. In *Neuroendocrinology, Vol. II*, L. MARTINI AND W. F. GANONG (Eds.), Academic Press, New York, pp. 61–99.

BAUM, M. J. (1974) Failure of perinatal administration of testosterone propionate to disrupt receptive behaviour in the female ferret. *J. Endocr.*, in press (abstract).

BAUM, M. J. AND GOLDFOOT, D. A. (1974) Effect of hypothalamic lesions on maturation and annual cyclicity of the ferret testis. *J. Endocr.*, **62**, 59–73.

BISSONNETTE, T. H. (1935) Modification of mammalian sexual cycles. *J. exp. Zool.*, **71**, 341–373.

DIAMOND, M., LLACUNA, A. AND WONG, C. L. (1973) Sex behavior after neonatal progesterone, testosterone, estrogen, or antiandrogens. *Horm. Behav.*, **4**, 73–88.

JOHNSON, D. C. (1972) Sexual differentiation of gonadotropin patterns. *Amer. Zool.*, **12**, 193–205.

KATONGOLE, C. B., NAFTOLIN, F. AND SHORT, R. V. (1974) Seasonal variations in blood luteinizing hormone and testosterone levels in rams. *J. Endocr.*, **60**, 101–106.

LINCOLN, G. A., GUINNESS, F. AND SHORT, R. V. (1972) The way in which testosterone controls the social and sexual behavior of the red deer stag *(Cervus elaphus)*. *Horm. Behav.*, **3**, 375–396.

PEPELKO, W. E. AND CLEGG, M. T. (1965) Influence of season of the year upon patterns of sexual behavior in male sheep. *J. Anim. Sci.*, **24**, 633–637.

POOLE, T. B. (1967) Aspects of aggressive behaviour in polecats. *Z. Tierpsychol.*, **24**, 351–369.

Rust, C. C. and Shackelford, R. M. (1969) Effect of blinding on reproductive and pelage cycles in the ferret. *J. exp. Zool.*, **171**, 443–450.

Verjans, H. L., Cooke, B. A., de Jong, F. H., de Jong, C. M. M. and van der Molen, H. J. (1973) Evaluation of a radioimmunoassay for testosterone estimation. *J. Steroid Biochem.*, **4**, 665–676.

Wilson, J. G. and Wilson, H. C. (1943) Reproductive capacity in adult male rats treated prepuberally with androgenic hormone. *Endocrinology*, **33**, 353–360.

Hormonal Influences in the Evolution and Ontogeny of Imprinting Behavior in the Duck

JAMES T. MARTIN*

Max Planck Institut für Verhaltensphysiologie, Seewiesen (G.F.R.)

Two major processes mold the behavior patterns of an organism. The first of these, evolution, represents the interaction of the species with its environment while the second, ontogeny, constitutes the individual's interaction with its environment. Evolution and ontogeny are difficult to study experimentally because both are dynamic time-dependent processes in which every event is dependent on the preceding one. Darwin first suggested that domestication might represent a simplified model for studying evolution. Domestication is, however, a subject worthy of study in its own right. Domestication may be defined as an adaptation of an animal or plant to life in intimate association with and to the advantage of man. Two major adaptations in the biology of the organism seem to characterize most domesticated animals — a reorganization of the reproductive function away from seasonal dependence and a reduction in the general "fearfulness" and reactivity in the animal. Evolution and especially ontogeny are limited with regard to the number of physiological means available to accomplish adaptive ends. It is well known that hormones are structurally conservative elements which may take on different functions depending on the evolutionary or ontogenetic needs of the organism. This paper deals with the role which hypothalamic–pituitary–adrenal hormones may play in mediating imprinting behavior in the neonatal duckling.

Imprinting is the process occurring in certain nidifugous birds through which the young bird develops an attachment to its parent(s). Lorenz (1935) originally drew attention to the phenomenon, and notable recent reviews are those of Bateson (1966) and Hess (1973). Development of this early attachment proceeds rapidly and without apparent reinforcement during the first two days after hatching. Elicitation of approach and following behavior becomes increasingly difficult after this early period, and instead the animal increasingly withdraws from all unfamiliar stimuli. The stimuli which will subsequently elicit withdrawal is, therefore, highly dependent on the length of this "sensitive period". This sensitive period for approach is also concomitant with a period of maximal receptivity to exposure learning as expressed by a discrimination test at a later age. The sensitive period in learnability has been described by Hess (1959) for mallard ducklings, and he reported maximum receptivity to his imprinting

* Present address: Department of Animal Science, University of Minnesota, St. Paul, Minn. 55101, U.S.A.

References p. 365–366

models at about 15 hr post-hatch. Considerable evidence suggests that the Pekin, a domestic counterpart of the mallard, has a longer and less sharply defined sensitive period (Gottlieb, 1961; Martin, 1973). Some insight into the physiological mechanisms mediating the sensitive period may be gained by examining the wild and domestic forms. Since behavioral differences exist between these forms, any relevant physiological concomitants would also be expected to covary in the two forms.

A number of lines of evidence suggest that adrenocortical hormones are involved in the imprinting process. Both ACTH and corticosterone are known to affect extinction of learned avoidance responses in rats (de Wied, 1966; Brain, 1972). Van Delft (1970) found a strong negative correlation between plasma corticosterone basal levels and the performance in a conditioned avoidance paradigm, hence suggesting a physiological role for glucocorticoids in learning processes. Moreover, Henkin (1970) has pointed out that alterations in glucocorticoid levels within a physiological range may exert marked effects on sensory and perceptual processes. In order to determine if a relationship between the hypothalamic–pituitary–adrenal system and the imprinting sensitive period existed, the following experiments were conducted.

Eggs from free-living mallards were gathered from nest boxes on the institute grounds approximately 5 days before hatching and placed in an incubator. After hatching the ducklings were individually marked and placed in a 121 cm × 71 cm × 65 cm holding pen with 3–6 other ducklings. Individual ducklings were decapitated at various intervals after hatching, and the blood was collected for hormone analysis. In a parallel experiment 48 ducklings of the domesticated Pekin strain were obtained

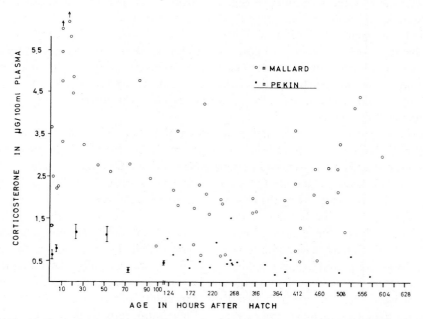

Fig. 1. Developmental course of basal levels of plasma adrenocorticoids in wild and domestic ducks in the early post-hatch period. Each data point represents the mean of duplicate assays on individual plasma samples except where standard errors are shown in which case the sample size is 8.

within 1 hr of hatching from a local breeder. These animals were moved to the institute and held in a lighted holding pen with food and water. Eight animals were decapitated at 4, 8, 24, 56, 72 and 120 hr of age. The plasma of all animals was stored at $-20\,°C$ for corticosterone analysis using a competitive protein binding method (Martin, 1973). Fig. 1. clearly indicates that the plasma total adrenocorticoids rise sharply after hatching and then fall back to the basal level in a manner remarkably similar to the time course of the behavioral-sensitive period. The peak of the mallard curve appears to be very sharply defined with an apex at about 15 hr post-hatch. This correlates well with the data of Hess (1959) who reported maximum sensitivity to an imprinting surrogate at 16 hr post-hatch. The rise in plasma adrenocorticoids among the Pekins is not so sharply defined as in the wild strain, and this corresponds to the less sharply defined sensitive period for imprinting in this strain. What function, if any, the activation of the adrenocortical system serves in the behavioral process of imprinting cannot be determined from these data.

It would seem plausible that an activation of the hypothalamic–pituitary–adrenal system could facilitate incorporation of the initial imprinting experience. In order to test this possibility two groups of ducklings were treated with a short-acting solution of 1 I.U. porcine ACTH 20 min before exposure to an imprinting model. The behavioral set-up and testing procedures have been described in detail elsewhere (Martin and Schutz, 1975). Briefly, the duckling is removed from the incubator and placed under the imprinting model in the dark. The model, which is either a 20-cm diameter blue ball or 21-cm square red cube, is equipped with a loudspeaker that emits a rhythmic "komm-komm" call and moves along a runway suspended from a track on the ceiling. The discrimination test which is given 8 days after this initial exposure employs both models, and the subject's preference for the imprinted model is measured. Table I illustrates that those animals which had received exogenous ACTH before the initial exposure to the blue ball performed better in a choice test 8 days later, *i.e.*, the peptide-treated ducklings preferred their imprinting model more strongly than controls. These results must be qualified in that 7 of 20 control animals

TABLE I

IMPRINTING BEHAVIOR IN PEKIN DUCKLINGS GIVEN ACTH 20 min BEFORE EXPOSURE AT 20 hr OF AGE TO A BLUE BALL MODEL

μ = mean; n = number of ducklings.

Behavior	Treatment					
	1 I.U. ACTH			Saline		
	μ	S.E.M.	n	μ	S.E.M.	n
Training						
Latency to approach in sec	105	$\pm$25.4	18	98	$\pm$23.7	19
Following time in 10 min of exposure to blue ball in sec	395	$\pm$22.6	18	347	$\pm$24.1	19
Choice test						
Time spent following blue ball in 10 min of exposure	370	$\pm$33.8	19	337	$\pm$36.0	20
Time spent following red cube in 10 min of exposure	98	$\pm$15.8	15	180	$\pm$30.6	13

References p. 365–366

failed to follow the unfamiliar red cube while 4 of 19 experimentals failed to follow that model. It is unclear what mechanism is involved in the improved performance. The data collected during the initial imprinting training period suggest that the peptide treatment increased the amount of following of the model during the 10 min of exposure. The increased attention or exposure to the model rather than a direct effect of the peptide may, therefore, be the cause of the improved performance in the choice test. Nevertheless, it seems rather likely that the endogenous release of ACTH evident from the data of Fig. 1 functions similarly to improve retention of the impending or ongoing imprinting experience.

Gene action during development

The post-hatch differences in both behavior and hormone levels between wild and domesticated forms can be traced to differential gene action in the embryo. Variance attributable to maternal factors or prior experience is negligible since the animal is in a highly buffered closed system until shortly before its performance in the experimenter's testing device. The primary question is, therefore, what physiological and biochemical processes have become genetically rearranged during domestication to produce these behavioral differences. Results from a previous experiment at the University of Connecticut (Martin, 1971) suggest that relatively few factors are responsible for substantial changes in post-hatch behavior.

Four strains of ducklings were obtained as eggs and hatched in a large forced-air incubator. The strains differed in the number of generations which the parent stock had been held in captivity. Group I was essentially wild having been outbred to wild-trapped birds for 5 generations. Group II had been in captivity for approximately 10 generations with no outbreeding to wild stock for at least 5 generations. Group III

TABLE II

PERCENT OF POPULATION RESPONDING IN 4 STRAINS OF 110-hr-OLD DUCKLINGS SUBJECTED TO A NOVEL "OPEN FIELD" AND "HAWK STIMULUS"

Strain characteristics are described in the text. n = number of ducklings.

Behavior	Strain			
	I (n = 49)	II (n = 49)	III (n = 25)	IV (n = 56)
Move less than 1.39 m in open field in min before hawk stimulus	36	47	57	70
Move more than 4.14 m in open field in min before hawk	40	48	30	12
Freeze in response to hawk stimulus	8	10	12	4
Increase movement $> 10\%$ in min after hawk stimulus	35	29	28	21
Decrease movement $> 10\%$ in min after hawk stimulus	18	24	12	9
Show $< 10\%$ change in movement in min after hawk	37	37	48	62
Vocalize before hawk stimulus	75	83	73	62
Vocalize after hawk stimulus	63	69	59	61

had been in captivity for 20–30 generations. Group IV was composed of domesticated Pekins which have been in captivity for 500–1000 years or more. At 110 hr of age the ducklings were placed individually in a large rectangular "open field" chamber, and their locomotor activity and vocalizations measured before and after a shadow of a hawk was passed over the enclosure. Table II indicates that those groups which had been subjected to the least amount of artificial selection, i.e., had been in captivity for the shortest time, demonstrated the strongest reaction to the hawk stimulus. The fact that the changes resulting from captivity and artificial selection are discernible within 20 generations suggests that the behavioral substrate is under the control of relatively few genes.

It is clear that adrenocortical function differs in wild and domesticated strains shortly after hatching (Fig. 1). Since the strong post-hatch elevation in adrenal function is much less dramatic in the domestic Pekins, it was hypothesized that the hypothalamic–pituitary–adrenal system of domesticated strains is also depressed during embryogenesis and that this depression affects the developing central nervous system. Artificial selection resulting from captivity may have acted to retard the onset or to suppress the level of hypothalamic–pituitary–adrenal function in the embryo. Experiments were designed to determine whether this hypothesis could account for some of the differences observed between wild and domesticated strains.

The eggs of Pekin ducklings were injected at days 15, 19 and 23 of embryonic development with either corticosterone, aminoglutethimide (an inhibitor of steroid synthesis) or vehicle control solutions. Following hatching, the effects of these treatments were evaluated upon performance in the imprinting situation and upon the adrenal response to immobilization stress at 16 days of age. Immobilization stress was accomplished by tying to a board for 65 min; blood samples were withdrawn at 0, 8 and 65 min and stored for corticosterone analysis. It is difficult to predict the true amount of hormone or drug reaching the embryonic circulation from the injection procedure. It is most likely that only a fraction of the injected material reached the embryo in an active form. Adjovi and Idelman (1969) indicated that a dosage of aminoglutethimide comparable to that used here was sufficient to suppress adrenal

TABLE III

EFFECT OF 3 EMBRYONIC CORTICOSTERONE INJECTIONS ON DUCKLING'S TENDENCY TO FOLLOW AN IM-
PRINTING MODEL AT 24 hr POST-HATCH

Treatment	Number of ducklings	
	Followers	Non-followers
Corticosterone		
50 + 50 + 50 μg	3	5
10 + 10 + 20 μg	9	6
(Treatments combined)*	12	11
Saline 25 μl	14	2

* Differs from saline control, $\chi^2 = 5.18$; $P < 0.025$.

TABLE IV

EFFECT OF 3 EMBRYONIC CORTICOSTERONE INJECTIONS ON IMPRINTING BEHAVIOR IN THE DUCK

Treatment	Behavioral test measure				
	Training latency in sec	Following time in sec	Choice test latency (median)	Following time in choice test	
				RC	BB
Corticosterone					
50 + 50 + 50 μg	76.7	317.6	0	507.6	386.0
	(3)§	(3)	(5)	(5)	(5)
10 + 10 + 20 μg	56.0*	517.3**	0	576.3	388.0
	(7)	(6)	(7)	(6)	(6)
(Treatments combined)	62.2	450.7	0***	—	—
Saline (25 μl)	139.0	428.5	47.5	407.4	393.9
	(7)	(8)	(8)	(7)	(7)

* Differs from saline control, "t_{12}" = 2.53, $P < 0.05$.
** Differs from saline control, U = 42, $P < 0.05$.
*** Differs from saline control, U = 74.5, $P < 0.025$.
§ Denotes sample size.

function in the chick embryo. Table III depicts the amount of corticosterone given over the 3 injections and its effect on the approach tendency. A significantly smaller proportion of corticosterone-treated ducklings followed the imprinting model. Those which did follow began following more quickly and followed longer (Table IV). During the choice test 9 days later, the corticosterone-treated ducklings once again responded more quickly to the model, but they failed to show better discrimination of the model. These results are striking in their relation to the behavior of mallards in the same imprinting situation. The treated birds resembled mallards in their behavior in two respects. Only about 67 % of all wild mallards exposed to the models approach them (Martin and Schutz, 1975); a similarly low proportion of cortico-

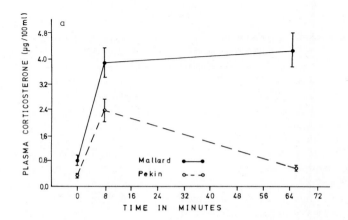

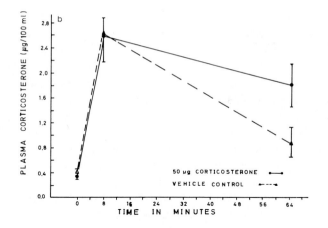

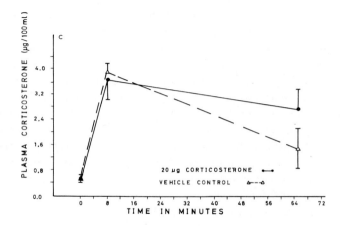

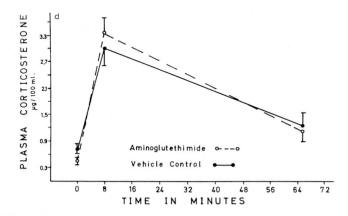

Fig. 2. Plasma adrenocorticoid response to acute immobilization stress in 16-day-old ducklings. a: untreated animals, n = 8; b: embryonically treated with corticosterone, n = 6 for experimentals and n = 9 in controls; c: embryonically treated with corticosterone, n = 5 for experimentals and n = 8 in controls; d: treated embryonically with aminoglutethimide.

sterone-treated Pekins followed the model. Secondly, mallard ducklings which follow usually do so quite closely, and the same situation appeared to characterize the treated Pekins.

Embryonic treatment with the steroid inhibitor aminoglutethimide in 3 doses of 1.25 mg of the phosphate salt failed to affect any imprinting parameters although the post-hatch weight was reduced.

The resemblance of the embryonically corticosterone-treated Pekins to mallards becomes more striking when one observes the stress response patterns. Fig. 2a depicts the adrenal response to immobilization stress in untreated mallards and Pekins at 16–18 days of age. Clearly the mallard, unlike the Pekin, sustains a high rate of release of corticosterone under stress. Fig. 2b and c indicate that treatment of Pekin embryos with corticosterone results in a shift in the capability of the adrenal to sustain secretion during stress, and this shift seems to be dose-dependent with the 50 μg dose producing the greatest shift toward the wild phenotype. Depression of the embryonic adrenal output with aminoglutethimide (Fig. 2d) produced only a small reduction in the basal level at 16 days of age and no change in the stress pattern.

The hypothesis proposed by Levine and Mullins (1966) and elaborated by Denenberg and Zarrow (1971) that early handling causes reduced adult adrenal response to stress via an increase in neonatal adrenal steroids could not be confirmed in these experiments. Rather, early stimulation of the system resulted in a more sustained response to an immobilization stress. Suppression of the system appeared to have no effect on the dynamics of the stress response. The results of these experiments do provide preliminary support for the hypothesis that the hypothalamic–pituitary–adrenal system is a factor controlling imprinting behavior. Further experiments utilizing physiological doses of a long-acting ACTH preparation for injection during embryogenesis also confirmed that early stimulation of the system can intensify the following response during imprinting. The effects resulting from altering embryonic levels of these hormones appear to be different from those of acute alteration in hormone level. No improvement in the learning component of imprinting was found from embryonic treatments; however, acute administration of ACTH did appear to improve retention. The dosage of ACTH used in the acute experiments was quite high (1 I.U.), and the possibility remains that the results may not reflect physiologically important events.

The results reported here also support the contention that domestication processes involve a suppression of pituitary adrenal function during early periods of development. Richter (1952, 1954) first suggested that domestication was accompanied by a suppression of adrenocortical function and a shift toward elevated gonadal function. A study by Pasley and Christian (1972) indicates that high levels of ACTH inhibit reproductive function in *Peromyscus*. Meier (1972) suggests that the circadian phase relationship of adrenal steroids and prolactin controls development of the reproductive system in a variety of animals. This information along with the experiments reported here suggests that suppression of early pituitary–adrenal function could contribute to the domestication process in the duck in two ways. Animals with low early glucocorticoid levels fail to sustain a high glucocorticoid secretion under stressful conditions and hence may be less likely to experience reproductive blockage from stress. Animals with low circulating glucocorticoid levels during development exhibit imprinting or social attachment behavior over a more extended time span and/or to a wider range of objects. Both these properties would facilitate the animal's adaptation to captive conditions and would accelerate the domestication process. It would be oversimplifying the matter to suggest that selection for reduced adrenocortical function alone results in domestication; nevertheless, this process appears to have been an important factor in the evolution of the domesticated duck, and considering the present results, a more intense and comprehensive examination of this question in the duck as well as other forms seems warranted.

SUMMARY

The imprinting sensitive period is accompanied by a strong rise in the basal level of plasma adrenocorticoids. The question of whether elevated adrenal activity during that time serves to facilitate the imprinting experience was examined by testing ducklings treated with ACTH before exposure to their imprinting model. ACTH-treated animals demonstrated better retention in a subsequent discrimination test. Differences in early imprinting and avoidance behavior between wild and domesticated forms of the duck, *Anas platyrhynchos*, were hypothesized to be attributable to differential adrenal system function in the two forms during embryogenesis. Injection of domesticated Pekin embryos with corticosterone resulted in young ducklings which were apparent phenocopies of the wild strain in their imprinting behavior and adrenal stress response. Suppression of hypothalamic–pituitary–adrenal activity in early stages of development may have played an important role in the domestication process.

ACKNOWLEDGEMENTS

This research was supported in part by grants from the Max-Planck Gesellschaft and the McGraw Wildlife Foundation.

Aminoglutethimide was a gift of Dr. K. Scheibli and the Ciba–Geigy AG, Basel.

REFERENCES

ADJOVI, Y. ET IDELMAN, S. (1969) Action d'un inhibiteur de la stéroidogenèse, l'élipten, sur la cortico-surrénale de l'embryon de poulet (Leghorn blanc). *C.R. Soc. Biol. (Paris)*, **163**, 2588–2593.
BATESON, P. P. G. (1966) The characteristics and context of imprinting. *Biol. Rev.*, **41**, 177–220.
BRAIN, P. F. (1972) Mammalian behavior and the adrenal cortex — a review. *Behav. Biol.*, **7**, 453–479.
DENENBERG, V. H. AND ZARROW, M. X. (1971) Effects of handling in infancy upon adult behavior and adrenocortical activity: suggestions for a neuroendocrine mechanism. In *Early Childhood*, D. N. WALCHER AND D. A. PETERS (Eds.), Academic Press, New York, pp. 39–50.
GOTTLIEB, G. (1961) The following response and imprinting in wild and domestic ducklings of the same species *(Anas platyrhynchos)*. *Behaviour*, **18**, 205–228.

HENKIN, R. I. (1970) The effects of corticosteroids and ACTH on sensory systems. In *Pituitary, Adrenal and the Brain, Progress in Brain Research, Vol. 32*, D. DE WIED AND J. A. W. M. WEIJNEN (Eds.), Elsevier, Amsterdam, pp. 270–295.

HESS, E. H. (1959) Imprinting. *Science*, **130**, 133–141.

HESS, E. H. (1973) *Imprinting: Early Experience and the Developmental Psychobiology of Attachment*, Van Nostrand Reinhold, New York, p. 473.

LEVINE, S. AND MULLINS, JR., R. (1966) Hormonal influences on brain organization in infant rats. *Science*, **152**, 1585–1592.

LORENZ, K. (1935) Der Kumpan in der Umwelt des Vogels. *J. Ornithol.*, **83**, 137–214, 289–412.

MARTIN, J. T. (1971) *A Laboratory Study of Wildness in the Duck, Anas platyrhynchos*, M.S. Dissertation, University of Connecticut, Storrs.

MARTIN, J. T. (1973) *The Role of the Hypothalamic-Pituitary-Adrenal System in the Development of Imprinting and Fear Behavior in the Wild and Domesticated Duck*, Doctoral Dissertation, Universität München, München.

MARTIN, J. T. AND SCHUTZ, F. (1975) Arousal and temporal factors in imprinting in mallards. *Develop. Psychobiol.*, **8**, 69–78.

MEIER, A. H. (1972) Temporal synergism of prolactin and adrenal steroids. *Gen. comp. Endocr.*, **Suppl. 3**, 499–508.

PASLEY, J. N. AND CHRISTIAN, J. J. (1972) The effect of ACTH, group caging and adrenalectomy in *Peromyscus leucopus* with emphasis on suppression of reproductive function. *Proc. Soc. exp. Biol. (N.Y.)*, **139**, 921–923.

RICHTER, C. P. (1952) Domestication of the Norway rat and its implications for the study of genetics in man. *Amer. J. hum. Genet.*, **4**, 273–285.

RICHTER, C. P. (1954) The effects of domestication and selection on the behavior of the Norway rat. *J. nat. Cancer Inst.*, **15**, 727–738.

VAN DELFT, A. M. L. (1970) The relation between pretraining plasma corticosterone levels and the acquisition of an avoidance response in the rat. In *Pituitary, Adrenal and the Brain, Progress in Brain Research, Vol. 32*, D. DE WIED AND J. A. W. M. WEIJNEN (Eds.), Elsevier, Amsterdam, pp. 192–199.

WIED, D. DE (1966) Inhibitory effects of ACTH and related peptides on extinction of conditioned avoidance behavior in the rat. *Proc. Soc. exp. Biol. (N.Y.)*, **122**, 28–32.

Free Communications

The role of hormonal steroids in the differentiation of sexual and aggressive behavior in birds

R. E. HUTCHISON — *MRC Unit on the Development and Integration of Behaviour, University Sub-Department of Animal Behaviour, Madingley, Cambridge (Great Britain)*

Androgen is involved in the sexual differentiation of the reproductive tract, pituitary–gonad system and certain aspects of behavior in mammals. In birds, estrogen is implicated in the sexual differentiation of the reproductive tract and plumage. However, the sexual differentiation of behavior has not been studied in detail. The effects of estrogen and androgen therapy in neonatal Japanese quail *(Coturnix coturnix japonica)* will be discussed with a view to showing the relative effects of these steroids on the development of sexual and aggressive behavior.

Sensitizing effects of androgen and photoperiod on hypothalamic mechanisms of sexual behavior

JOHN B. HUTCHISON — *MRC Unit on the Development and Integration of Behaviour, University of Cambridge, Madingley, Cambridge (Great Britain)*

Significantly more intramuscular TP is required to restore sexual and aggressive patterns of pre-copulatory courtship in long-term than in short-term castrated male doves. To investigate whether this was due to a difference in responsiveness of hypothalamic as opposed to peripheral mechanisms of sexual behavior, the effectiveness of anterior hypothalamic implants of TP in restoring behavior was measured at different periods after castration in groups maintained on long or short photoperiods. The effects of implants were inversely related to the period between castration and implantation irrespective of photoperiod. Behavioral deficits were greater in long-term castrates on a short photoperiod. The effects of prolonged androgen deficit were completely reversed by large doses of intramuscular TP. But the number of doses was proportional to the period between castration and onset of treatment. After castration, there is a rise in the threshold of response of hypothalamic mechanisms of sexual behavior to testosterone. This effect is facilitated by short photoperiod. High levels of androgen reverse the threshold change in long-term castrates after a latency proportional to the castration period, suggesting that cells in the anterior hypothalamus require the sensitizing effects of androgen before the behavior is mediated by the brain.

Light and social exposure: complimentary effect on pituitary gonadal function

MEI-FANG CHENG — *Rutgers – The State University, Institute of Animal Behavior, Newark, N.J. 07102 (U.S.A.)*

Testicular hypertrophy response was used as a measurement for relative effect of light and social effect on neurosecretory activity in hypothalamo–hypophysial complex.

Right testis (larger of the two) were removed from male doves and were weighed. Birds were then assigned to various combination of (1) short *vs.* normal light cycle, and (2) isolation *vs.* social stimulation. At the end of 4 weeks all birds were laporato-mized. The left testis was removed, weighed and expressed in percentage weight of right testis for each bird. The main results are (1) testicular hypertrophy is complete in 4 weeks in 14 h light cycle. This response is absent for birds kept in 8 h light cycle — testes were even smaller than their pre-castration size. However, this in-sufficient pituitary response to unilateral castration in short light group can be facilitated by periodic exposure to stimulation female. This effect is not attributable to added light exposure associated with female-exposure period. The results were discussed in terms of existing hypothalamic neurosecretory system.

Inhibition effects of "neo-natal" estrogenization on the sexual behavior of the male rat and modifications of the genital tract

A. SOULAIRAC AND M. L. SOULAIRAC — *Department of Psychophysiology, Faculty of Sciences, University of Paris VI, Paris (France)*

Young rats given 10 μg estradiol benzoate between the 2nd and 5th days after birth present a very striking inhibition of sexual behavior at adulthood. The greatest effect is seen when estradiol is administered on postnatal days 4 and 5. The inhibition is not abolished by testosterone administration, but some positive behavioral responses are obtained using neurostimulating drugs (for example, caffeine).

In these animals, development of the genital tract is markedly impaired; spermato-genesis is suppressed, mainly following administration on postnatal days 4 and 5, but androgenic interstitial activity is maintained.

The possibility of an elective injury of some nervous structures by estrogen at some especially critical periods of central nervous system development is discussed.

The role of growth hormone in brain development and behavior

V. R. SARA AND L. LAZARUS — *Garvan Institute of Medical Research, St. Vincent's Hospital, Sydney 2010 (Australia)*

The factors regulating *in utero* brain growth have yet to be determined. Variation in the timing of critical periods for different organs reveals that the response to any growth stimulus will be a function of the time it is applied. It is therefore proposed that factors regulating somatic growth postnatally will affect brain growth and subsequent function when applied prior to birth. This study investigates the role of growth hormone in brain development and behavior.

Growth hormone was administered to pregnant rats and the brain growth and behavior of progeny examined. The results showed a significant increase in brain weight and cortical neuron number as determined by the incorporation of labeled thymidine into DNA and subsequent autoradiography. At maturity, learning performance on a series of conditional discrimination tasks was found to be enhanced. These data indicate that maternal administration of growth hormone produces offspring with an increase in brain size due to elevated cellular content and consequently enhancement of learning ability.

Preliminary report on behavioral (Beh) change in a 2-year-old boy with precocious puberty (PP) following L-DOPA (D) treatment

CHANDRA M. TIWARY AND JERRY E. DYKSTERHUIS — *Department of Pediatrics, University of Nebraska Medical Center, Omaha, Nebr. (U.S.A.)*

An 18-month-old white boy was evaluated in October 1973 for PP; no cause was found. His social age was 2.7 years (Vineland) and mental age 2.4 years (Peabody). He was emotionally labile, behaviorally unpredictable and physically aggressive. We serendipitously observed serum LH decreased during 60 min of D test* and his Beh improved following testosterone propionate** (T) injection (given for evaluating the integrity of hypothalamic–pituitary–gonadal axis). The preliminary results of the Beh change for the first 6 weeks after D follow.

100 mg of D was begun on March 3, 1974 and raised 100 mg each week. The parents were instructed to record daily the following Beh pinpoints: (1) number (no.) of times he hit another person during the entire waking day; (2) no. of attention changes during a 10-min period after supper; (3) no. of demands for mother's attention for 10-min period, 1 h prior to bedtime. Other Beh counted included no. of times awake each night and the amount of time slept at night and during naps. No advice on Beh management and change was offered. The weekly means of the data during each observation period show: (1) aggressive Beh decreased from 2.71/day during week 1 to 0.28/day during week 3 and none thereafter; (2) distractions decreased from 5.42/sample during week 1 to 2.83/sample during week 6; (3) demands for attention decreased from 4.57/sample during week 1 to 2.60 during week 6. His nap and night

---

* Decrease in luteinizing hormone (LH) by L-DOPA in isosexual precocious puberty (IPP); possible relation of LH to behavior (C. M. TIWARY, *Clin. Res.*, in press).
** Behavioral change occurring in a young child following testosterone injection (C. M. TIWARY, Letter to *Lancet*, in press).

sleep patterns remained relatively unchanged except for less daily variability during the last 3 weeks. Additionally, parents reported remarkably improved general Beh, similar to that experienced post T. Serum LH decreased after 3 weeks of D treatment but serum T level remained elevated. We suggest that D caused a fall in LH-RH resulting in Beh change and also a drop in LH levels.

Psychoendocrine problems in patients with a late diagnosis of congenital adrenal hyperplasia: observations in a case of bilateral pseudocryptorchidism (female pseudohermaphroditism)

J. J. LEGROS, A. BAUDUIN AND M. VERFAILLE — *Institute of Medicine and Institute of Pediatrics, University of Liège, Liège (Belgium)*

Congenital hyperplasia of the adrenals is the most common cause of female pseudohermaphroditism. Although some cases are detected at birth, others are so similar morphologically to males that recognition of true sex may be made only in childhood or even adolescence. These latter cases present difficult problems in the definitive assignment of sex and only a multidisciplinary approach, such as we described previously[1], makes it possible to carry out psychoendocrine treatment.

In this presentation, we will emphasize particularly on the psychologic disturbances as they were shown by different tests. This is of importance since our patient (6 years old, genotype: female, phenotype: male) was massively impregnated by androgens (plasmatic testosterone: 3.529 ng/100 ml) since the first weeks of fetal life and would then have had few psychological disturbances.

In fact, even in the presence of androgenic hormones, our patient presents the "hermaphrodite identity" as described by Stoller[2]. This suggests that early hormonal impregnation and sociological impacts are not the only two factors which cause the male psychological differentiation in man.

1 LEGROS, J. J., VAN CAUWENBERGE, H., LAMBOTTE, R., BAUDUIN, A., FRANCHIMONT, P. ET LEGROS, J. Problèmes psycho-endocriniens posés par un cas d'hyperplasie, surrenalienne congenitale reconnu tardivement. *Rev. Méd. Liège*, 29 (1974) 73–80.
2 STOLLER, R. J., *Sex and Gender*, Science house, New York, 1968.

Session VII

MISCELLANEOUS

Free Communications

Glucose–insulin metabolism in chronic schizophrenia

F. Brambilla, A. Guastalla, A. Guerrini, F. Riggi, C. Rovere, A. Zanoboni and W. Zanoboni-Muciaccia — *Ospedale Psichiatrico Paolo Pini, Milan and Ospedale Psichiatrico Antonini, Milan Limbiate and Patologia Medica II, Università di Milano, Milan (Italy)*

The present study deals with possible connections between the schizophrenic syndrome and alterations of glucose–insulin metabolism.

Data have been obtained in 18 patients, 9 males and 9 females, aged 22–62 years, suffering from chronic schizophrenia of 5–29 years duration. The patients were treated with haloperidol for 30 days, 6 mg/day i.m. to a total dose of 180 mg. We also examined 12 physically and mentally healthy controls, matched for age and sex. Glucose metabolism was examined by a glucose tolerance test (GTT, with a glucose load of 100 g p.o.) and an insulin tolerance test (ITT) with 0.1 I.U./kg body weight.

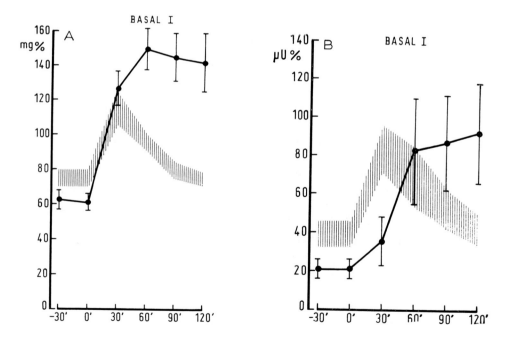

Fig. 1. Effect of schizophrenia on glycemic (A) and insulinemic (B) levels under glucose load. The drawn line refers to the average obtained from schizophrenics. The band refers to data obtained from controls.

Insulin levels were examined after the glucose load by the radioimmunological assay of Hales and Randle. The psychopathological features were examined through a Wittenborn Rating Scale. The metabolic and psychological examinations were performed twice before the beginning of the therapy, at 48 h intervals, and then after 10, 20 and 30 days of therapy.

The results are indicative of the presence of a chemical diabetes in a significantly high percentage of patients, as demonstrated by markedly elevated insulinemic and glycemic peak values, delayed insulinemic and glycemic peak values, and prolonged hyperglycemia and hyperinsulinemia (Fig. 1A and B). The response to exogenously administered insulin was normal rather than excessive. Haloperidol treatment did not modify these results. The biochemical data seem to correlate with the presence of specific psychopathological symptomatology, such as severe mental deterioration, apathy and withdrawal from reality.

A possible common basis for both the biochemical and psychological impairments is proposed.

A noradrenaline insufficiency, which may be related to the presence in the CNS of an excessive amount of 6-OHDA, could explain the reported pathological data.

Metabolism of cerebral peptides of physiological importance

ABEL LAJTHA AND AMOS NEIDLE — *New York State Research Institute for Neurochemistry and Drug Addiction, Ward's Island, New York, N.Y. 10035 (U.S.A.)*

Peptides with even a small number of amino acid residues present an almost unlimited array of sizes, shapes, and electrical charge distributions. Small peptides with such properties could play an important role in information transfer in brain by interaction with appropriate receptors. The observations that hypothalamic releasing factors can influence mood and behavior without endocrine mediation support this concept. We have shown that endogenous peptidase activity might be involved in the release and inactivation of these agents. Another example of peptide specificity has been recently reported[1]. Carnosine (β-alanylhistidine) is present in the olfactory bulb of the mouse at about 2 μmoles/g, a concentration 100-fold higher than its γ-aminobutyryl analog, homocarnosine. This is in marked contrast to other brain areas in which homocarnosine predominates. A similar distribution was found in rat brain. In a single sample of human bulb, carnosine and homocarnosine were present in nearly equal concentration. Experiments with radioactive precursors *in vitro* indicate that carnosine is synthesized in olfactory bulb by an enzyme which incorporates β-alanine, but not GABA, into peptide linkage. Therefore, this enzyme appears different from the homocarnosine synthetase of cerebral hemisphere which does not distinguish between these two substrates. The preferential distribution of carnosine as well as its rapid turnover in bulb suggests an important functional role for this dipeptide. Such a role has been independently proposed[2] based on the decrease of the carnosine concentration in mouse olfactory bulb following chemical ablation of the afferent olfactory neurons of the nasal mucosa.

1 *Proc. Amer. Soc. Neurochem.*, 5 (1974) 169.
2 MARGOLIS, F. L., *Science*, 184 (1974) 909.

Delta-9-tetrahydrocannabinol action and neuronal membrane-bound enzymes

J. J. GHOSH, M. K. PODDAR, D. NAG AND B. BISWAS — *Department of Biochemistry, University College of Science, Calcutta University, Calcutta-19 (India)*

Delta-9-tetrahydrocannabinol (Δ-9-THC), the major pharmacologically active component of cannabis, produces characteristic changes in the activities of membrane-bound enzymes of rat brain, under both *in vivo* and *in vitro* conditions. Acute Δ-9-THC administration (10 mg and 50 mg/kg, i.p.) produced stimulation of acetylcholine esterase and glutamine synthetase activities in both synaptosomal and microsomal fractions, whereas the Na^+-K^+-ATPase activity in synaptosomes was inhibited and in microsomal fractions was stimulated under the same experimental conditions. Chronic treatment (10 mg/kg, i.p., 30 days) produced no significant changes in the activities of these enzymes.

In vitro treatment with Δ-9-THC (10^{-5} M and 10^{-4} M) produced inhibitory effects on both synaptosomal and microsomal Na^+-K^+-ATPase activities, stimulatory effects on synaptosomal activities, and stimulatory effects on synaptosomal and microsomal glutamine synthetase activities. The activity of acetylcholine esterase was stimulated in synaptosomes and inhibited in microsomal fractions.

The effect of exposure to two odorous compounds (pheromones) on an assessment of people test

J. J. COWLEY AND B. W. L. BROOKSBANK — *Department of Psychology, The Queen's University, Belfast (N. Ireland)*

Work has been carried out on the effect of exposing people, for a short period of time, to a mixture of short-chain fatty acids and to androstenol (5-androst-16-en-3-ol). The compounds were selected as they have been reported as having pheromone-like properties. Subjects were exposed to one or other of the compounds, and a third sample acted as a control. A test was designed which required participants to express favorable or unfavorable opinions about the suitability of a number of applicants, of both sexes, for a position of responsibility. A brief character sketch was provided as a basis for making judgments. The results show that women exposed to the presence of the fatty acids and the androstenol are not affected in their assessments of applicants of their own sex, but that exposure is accompanied by a change in their assessment of male applicants. Further, marked sex differences are present between men and women in their judgments, and there is an interaction between sex and the characteristics of the applicants. Males were little affected by the compounds, but there was some evidence to suggest that they reacted differently when assessing men and women. The investigation shows that people can be influenced in their judgments by exposure to androstenol and a mixture of free fatty acids. One does not know what particular traits influence the judgments, but as there are differences between the experimental treatments and the control condition, one is inclined to reject the suggestion that it is simply a response to odor, as such.

The effect of epinephrine on liver 5-nucleotidase

A. N. GRANITSAS AND S. A. HITOGLOU — *Department of General Biology, Medical School, Aristotelian University, Thessaloniki (Greece)*

In a previous series of experiments it was found that adrenaline produces a significant increase on the excretion of purine derivatives in rats. In the present series of experiments the effect of catecholamines on the liver ribonucleic acids and 5-nucleotidase was studied. It has been found that after administration of adrenaline the activity of liver 5-nucleotidase is increased, while there is no change on the concentration of purines or ribonucleic acids. When adrenaline was added in liver homogenates the activity of 5-nucleotidase and the level of purine derivatives was increased.

There is also an increased breakdown of ribonucleic acids, although a concomitant increase of liver ribonuclease activity was not observed. The mechanism of the observed action of adrenaline is obscure. There is evidence, however, that this effect could be due to formation of cyclic AMP.

Subject Index